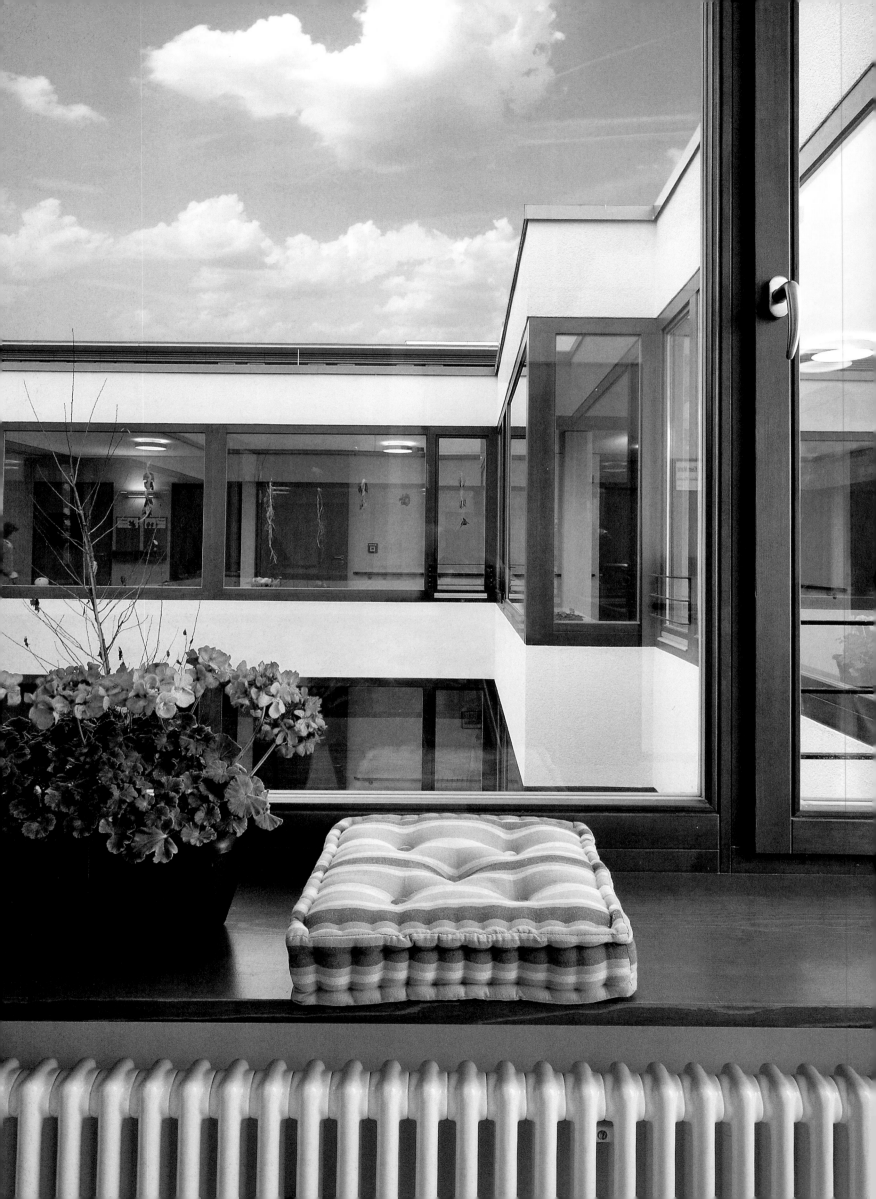

A DESIGN MANUAL

Living for the Elderly

Eckhard Feddersen
Insa Lüdtke

CONTRIBUTIONS BY

Helmut Braun

Stefan Dreßke

Maria B. Dwight

Dietmar Eberle

Angelika Hausenbiegl

Bernhard Heiming

Matthias Hürlimann

Katharina Hürlimann-Siebke

Marie-Therese Krings-Heckemeier

Yasmine Mahmoudieh

Johanna Myllymäki-Neuhoff

Georg W. Reinberg

Beth Tauke

Nikolaos Tavridis

Rudolf Welter

Harms Wulf

Birkhäuser
Basel • Boston • Berlin

The authors and the publisher wish to thank the following institutions and companies
for their participation in this book:

Robert Bosch Stiftung GmbH

BOS GmbH Best of Steel

Forbo Flooring GmbH

FSB – Franz Schneider Brakel GmbH + Co KG

Gira Giersiepen GmbH & Co. KG

IMMAC and IMMAC Sozialbau GmbH

Franz Kaldewei GmbH & Co. KG

Herbert Waldmann GmbH & Co. KG

Layout and cover design: Oliver Kleinschmidt, Berlin

Translation from German: Julian Reisenberger, Weimar
copyedited by Michael Wachholz, Berlin

Editor: Christel Kapitzki, Berlin

Organisation and research: Claudia Jäger, Berlin

Editor for the publisher: Andreas Müller, Berlin

Lithography: Licht & Tiefe, Berlin

Printing: Medialis, Berlin

Cover: "Wohnfabrik Solinsieme", St. Gallen, Switzerland
Photographer: Urs Welter, Oberbüren

This book is also available in German:
ISBN 978-3-7643-8870-6

A CIP catalogue record for this book is available from
the Library of Congress, Washington D.C., USA

Library of Congress Control Number: 2009924663

Bibliographic information published by The Deutsche Nationalbibliothek
The Deutsche Nationalbibliothek lists this publication in the Deutsche
Nationalbibliografie; detailed bibliographic data is available in the
Internet at http://dnb.ddb.de.

© 2009 Birkhäuser Verlag AG
P.O.Box 133, CH-4010 Basel, Switzerland
Part of Springer Science+Business Media

Printed on acid-free paper produced from chlorine-free pulp. TCF ∞

Printed in Germany
ISBN 978-3-7643-8871-3

www.birkhauser.ch
9 8 7 6 5 4 3 2 1

Living for the Elderly – Principles and Processes

Living for the Elderly – Typologies and Projects

LIVING CONCEPTS FOR SPECIFIC USER GROUPS

LIVING CONCEPTS FOR PEOPLE WITH DEMENTIA

INTEGRATED HOUSING AND NEIGHBOURHOOD CONCEPTS

APPENDIX

Preface

The design of housing for the elderly is not generally regarded by architects as a glamorous task. The temples of global society have been and continue to be museums of different cultures, the headquarters of powerful financial institutions or showpieces for leisure and culture. The fame of architects such as Gehry or Libeskind, Foster or Ando cannot be attributed to their housing projects and housing does not feature prominently in their work. Instead, technically innovative solutions, spectacular dramatics and event architecture have eclipsed the comparatively everyday phenomenon of living.

This situation changes, however, as soon as we begin to reappraise society's actual needs, to focus less on wealth and luxury in society and more on bringing real needs into the foreground. It becomes immediately apparent that there is no greater or more urgent task than to address the living requirements of young people, of families and of ever older generations.

The most important and objective indicator for the pursuit of happiness of a person born today is their life expectancy. This indicator tells us, for example, whether or not there is a high instance of death in infancy and whether food and nutrition is abundant and clean. Life expectancy reflects the environmental hygienic condition of air and water, the availability and quality of health care provisions, pension systems and working conditions. This indicator is a more fundamental explanation for the migration of millions of people from south to north than any number of individual parameters.

The average life expectancies in central and northern Europe as well as in Japan are the highest in the world, even when some other populations have a particularly high proportion of elderly people who reach an advanced old age. The average is highest in western central Europe. It is therefore no surprise that a greater than average proportion of good examples featured in this book are to be found in Switzerland and neighbouring countries. Yet old age is not a territorial or national phenomena but a global issue. The whole world would like to live as long as one already lives in central Europe. Our topic will become increasingly important in coming decades in regions of the world outside of the highly industrialised nations, although this may apply only to particular sections of society. Even in China and India, families are already increasingly paying outside providers to assist the family with "services" that they in the past provided themselves. The only realistic alternative to the variety of forms, typologies and concepts for housing old people shown in this book is the Scandinavian model. Here, elderly citizens are provided with outpatient care in their own homes, and special facilities and homes for the elderly are only rarely built. This, however, requires even greater investment and involvement and is only possible with a corresponding political commitment.

Living means "to feel comfortable". For each individual to feel comfortable, a myriad of minute factors have to be fulfilled. Among the many functional means of addressing these factors, we architects feel particularly driven to provide the appropriate design frame for this sense of well-being. In the process, we need to be aware that in old age, one is still very much able to judge what one likes and dislikes. The attraction of unnecessary frippery fades with age in favour of more "essential" aspects, items of actual worth, clarity of expression and fitness of purpose. We hope with this book to convey something of this message.

Eckhard Feddersen and Insa Lüdtke
Berlin, March 2009

Universal Design:
a declaration of independence

BETH TAUKE

One of the most significant changes in our world today is the shift in population demographics. The people of the world are getting older. In 2000, there were 600 million people aged 60 and over; there will be 1.2 billion by 2025 and 2 billion by 2050.[1] By 2050, the number of older persons in the world will exceed the number of young for the first time in history.[2]

People are living longer today for several reasons including advances in medical science, technology, health care, nutrition, and sanitation. An important consequence of this progress is that those aged 80 or older are the fastest growing age group in the world.[3] Although this larger older population is in better health than ever before, they have some modified abilities. Sensory, cognitive, and physical health, mobility and dexterity changes are prevalent among older persons, and raise many questions about the ways that we think about human-environment interaction.

Attendant to this historic demographic shift is enormous social change. Throughout their lives, this older population, particularly the baby boomer generation of the 1960s, has been a force for social justice and transformation. They have used their numbers to initiate changes in civil rights, women's rights, workers' rights, gender identity rights and the rights of those with disabilities. Without question, they are leading changes in the rights of older persons to lead independent lives as full participants in all aspects of our contemporary culture. On the practical level, this includes changes in attitudes and policies on ageing, accessibility, safety, health care, employment, living arrangements, community planning, maintenance of independence and life quality. The rights of older persons are a key component of social sustainability, which "is focused on the development of programmes, processes, and products that promote social interaction and cultural enrichment. It emphasizes protecting the vulnerable, respecting social diversity and ensuring that we all put priority on social capital. Social sustainability is related to how we make choices that affect other humans in our 'global community'."[4]

Where and how people live is one of the primary elements of social sustainability. In the development of the United Nations Principles for Older Persons (resolution 46/91), the UN General Assembly recognised the importance of living conditions and housing for the elderly, and infused it throughout all five categories relating to the status of older people: independence, participation, care, self-fulfilment and dignity. Key principles related to housing for the aging population include:
• Access to adequate food, water, shelter, clothing and health care through the provision of income, family and community support and self-help;
• Ability to live in environments that are safe and adaptable to personal preferences and changing capacities;
• Ability to reside at home for as long as possible;
• Ability to utilise appropriate levels of institutional care providing protection, rehabilitation and social and mental stimulation in a humane and secure environment;
• Ability to enjoy human rights and fundamental freedoms when residing in any shelter, care or treatment facility, including full respect for their dignity, beliefs, needs and privacy and for the right to make decisions about their health care and the quality of their lives.[5]

These principles have the primary goal of promoting active and independent living for as long as possible. While many older people prefer to stay in their own homes or apartments because they have close ties that are connected to where they have been living, others are interested in or might need new modes of living or places that provide more amenable weather conditions, community conveniences, services and health care.

Unfortunately, most typical housing design caters to younger sectors of the population, and can pose obstacles to those with sensory, mobility or cognitive limitations. As a result, new thinking about housing for older persons that provides better choices for ageing has been emerging during the past few decades. Innovative ideas about living full lives for as long as possible involve both living arrangements (i.e., inter-generational housing, co-housing, etc.) and the redesign of housing itself to support a wider range of abilities. Concepts of universal design are at the core of these explorations, and provide a basis for "increased accessibility, safety and health for a diverse population."[6]

Universal design is essential in the development of all new senior housing concepts. It maps well onto the United Nations Principles for Older Persons and goes further, defining more clearly the practices necessary to transform the everyday environment into one that can accommodate those with different needs. Not only does this approach involve "the design of products, information, environments, and systems to be usable to the greatest extent possible by people of all ages and abilities",[7] but it is also a "socially focused design process grounded in democratic values of non-discrimination, equal opportunity and personal empowerment."[8] With roots in the Civil Rights Movement,[9] universal design emerged from the idea of "barrier-free" or "accessible design".[10] However, it moves beyond concepts that are based solely on physical function, and includes the comprehension and sensory enhancement of products, environments and systems. It offers seamless solutions that are not stigmatising, but, instead, are mainstream components of our built world. According to Dr. Edward Steinfeld, director of the Center for Inclusive Design and Environmental Access (IDEA) at the University at Buffalo – State University of New York, "Universal design does not claim to accommodate everyone in every circumstance. Rather, it continuously moves toward this goal of universal usability. Consequently, a more appropriate term may be universal designing, a verb rather than a noun."[11]

By designing for a diverse population, universal designers integrate usability by everyone into their work on a routine basis. This approach leads to greater inclusion for many groups often neglected in the design process including older persons, people of small stature, frail people, etc.[12] If independence is the 'what', universal design is the 'how'. The Seven Principles of Universal Design, developed in 1997,[13] point the way to the implementation of this approach, and can be adapted to any design situation. When considering housing for older persons, the principles can be applied to specific situations as demonstrated in the following examples.

Principle One: Equitable Use[14] – Housing is usable by anyone, and does not disadvantage, stigmatise, or privilege any group of users. No-step entries are an example of an equitable feature that allows all people to enter the dwelling in the same way.

Principle Two: Flexibility in Use – Living environments accommodate not only a wide variety of individual choices, but also adapt to user's varying functional abilities. For example, placing kitchen counters at various heights permits people who are of tall or short stature or those who are in seated positions to prepare food in a comfortable manner.

Principle Three: Simple and Intuitive – All aspects of the domestic environment are easy to understand regardless of the inhabitant's experience, knowledge, language skills or concentration level. Bathroom taps that make operation apparent and that clearly indicate temperature levels are an example of a universally designed solution. Light switches that are consistently located in relation to room entrances and that contain uniform "on/off" indicators help people to intuit lighting operation.

Principle Four: Perceptible Information – The housing communicates all necessary information effectively to all users regardless of ambient conditions or the user's varying cognitive or sensory abilities. Both auditory and visual warnings on appliance buzzers and security alarms alert people to important information, and circumvent negative situations that might occur because of low vision, hearing limitations, environmental noise, and dark or clouded spaces.

Principle Five: Tolerance for Error – The design of residences minimises hazards and adverse consequences of accidental or unintended actions by all users. Built-in shower seats are an example of a universally designed feature that can prevent slips and falls while bathing. Niches for keys and other items near every entrance door help users to remember where they locate items that are often misplaced.

Principle Six: Low Physical Effort – Everyone can use the dwellings efficiently, comfortably and with minimal fatigue. Locating all basic living requirements on one entrance grade level reduces effort for those with mobility difficulties.

Principle Seven: Size and Space for Approach and Use – Housing provides appropriate size and space for approach, reach, manipulation and use regardless of the user's body size, posture or functional abilities. For example, wide doorways and passageways provide a clear path of travel throughout the dwelling for all inhabitants. Reachable cabinets give users access to all stored items.

As demonstrated in these examples, universal design is common sense design that is human-centred. It is a set of ideas, principles and practical solutions to a complex set of issues that directly affect the quality of life not only for older persons, but for everyone.

Whatever benefits universal design ultimately brings to society, the biggest winners will be older people. There are few approaches to housing that will do more for seniors than universal design. It is an option that is both sensible and economically possible, especially now given major advances in technology that make mass customisation and digitised solutions more feasible than ever before. In addition, people are beginning to understand that universal design can promote conditions in which older people can minimise their dependence and instead flourish as active members of their communities. They are realising that universal design gives older persons options to lead the kind of lives they choose by giving them built environments that support a wider range of abilities. They are recognising the enormous potential of this once quiet movement to build a more socially just world by bringing equity and independence into their daily lives. Now that universal design is becoming part of social consciousness, there is no going back.

Notes

1 World Health Organization, "Ageing and the Life Course", www.who.int/ageing/en/ (accessed 1st June 2008).

2 Department of Economic and Social Affairs Population Division – United Nations, *World Population Ageing: 1950-2050*, New York: United Nations Publications, 2002, p. xxviii.

3 Ibid, p. xxix.

4 Interface Sustainability, "Social Sustainability", www.interfacesustainability.com/social.html (accessed 1st June 2008).

5 Towards a Society for All Ages: International Year of Older Persons, "The United Nations Principles of Older Persons", www.un.org/NewLinks/older/99/principles.htm (accessed 15th June 2008). The United Nations Principles of Older Persons was adopted in 1991 and the International Year of Older Persons took place in 1999.

6 E. Steinfeld, "The Nature of Barriers", lecture presented in Diversity and Design course, University at Buffalo, State University of New York, USA, 15th April 2008.

7 R. Mace, G. Hardie and J. Plaice, "Accessible Environments: Toward Universal Design" in: *Design Intervention: Toward a More Humane Architecture*, (eds.) W. F. E. Preiser, J. C. Vischer and E. T. White, New York, NY: Van Nostrand Reinhold, 1991, p. 156.

8 Steinfeld, "The Nature of Barriers", op. cit.

9 P. Welch (ed.), *Strategies for Teaching Universal Design*, Boston, MA: Adaptive Environments Center, 1995, p. 8.

10 S. Keithler, "Selling Points: Universal Design Can Benefit All" in: *Multi-Housing News*, vol. 42, issue 8, August 2007, p. 33.

11 E. Steinfeld, "Introduction: Universal Design Defined," in *Universal Design: New York*, (eds.) G. S. Danford and B. Tauke, New York: Mayor's Office for People with Disabilities, 2000, p. 2.

12 Ibid, p. 1.

13 B. R. Connell, M. Jones, R. Mace, J. Mueller, A. Mullick, E. Ostroff, J. Sanford, E. Steinfeld, M. Story and G. Vanderheiden, *The Principles of Universal Design: Version 2.0* (Raleigh, NC: The Center for Universal Design, 1997). Funding for this project was provided by the U.S. Department of Education's National Institute on Disability and Rehabilitation Research (NIDRR).

14 Pictograms of the Principles of Universal Design were developed and are copyrighted by ©Beth Tauke, Center for Inclusive Design and Environmental Access (IDEA), University at Buffalo – State University of New York, 2000. They were published in Danford and Tauke, op. cit.

ECKHARD FEDDERSEN

One's bed, room and house in old age

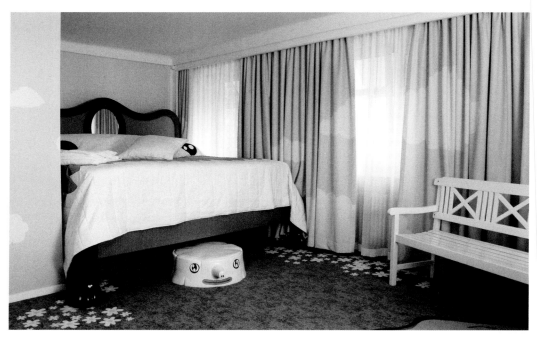

The bed as the heart of the home

Where are we most at home? Probably in bed. However much one likes being in other places, there reaches a point where one wishes for one's own bed. Everyone has experienced this physical and emotional process and it is widely accepted. One's own bed is the innermost part of one's house, the "nest" from which one flies every morning and to which one returns. For this reason, most people would like to die in their own bed, to gently fall asleep and never wake up.

This feeling we also apply to our entire home. With only very few exceptions, nobody wants to have to leave their home in old age. The longer one has lived there, the stronger one's desire to stay. One's home serves as an anchor, a place where one feels secure and that gives a sense of meaning to things. As long as I have my home I am the same person I have always been. To give up one's home, therefore, represents the loss of a part of one's self. This sense of loss is irrefutable and, given the anthropological development of mankind, will most probably always be the case.

It becomes problematic when, for a variety of reasons, segregative forms of living in old age result. The reasons are for the most part health-related, but can also result from social or economic circumstances or because the existing living environment is no longer being used. There are no homes that can "grow" and "shrink". However, very often it is not the home itself that necessitates a move but changes in the person's environment. For older people, it is much more important to feel safe in their surroundings than for younger people, and sometimes it is detrimental changes to local districts, even entire towns, that cause people to feel forced to move away.

In most cases, when old people give up their own home they move into a more isolated form of living, whether into an individual house with apartments especially for older people, high-quality "residences" for seniors or even entire "Sun Cities" as in the USA. Despite many advantages with regard to safety, comfort, acceptance or appropriateness, a certain stigma remains: the richness of life, of choice, is reduced. It is replaced by a select offering of specially designed products and living environments. Flats become sheltered flats for old people, visits to the cinema are reduced to occasional film evenings, living with children is reduced to isolated visits. We realise that what we actually want is to retain the vitality of our lives around us, even though we may make less and less actual use of it, and that if we are to move into a new home and cannot keep everything, we want to keep as much as possible. Above all, we must avoid aspects of life from falling away entirely, whether it is our personal availability, security or social relations.

How can we transpose "normal life" into this new, in a sense "fabricated" life? This is the key question: regardless of issues of money, health or family relations, it is the art of living, the way in which we lead our lives that constitutes our culture of everyday life. The problem is that this is different for each and every one of us. One of the greatest challenges for architects, urban planners and designers is to allow individual people to maintain their own everyday way of life, one that largely corresponds to their biographical background, and to provide a "substitute" or "vignette" of their life in as natural a form as possible, even if it may appear nonsensical to us. The sole governing criteria for the design of living environments for the elderly should be the well-being of the resident.

If one subscribes to this opinion, a number of maxims follow. The most important of these is probably the freedom of choice within a diverse range of alternatives. The sophistication of everyday life does not level off with age but in fact becomes particularly apparent. As people grow older, they have a more precise idea of their preferences than younger people. They are also able to articulate these more strongly as they are less likely to expect sanctions, and furthermore are in most cases more realistic in their expectations and self-awareness. Accordingly, older people know very well what they like from the choices available, as well as what they can afford.

New developments in society, which can be seen around the world, in which society has grown older more or less en bloc – the section of society between 60 and 80 is growing fastest in comparison to all other age groups – mean that we can and will need to experiment greatly in order to cope with this comparatively new situation. In fact, it is not a case of can but of must. In this process, the better quality solution will always be the enemy of the cheap surrogate, and solutions that take a larger view will outstrip those with smaller aims. Larger and better often translate as more expensive. Then again, more investment in the search for the right culture of everyday life will help us to learn more. Similarly, an authentic solution takes more seriously than a surrogate.

In contrast to today's older generation, it is difficult to identify the needs of the coming generation of senior citizens. Today's over 50-year-olds find themselves in a transitional period from protective to leisure-oriented values. Like the rest of society, this target group – the so-called sandwich generation between 55 and 65 years of age – is separating into ever more micro-segments. The variety of lifestyles has never been so complex or contradictory. In addition, improved medical care has extended life expectancy and with it the period of "active old age". Trend researchers speak of the phenomenon of "down ageing": old people already feel ten to 15 years younger than they did 30 years ago. The third phase of life of "young old age" is for most people a productive and eventful period. The fourth phase of life now denotes the over 80-year-olds and is commonly characterised by more serious illness, dementia and ongoing nursing care, sometimes also multimorbidity.

The housing market for the elderly – especially for the third phase of life – will need to provide a wide variety of different offerings to cater for wide-ranging demands. In addition to flexible floor plan concepts, IT and household technology equipment (air climate control, security systems, internet and multimedia) as well as ecology will feature more heavily. In addition, younger pensioners will in future want to have a greater say in the form and organisation of alternative housing projects. For the operator, this means that for such projects they will need to factor in a longer preparatory period for their calculations. On the other hand, the operator can use this as a means of achieving greater customer loyalty.

Today's consumer generation is used to choosing between brand name products and service offerings on an everyday basis, using image as a key criteria of choice. Using a system comparable to the star grading of hotel facilities, nursing home care providers are increasingly implementing quality standards for their facilities. These denote the kind of floor plans, the quality of furnishings, materials and technology as well as the care and service concept. Similarly, housing providers may in future use corporate identity elements in their architecture, residential environment and concept to create "built atmospheres" to distinguish themselves

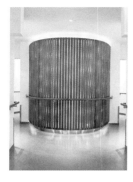
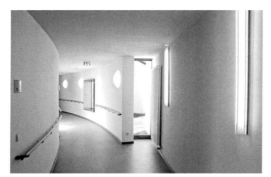
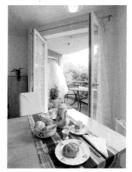
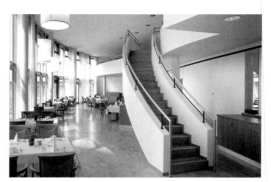

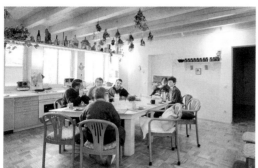
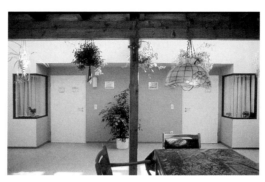
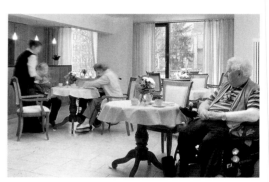

Corridors providing orientation | Light and friendly interiors | Communal living areas

from competitors in the market-place. Where such identities resonate with personal values, this may help create a sense of belonging and feeling at home for the residents.

A lifestyle oriented around wellness is becoming increasingly important – especially with regard to the growing relevance of self-sufficiency – for the "50 plus generation". Well-being is likewise the motto for the living environment. Wellness offerings are already becoming more and more part of everyday life. Co-operation with wellness centres, freelance personal trainers and the like in order to provide wellness offerings in the locality or at home can attract residents – and not just older residents. Furthermore, today's pensioners are more mobile than ever. Globalised work structures have brought with them the experience of life in transit with short stays in hotels or boarding houses. As more and more of the "greying society" choose to live part of the year in other countries with a more Mediterranean climate, or spend large parts of the year travelling, the home takes on a more temporary character. Housing providers for the elderly could respond to the needs of this group by providing assisted living in temporary housing units, coupled with service offerings (also when absent) provided by neighbouring hotels or senior residences.

New technologies, as used in so-called "smart houses", such as "voice butlers" and the like, make it easier for the "silver surfer" to manage everyday needs. Sensors and voice-controlled systems can control blinds and room temperature. Toilets with an internet connection are already available, which send the results of urine tests and fat analyses via email to the doctor's laboratory. Alongside the technology boom, one can also observe a growing ecological awareness, particularly among the age group of the early ecology movement, as well as a social conscience with regard to following generations. The increasing demand for ecologically-friendly building methods will in future also be pursued for economical reasons.

However, despite the demand for greater flexibility in old age, a fundamental need for a sense of place and of belonging still exists. According to a recent study by the trend researchers Trendbüro in Hamburg, the desire for a flexible dual residency arrangement goes hand in hand with a longing for "home sweet home". The dissolution of family structures and friends as relations spread around the globe can be compensated for through informal communal structures in one's local neighbourhood.

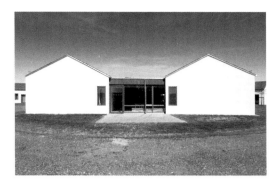

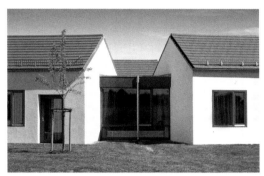

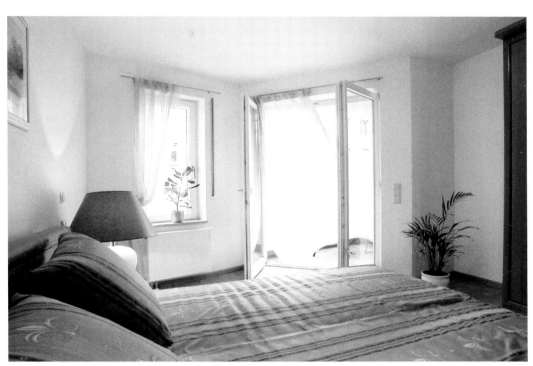

A house within a house: rural archetypes | Contact with the world outside from one's bed

Small wonder, then, that the best examples of housing for the elderly are to be found in the northern hemisphere of the world, in Western Europe, North America and in Japan. Anything else would be a surprise: in societies where the elderly are cared for in the family there are no new segregative forms of living – but there is also no freedom of choice to live one's own independent life. So where can the Americans, Swedes, Dutch or we ourselves expect to find the best examples, the most active experiments and the most precise architectonic expression? In those countries where projects are being built with the highest ideals and the necessary financial investment: in Switzerland for example. Here several factors come together – a land without fear of war, with democratic self-goverment in small communities and general prosperity accumulated over generations – that contribute to a notion of living in old age that comes close to that of "paradise in old age" in all its forms, including in its care for people with dementia.

The cultural differences between countries such as Holland with its strong sense of community, or a country like Sweden with a strong state welfare programme, result in systems for the care of the elderly with different characteristics: some, such as in Sweden, are more focused around outpatient care, others around in-patient care. In all countries, however, and particularly in more prosperous societies, there is an increasing awareness that the more old people are able to be cared for in the familiar surroundings of their own living environment the better. In some cases, in-patient care is relegated to little more than emergency care provision. But here too, the same applies: the more homely the environment the better. Regardless of the quality of medical and nursing care, elderly people must be given more than just a semblance of living; they should be able to retain as many aspects of their life as possible.

Perspectives on ageing across various cultures

ANGELIKA HAUSENBIEGL

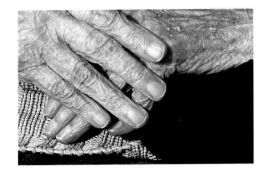

Demographic ageing as a global phenomenon

In all societies, population size and structure is determined by a combination of fertility rate, mortality rate and international migration. The current demographic ageing of societies will have a lasting and profound effect on population structures and accordingly on the respective societies themselves. In industrialised nations, the ageing of the population is already at an advanced stage compared with that of nations with emerging economies where the age of the population is on average younger, but still much older than in developing countries. These developments are due in part to improved economic and social living conditions, which have contributed towards a shift in the age distribution in different areas of life towards older people.

Within this group, a shift in the age structure can also be observed. Advanced old age, the section of society aged 80 years or older, currently represents 1.3% of the global population but is expected to rise to 4.3% by the year 2050. Even the number of 100-year-olds is predicted to rise in the next 40 years by a factor of 13: from 287,000 in 2006 to 3.7 million according to figures published by the United Nations Department of Economic and Social Affairs in 2007.

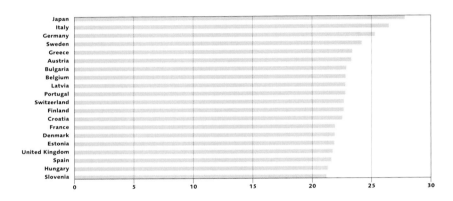

In 2050, 4.3% of the global population will be of an advanced old age.
A comparison of the percentage of people over 60 years of age in different countries; United Nations 2007, Economic and Social Affairs, Population Division

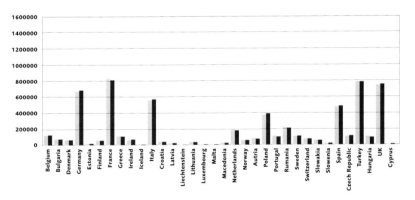

Number of births in Europe in 2006 (light) and 2007 (dark); Eurostat

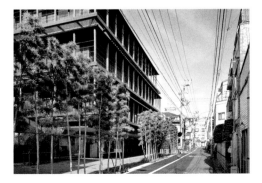

Kengo Kuma: Nezu Withus, Tokyo; residential and nursing home in a historical urban quarter

In worldwide statistics for 2007 published by the Population Division in the United Nations Department of Economic and Social Affairs, Germany, closely followed by Sweden, Greece and Austria, is among those countries with a high proportion of old people. Only Italy and Japan have a higher proportion of over 60-year-olds. Japan is a special case as the highly-developed industrial nation with the highest level of population ageing and sharply rising life expectancy – over 23,000 Japanese are older than 100 years – has been tackling the challenges of population ageing through social insurance system reforms for nearly 35 years. As a consequence of the country's continuing economic growth, professional life has slowly but steadily become ever more demanding so that fewer people are able to care for their parents. The traditional image of Japan, in which the elderly are looked after in the family, usually by the eldest child, is beginning to fade away. Very often there is little alternative to an old people's home, but this is still generally frowned upon in society. The result is an irreversible decline in communal living in large family structures, which in turn leads to the increasing isolation of many old people.

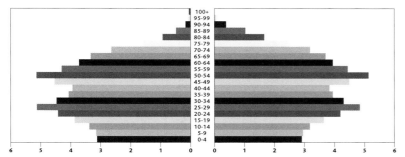

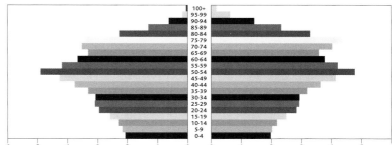

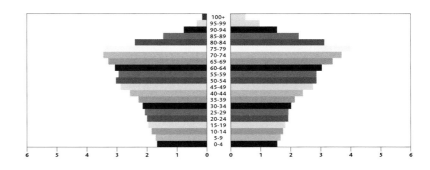

The age distribution pyramid in Japan in 2000 and prognosis for 2025 and 2050;
U.S. Census Bureau, International Database

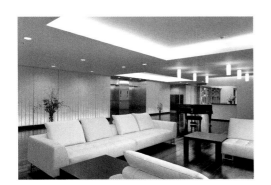

Kengo Kuma: Nezu Withus, Tokyo; hotel-like interior of
communal areas

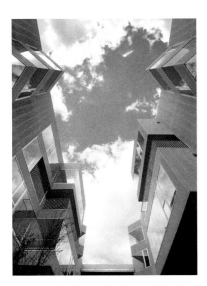

Muramatsu Architects: Idu Terrace, Shizuoka;
barrier-free housing project completed in 2008

How does **Japan** deal with this situation? The government responded by encouraging the building of nursing homes, day-care centres and the development of care at home programmes. According to the Japanese Ministry for Health, Employment and Social Affairs, in the year 2000, 349 private homes for the elderly catered for around 26,000 senior citizens. By July 2004, over 52,000 residents lived in 990 assisted residential schemes for the elderly, a tendency that continues to rise. A large number of hotel-like facilities with a luxurious character have since been built, such as the "Sun City Ginza East" in Tokyo. In recent years, however, more barrier-free residential complexes have been built, such as the "IDU Terrace" in Mishima, a modern and attractive complex completed in May 2008.

It goes without saying that the increasing number of older people results in a greater demand for care personnel. This demand cannot be adequately fulfilled, at least by European standards, partly because Japan has very few migrant workers. Technical aids are therefore being increasingly employed to address the care needs and loneliness of old people. As a country renowned for its creative use of entertainment electronics, Japan has turned to robotic social aids such as the robotic dog "Aibo", a replacement for a real four-legged friend, or "Paro", an artificial baby seal that serves as a pet for elderly people in residential homes. Hardly a month goes by without news of a new "social robot" on the market: even "humanoid" robots that can recognise their owner and can speak a vocabulary of 10,000 words. Wealthy working people buy such robots to "look after" their ageing parents. A further sector constitutes household service robots such as the "Wakamaru". Future generations of robots should be able to react sensitively to the needs of old people, help them with eating, remind them to take their medicine, even administer medicine and injections as well as attend to simple errands.

Has Japan succumbed to the attractions of technical possibilities? Does it run the risk of excluding or even dehumanising old people? Or is the development of robots just a logical consequence of demographic development? Maybe it really is about giving people greater independence. Would not assistive technology have the potential to save the state, as well as individuals, a considerable amount of money? One way or the other, the Japanese are much more used to the creative use of technology, and care robots are regarded from a far less ideological point of view than in Europe.

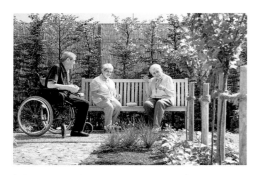

feddersenarchitekten: Competence Centre for People with Dementia, Nuremberg; the sheltered courtyard areas invite one to spend time outdoors

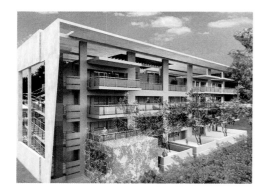

T-STUDIO: integrative high-tech, barrier-free housing project, Pesaro; planning stage

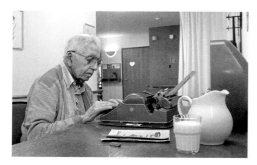

Competence Centre for People with Dementia, Nuremberg; maintaining remaining abilities

The ageing population as a challenge for society

In **Europe** the total population would fall significantly by 2050 were it not for migration. Germany, Spain, Greece and Italy are particularly affected by the low birth rate and rapid ageing of the population. But who will provide professional care for the increasingly older generations and the larger numbers of people in advanced old age? The care of old people is in general dependent on a number of different factors. These include cultural and contextual factors, the individual characteristics of parents and children, family structures and state welfare provisions. Empirical analyses[1] show that inter-generational care is most common in southern and central European countries where state support is available for children to care for their parents. In addition, in countries such as Greece, Italy and Spain, care for the elderly has traditionally been a matter for the family.

In northern European countries, old people are more commonly cared for by trained care personnel and state support is provided for professional home care services.[2] To improve the quality of life for these people, residential concepts are called for that integrate nursing home and residences into existing urban districts. This means the small-scale networking of home care services, of inpatient nursing and informal services and a good infrastructure with social meeting places, efficient public transport and sufficient local shopping opportunities. For such approaches to be successful, it is of vital importance that all the agents involved are consulted and included in the planning.

Italy, which occupies second place in the international ranking of ageing societies, is employing a series of quite different, often regionally-specific solutions. The spectrum ranges from the revitalisation of northern Italian villages (Tiedoli for example), where old people can live together with younger generations, to living in high-tech barrier-free residential buildings, such as those being built in Pesaro. In Italy, migrant workers from low-wage economies, so-called "badanti", are often employed to take care of the elderly.[3]

In **Greece** many women are no longer able to take care of the household and family in the same way as they used to as more and more women now wish to, or indeed have to, go to work. At the same time, old people are dependent on their families for care and support as most pensioners live beneath or just above the poverty line. Despite the irreconcilable nature of this problem, the traditional family model is still prevalent, even in the cities. As a result, young and old generations often live on different storeys of the same house. The resulting demand for larger apartments for more than three to four people is, however, not covered by the housing market.

The situation in **Russia** has changed markedly since the collapse of the Soviet Union. The loss of a fifth of the population, as reported in 2008 in the journal "Eurasisches Magazin", has resulted in far-reaching demographic changes. The booming Russian cities of Moscow, St. Petersburg and Nizhny Novgorad have attracted young people from all over the land, as wage earnings are higher than elsewhere. Outside the aforementioned cities, however, poor economic conditions mean that the younger generation usually lives with their parents. The grandparents very often take over childcare duties, not least because their very low pension means that they cannot afford to live outside the family unit. This is nevertheless preferable to living in an old people's home, which for many is their greatest fear. As there is no state support of any kind for taking care of one's relatives, solidarity within the family unit remains of crucial importance.

Finland, like several other countries, faces the dual problem of an ageing society and an uneven regional distribution of the population. The population of the country becomes increasingly sparse to the north, whereas in the southern provinces, particularly in the region of Helsinki, the population density rises. The provision of care for the elderly in outlying regions is considerably more difficult than in the conurbations. Old people in rural areas may often need to travel many kilometres to reach the required services. Although the state is traditionally responsible for social welfare, family and children play an important role. As a highly modernised country, Finland looks set to make increasing use of advanced technology in the foreseeable

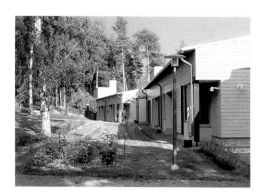

L&M Lievänen: Ulrika Eleonora, Loviisa; a residential and nursing home

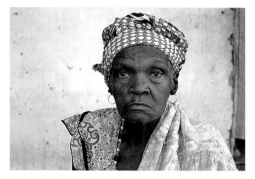

An almost 100-year-old African woman

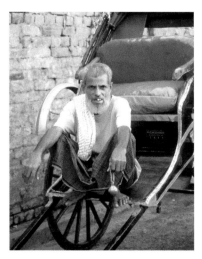

Elderly rickshaw driver

future to assist the older generation. Computers and the internet already augment the patient-doctor relationship, for example in the recording and transmission of blood pressure, heart rate and sugar levels. Studies have also revealed that four of every ten older people over 60 years feel lonely some of the time and one in ten constantly.[4] To counteract this development, in 2001 Finland introduced so-called "Elder's Stations", group therapy and community centres to counteract loneliness and isolation.

Demographic changes in **Africa** are far more turbulent than in the industrialised nations. Family support networks, which traditionally guaranteed social security in old age, are disintegrating. One reason is that young people are moving to the cities to benefit from better educational opportunities and higher earnings with which to support their families. Another reason is that the number of people, particularly younger people, at a reproductive age has reduced significantly as a result of the impact of Aids. The surviving older generation has to take over key tasks that they are largely unable to fulfil. Not only do they need to care for their grandchildren and great-grandchildren, but after a lifetime of work they are forced to continue working to cover the needs of their descendants. When old people fall ill themselves, they for the most part help one another. According to prognoses, Africa will, like other continents, also see a significant rise in the proportion of over 60-year-olds in the coming years. Women who are widowed face an even graver situation as they are both accorded a lower social status than men and have far fewer economic resources of their own. The ageing of the rural population will in particular have serious consequences. A major challenge will be to stimulate rural agricultural production to ensure a local nutritional basis and with it care and nursing for the elderly. The particular developments in family structures in Africa mean that it is important to strengthen the responsibility of the family and the community towards the elderly.

Only 25 years ago, **China** feared that it might have to care for too many children due to the high birth rate. Today the country faces the opposite problem. As a result of the success of the one-child-per-family policy, China's population will age dramatically, which in turn will lead to serious problems in the provision of care for the elderly. At present, Beijing and Shanghai already have more pensioners than children under 15.[5] Today, 144 million Chinese people are over 60 years old, representing 11 % of the population. According to estimates by the World Bank, this number will rise to 460 million by 2050. In China, old age is not a separate phase of life, marked for example by the end of one's working life as it is in Europe. The elderly switch back and forth between family and earning a living, often putting back their own interests. They rarely live alone and in most cases contribute significantly to looking after their grandchildren, easing the burden for their working children. However, the traditional generational bond that accorded old people in China value, respect and influence in the family has in many cases been reduced to one of economic convenience. Societal transformations are pervading the former emerging economy and China will need to develop ever more alternatives to elderly care in the family. The few private and state-funded homes for the elderly are of very different quality and for many old people and their families quite simply too expensive.

India, numbering 1,129,866,000 residents in the year 2007, is the second most populous nation on earth after China and is decidedly "young". Half of the population was born after 1980, making it an unusually large section of society. Consequently, each year 15 million new jobs are created. As an emerging country, India is, of course, not exempt from the accompanying transformations in society. The prevailing system of care and support in the family is declining continually, and the respect and esteem accorded to the older generation is likewise disappearing rapidly. As values shift from wisdom, experience and tradition to foreign languages and computer skills, older people find their dignity and authority increasingly undermined. The younger generation has fewer children, is more career-oriented and increasingly westernised. Is the extended family soon to become a thing of the past?

In order to ensure adequate care and support for the elderly, the relief organisation HelpAge India, a non-government organisation, is implementing homes and other support. According to management of HelpAge India, 2000 homes for the elderly are already in operation.[6] In view of the current situation, the federal government intends to raise the current very low level of pension provision.

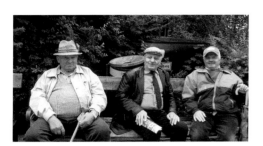

Getting to know one another, learning about one's differences

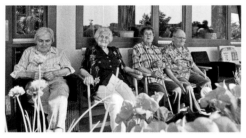

Competence Centre for People with Dementia, Nuremberg; enjoying the outdoors regularly helps improve one's sense of physical and mental well-being

Old people from migrant backgrounds

The number of older and elderly people among migrants is increasing too. This applies particularly to the first generation of immigrants. According to estimates, around 42 million immigrants live in the current European Union.[7] The majority of migrant workers who went to other countries, predominantly Germany, Austria and Switzerland, between the 1950s and the 1970s settled in the respective country and were later joined by relatives and partners. Now in the third or fourth generation, the chosen country has become their home and the centre of their lives. Although originally intending to return to their country of origin after the end of their working life, particularly as a sense of alienation can grow stronger in old age, most migrants decided to remain. On the one hand, after many years in the guest country, they are already subject to a conflict of identities; on the other, they do not want to give up health care, particularly in old age, the proximity to their children as well as the social network they have built up over many years.

In general, residents who originate from foreign countries are not very common in nursing homes and inpatient care facilities. This is primarily due to the fact that the number of older migrants is relatively low. A care centre in **Switzerland** has, for example, set up a so-called Mediterranean wing especially for Italian, Spanish and Portuguese guest workers, who are also cared for in their respective mother tongue. More recently, a rise in the proportion of care staff from multicultural backgrounds can also be observed.

In **Germany**, the first multicultural home for the elderly (Haus am Sandberg) was opened in 1997 in Duisburg. The pilot project "Care for the Elderly with Ethnic Backgrounds" was a joint project funded by the University of Duisburg and the Foundation for Social Welfare. The centre provides care and nursing that is sensitive to the cultural needs of other backgrounds. In the Sossenheim district of Frankfurt, a nursing home for Turkish and German senior citizens was opened in 2007. Germany's first nursing home for elderly people of Turkish origin was also opened in 2007 in Berlin-Kreuzberg.

Intercultural, trans-cultural, culturally-sensitive are a few of the many adjectives that describe the aim of providing suitable care and nursing for migrants. For a long time cultural integration activities gave little attention to the aspect of old age as the issue was not pressing. In the meantime, according to the German Federal Statistical Office, over 1.3 million foreigners living in Germany are over 60 years old, a number that will rise to 2.8 million by the year 2030. Numerous studies have underlined an urgent need for action, indicating that elderly migrants will be an increasingly important sector in care for the elderly. Most migrants are aware of nursing homes, but associate them primarily with loneliness and decrepitude. For a long time there were very few concepts for adapting care, living and nursing services to the needs of migrants. Very slowly, care facilities are showing a gradual awareness of the need to deal with this issue, particularly in view of the fact that more and more elderly migrants will need social, health and care facilities in the future. As a result of the historical separation of migrant work and care for the elderly, comparatively little is known about provisions and care for the elderly. Efforts should be made to intensify the link between policies for the elderly and migration. Furthermore, there is insufficient knowledge of cultural requirements for the adequate care of migrants in old age. For this reason, a systematic exchange of information at a regional level between facilities and projects who already have experience with the specific problems facing migrants as they grow older would be most desirable. In addition, migration should become anchored in social policy in order to integrate future generations of migrants from an early stage in the pre-existing culture of social care for the elderly.

In the south German city of Fürth, for example, many migrants from different backgrounds live for the most part in their own cultural groups and organisations. An attempt at counteracting this tendency has been made through the creation of an "intercultural garden". A promenade along the banks of the River Rednitz serves as an important bridge between the cultures and is intended to become a meeting point for people from various cultural backgrounds.[8] Through the inclusion of facilities for the elderly and inter-generational recreational areas, this kind of garden could be a constructive way of enriching and transforming life in old age.

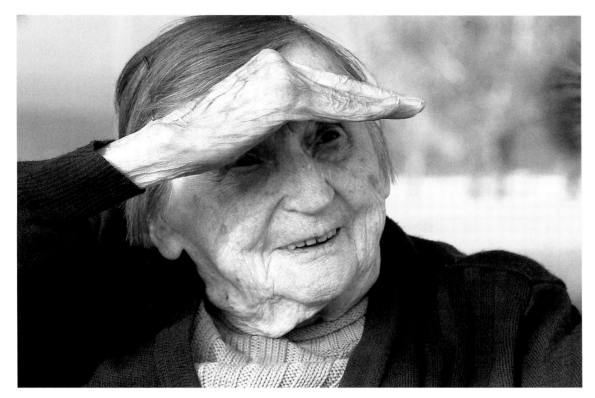
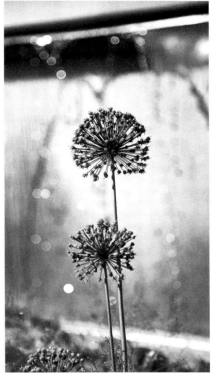

Outlook

Political, economic and societal transformations will continue to influence the development of life expectancy, but the transformations resulting from the ageing of society are already visible and can no longer be ignored. While the topic has had a degree of public exposure, the issue needs to be reconsidered from the point of view of society as a whole; in addition to numerical factors, greater consideration has to be given to environmental factors and cultural, social and psychological aspects. Furthermore, society has to work towards developing a more positive attitude towards older generations. All too often pensioners are regarded as a group that primarily costs money. It is indicative that around the world, only Japan has a day – the 15th September – dedicated to respecting the elderly.

Notes

1 *Survey of Health, Ageing and Retirement in Europe.*

2 K. Haberkern, M. Szydlik, *Kölner Zeitschrift für Soziologie und Sozialpsychologie*, 2008.

3 Ibid.

4 S. Tschirpke, *Gemeinsam statt einsam: Die Seniorenhaltestelle* (http://gesundineuropa.radio.cz/), 2006.

5 R. Lorenz, *Der Spiegel*, Sep. 2005.

6 H. Kazim, *Spiegel Online*, Feb. 2008.

7 R. Münz, *Migration in Europa: Rückblick auf das 20. Jahrhundert, Ausblick auf das 21. Jahrhundert, Konsequenzen für die politische Integration*, 2006.

8 www.iska-nuernberg.de/zab/ (accessed 05/2008).

MARIE-THERESE KRINGS-HECKEMEIER

New forms of living for the elderly

New challenges arising from demographic change

In all European nations, the population will grow steadily older in the coming years.[1] In addition, longer life expectancy means that there is a greater proportion of people of an advanced old age. As the risk of becoming dependent on ongoing nursing care increases disproportionately with age, the level of care and support facilities for the elderly will change, both in terms of quantity and quality, to a degree that is generally still underestimated today.

Societal conditions are changing. In Germany, the greater proportion of all care for the elderly is undertaken by families, sometimes by friends and neighbours in conjunction with external services. In Europe, the level of support provided by families and relatives will change in the coming years as fewer children are being born[2] and because many have moved away from their home environment to find work, while the older, less mobile generation remains where they are. In addition, the proportion of women who work has risen, resulting in less capacity for informal assistance.

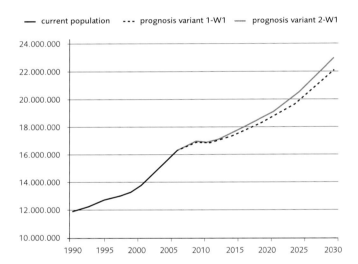

Projection of the old-age-dependency ratio (65 years and older) in Germany
Source: German Federal Statistical Office, 11th coordinated population projection, in part interpolated (2006); *empirica*

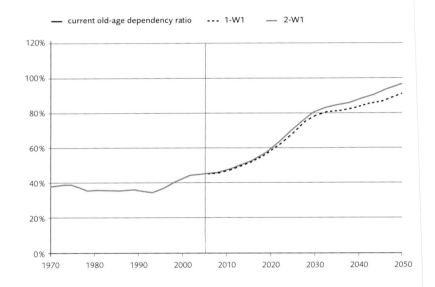

Old-age dependency ratio
The old-age dependency ratio describes the ratio of people aged 60 years and older to 100 people aged between 20 and 59 years. Dataset: Germany overall (values prior to 1990 are mean values for GDR and BRD).
Source: German Federal Statistical Office, 11th coordinated population projection, in part interpolated (2006); *empirica*

Excursus: 11th coordinated population projection
In the current coordinated population projection by the German Federal Statistical Office (11th projection, 2006), the statisticians have calculated twelve relevant prognoses which differ according to long-term external migration, birth rate and life expectancy scenarios. The diagrams show the prognoses 1-W1 and 2-W1, which represent the middle projection for birth rate (1.4 children per woman, consistent with the past) and a migration balance of 100,000 (W1) for external migration. In view of the falling and lower net immigration rates in the last five years (from 2003-2007 on average 74,000 persons per year), the 200,000 migration balance prognosis is probably too high.
In terms of different life expectancy scenarios, variants 1 and 2 are both shown. Variant 1 predicts the life expectancy of a new-born boy in 2050 to be 83.5 years and the continuing life expectancy of a 60-year-old man to increase to 25.3 years. The life expectancy of a new-born girl will increase to 88.0 years in 2050 and the continuing life expectancy of a 60-year-old woman to 29.1 years. Variant 2 predicts the life expectancy of a new-born boy in 2050 to be 85.4 years and the continuing life expectancy of a 60-year-old man to increase to 27.2 years. The life expectancy of a new-born girl will increase to 89.8 years in 2050 and the continuing life expectancy of a 60-year-old woman to 30.9 years.

It is foreseeable that the cost of services for the elderly will escalate rapidly, caused by an increased demand for affordable care and support services coupled with unfavourable conditions. The aging of society in general will be accompanied by a parallel decline in the level of support provided by families, resulting in a contradiction for service providers: the number of elderly people dependent on help and services of various kinds will rise; at the same time the cost of these services will rise disproportionately as increasing demand leads to bottlenecks in supply and higher prices.

In the interests of the elderly and of the public sector, the changes described make it essential to develop new, innovative forms of living that foster self-organised arrangements and integrate forms of mutual assistance. In addition, it will be necessary to develop a variety of different offerings so that people with different needs can find an option appropriate to their requirements: the ability to remain independent for as long as possible and to make use of care and support only where absolutely necessary.

Forms of living for the elderly

The great majority of old people – in Germany over 90% of over 65-year-olds – live in private households. In Germany, of those in need of ongoing care, nearly a third live in nursing homes and around half are cared for by relatives. In addition to nursing homes, there are a number of professionally-run alternative forms of housing with combined care and support services.

Assisted living / serviced apartments

Assisted living or sheltered housing facilities with outpatient nursing and health care has existed for several years and increased since the introduction of long-term care insurance. The basic principle is that each person lives in "their own four walls" – whether as tenant or owner – and leads their everyday life more or less how they wish. The design and fittings are conceived with the needs of old people in mind, for example taking into account possible mobility restrictions, so that they can still live independently even when in need of ongoing care and assistance. This is complemented by a series of professional services (including nursing care) which can be taken advantage of as needed and are payable only when used. Ancillary services are provided in different combinations and extents and are usually covered by a service fee. The concept of sheltered housing/assisted living is provided in a whole variety of different constellations:
- Housing schemes employing external service providers including outpatient health care and nursing;
- Housing schemes with their own staff who provide outpatient care;
- Housing schemes with their own dedicated nursing facilities;
- Housing schemes alongside a nursing home.

Retirement homes and senior residences

Retirement homes and senior residences are privately financed, well-equipped housing schemes consisting predominantly of suites as well as small apartments. Care and support is provided at home; sometimes additional inpatient care in a separate part of the complex is part of the comparably exclusive service.

Retirement homes and senior residences often have a hotel-like character with a café and/or restaurant. In most cases basic services are provided, such as lunch, cleaning services and general support services. Retirement homes and senior residences offer a series of more or less generous common areas. These can include an appropriately generous entrance lobby, a library, swimming pool, well-equipped common rooms such as a club room or fireside room, and a sun terrace. In addition, they offer recreational and cultural activities from readings to courses, visits to the theatre and even holidays, at additional cost depending on the activity. Residents typically enter into a contractual agreement covering overall board and lodgings.

Communal flats, co-housing and communities

In addition to self-organised communal housing projects, an increasing number of professionally-run housing projects with a communal arrangement are appearing on the market. In some communal projects, each resident has their own apartment and lives in close quarters with others, for example in a shared house or a community of neighbours. In communal flats, each resident has their own living area rather than a distinct apartment. Communal flats are often shared by older, less able-bodied people, for example as an alternative to a nursing home for people suffering from dementia.

Urban-scale alternatives: neighbourhoods for young and old

For the future, the development of existing and new urban quarters as inter-generational neighbourhoods for young and old and the funding of community housing projects will gain increasing importance. Without such innovative solutions, local municipalities will be faced with the negative consequences of demographic change, for example the ageing of entire neighbourhoods without the necessary supporting infrastructure or the increasing financial burden of care provisions for the elderly. A study undertaken in 2006 shows that the current and, even more so, the next generation of pensioners are willing to consider new forms of living.

Current discourse focuses on forms of living in old age that not only make use of paid services provided on the market but also integrate means of informal support. In Germany in particular, sustainable urban development policies are accorded increasing importance. A German government report on the urban environment[3] emphasises the importance of cities as a living environment for all generations.[4] Housing policy aims need to be aligned with those of urban development.[5] Following this initiative by the federal government, a series of municipalities throughout Germany have implemented new approaches to local neighbourhoods,[6] promoting urban developments that give residents the chance to continue living in their neighbourhood until they die. The urban quarters are organised in such a way that informal support structures complement professional care services.

To encourage the development of neighbourhoods as places for young and old alike, it is necessary to undertake both built projects as well as social initiatives. For new building projects as well as conversions of existing buildings, the following principles are relevant:

• New housing projects for old people or major alterations to existing structures should strive for flexible solutions that make it possible to use or convert normal apartments so that their inhabitants are able to receive nursing care at home ("from living to nursing").

• As one cannot expect to cover the increasing demand for care and support through paid services alone, it is necessary to encourage and promote networks based on mutual assistance. It is important to mobilise the help old people can give to other old people: "younger pensioners" are a potentially valuable source of voluntary help and have sometimes ten to 20 years "time on their hands". Mutual support will only come about with the help of a formal structure and staffing, such as a residents' association.

• New housing projects should ensure that services are available in the vicinity. To avoid unnecessary costs, each individual scheme does not need to have its own expensive-to-run services. Urban quarters can be organised in such a way that a "common care centre" can provide affordable services and round-the-clock cover, which can be called upon by the entire neighbourhood.

• The integrative approach of multi-generational neighbourhoods represents a model for the future: combinations of different housing options together with an easily accessible living environment (following the principles of Universal Design). Neighbourhood housing should be arranged so that it encourages the exchange of services between young and old.

• Housing schemes for old people that are integrated into local neighbourhoods can represent a focal point from which additional services for members of the local community in need of care can be based. They can provide, for example, a midday meal for young and old alike as well as different forms of recreational activities.

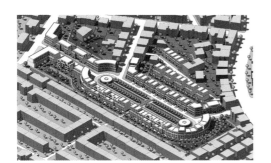

New housing quarter for young and old in Braunschweig

Notes

1 Life expectancy of a new-born boy in the year 2002/2004: 75.9 years; 60-year-old man, 20 years.

2 Life expectancy of a new-born girl in the year 2002/2004: 81.5 years; 60-year-old woman, 24.1 years.

3 Representative survey conducted by *empirica* among the 50 plus generations: "Die Generationen über 50 – Wohnsituation, Potenziale und Perspektiven", commissioned by the national headquarters of the Landesbausparkassen im Deutschen Sparkassen- und Giroverband, 2006. Download: www.lbs.de/publikationen.

4 "Nachhaltige Stadtentwicklung – ein Gemeinschaftswerk", Städtebaulicher Bericht der Bundesregierung, 2004.

5 "Innovationen für familien- und altengerechte Stadtquartiere", ExWoSt-Informationen Nr. 32/1 - 03/2007, Bonn.

6 Model project "Innovationen für familien- und altengerechte Stadtquartiere", www.stadtquartiere.de.

7 Special report "Innovationen für familien- und altengerechte Stadtquartiere – europäische Fallstudien", European case studies conducted by the University of Stuttgart, Städtebau-Institut, Fachgebiet Grundlagen der Orts- und Regionalplanung, publication forthcoming in 2009.

8 A project as part of the research programme on experimental housing and town planning ("Experimenteller Wohnungs- und Städtebau") by the Federal Ministry of Transport, Building and Urban Affairs and the Federal Office for Building and Regional Planning.

9 www.woonservicewijken.nl, www.moerwijk.nl, www.woonzorgzone.nl, www.moerwijker.nl.

10 www.braunschweig.de/stleonhardsgarten/index.html.

Innovative urban quarters in Europe for families and old people

A series of European case studies[7] undertaken as part of the model project "innovative urban quarters for families and old people"[8] describe approaches from different countries which focus on the integration of young and old at the level of the neighbourhood.

In the Netherlands, so-called residential care zones ("Woonzorgzone") have been initiated since the turn of the century. These are neighbourhoods, settlements, sometimes villages which offer optimal conditions for assisted living. The aim is that the residents can continue to live their own lives as they grow older and when they become less mobile. Since the realisation of the first residential care zones, the term and concept of this form of accommodation has changed. They are now termed residential serviced settlements or quarters ("Woonservicewijken"). In this revised concept, care and support services are no longer solely for senior citizens but for all inhabitants in the neighbourhood. An example of such a settlement is the Woonzorgzone Moerwijk in The Hague.

In Denmark too, there is a long tradition of urban and housing policies aimed at social integration where old people can live in normal apartments. For this reason no dedicated housing schemes for old people have been built since 1987. The idea that older people live alongside younger people in their home neighbourhoods has been accorded high priority and is anchored in legislation. Housing for the elderly (which is accessible, equipped with alarm systems and so on) is eligible for grant funding and schemes are scattered throughout existing quarters.

In Germany, current initiatives are examining how lessons from the aforementioned model projects can be transferred. In Braunschweig a former tram depot in the city centre is being converted into a new housing quarter for young and old.[10] From the very beginning, a series of events, surveys and activities were employed to involve interested parties in a multi-phase competition. The end result encourages different generations to live together, and the architectural design of the scheme is planned so as to adapt to the changing structure of generations in the years to come.

The experiences of the model projects throughout Europe can serve to elaborate new directions for sustainable urban development. Urban qualities and housing tailored to the needs of the people can contribute towards strengthening communal living for all generations.

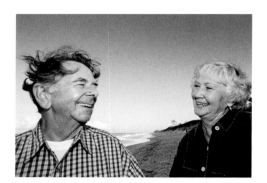

MARIA B. DWIGHT

From retirement-communities of care to communities of meaning

Introduction

Every society in every country has its own special considerations and will seek its own appropriate solutions to improve and maintain the quality of life for its older citizens. Every culture has its very special nuances. Every individual has a personal set of values and expectations. But people everywhere are seeking a quality of life that transcends just the need for medical care and shelter. There is no best or correct model, but rather a multiplicity of appropriate responses which, when thoughtfully combined, will make the most appropriate model for that specific time, in that specific place.

As populations continue to expand and new generations of people enter late life in an increasingly techno-logical and global community, the options and models will need to be flexible to respond to market factors. The demands for less costly, less institutional responses will continue to drive the private and public sectors towards consumer-driven innovation.

The traditional models

In the last 60 years, the major providers of housing and care for the elderly in the United States have fo-cused their energies on emulating two diverse and equally inappropriate models. The retirement housing segment looked for cues within the collegiate model of campus and dormitory. The health care component, driven by the advent of the federal insurance programmes of Medicare and Medicaid, followed the medical model as exemplified by the acute care hospital. Within the rigid boundaries of such diverse environments, we have tried to develop continua of care, which have historically required the consumers to physically move from living space to health care space, depending upon their level of frailty.

The management concepts developed over this period were based on a hierarchical structure, with a pater-nal attitude towards residents and families. Loyalty to the sponsoring organisation was assumed, through brand names or religious or fraternal memberships. The rigidity of the rules and daily schedule was not ques-tioned. The flow of information was controlled and narrow. The focus was "we are taking care of you".

The new forces

Within the last decade we have seen the unravelling of this model. There has been a dramatic change in expectations and demands among older people. They are seeking a different philosophy and new poli-cies that encourage and support healthy ageing. They refute the concept that old age is a disease. There are diseases common to late life and the ageing process, just as there are those common in childhood and adolescence. These geriatric diseases are overwhelmingly chronic, are often multiple and are usually treat-able, but not necessarily curable. This reality means that older people are aware that their lifestyles do and will play an important role in their health and in the quality of life in their later years. They are looking for the services that will help them to stay mentally and physically active, and not simply for services to care for them when they are ill.

They are also looking for continued control over their lives, maintaining the dignity and autonomy that comes with self-direction and decision-making. This is true throughout the age spectrum and should affect the operations of nursing centres as well as assisted living and retirement communities.

There is power in information. Older people are finding access to information through new and varied con-duits. The net and the web have opened up new avenues. Alternative and/or complimentary medicine has augmented or sometimes replaced traditional "Western" medicine. The use of vitamins, herbs and hormo-nal supplements is commonplace among the older population, as is the demand for therapeutic massage, and stress-reducing exercise and meditation. The concept of healing has taken on new dimensions that in-clude spiritual as well as physical manifestations.

There is accessible information about all facets of life besides health care. The knowledge of where to ac-cess reliable and valued services is available, as well as costs, quality measures and consumer satisfaction levels. Our research shows us that older people are primarily seeking accessibility to, and quality of, services, to help them help themselves. The old constituent loyalties are gone, having been replaced by the pursuit of quality.

This bursting forth of technology as an information source has had another profound effect on the future of service delivery among the elderly. Most older people prefer to remain in their own homes until they die. It is not an unreasonable expectation, which is now made more possible through the plethora of medical procedures that can be delivered in the home setting. Adaptive and new technologies are being beta-site tested now, to make the homes of the future into intelligent environments, providing unobtrusive security, health monitoring and safety features.

This combination of forces, a new consumer cohort with new demands and new technologies with innovative applications, is creating cracks of significant proportion in the traditional models of care and service for older people. However, we see builders and service providers perpetuating the old order, resorting to the comfortable past, controlling the information flow and maintaining systems that discourage consumer participation and decision-making. To exacerbate the situation, the health insurance industry has another agenda, which is to reduce costs through reduced utilisation. If all of these forces were to come together in a reasoned fashion, we might construct a new policy and an intelligent approach to serving the needs of the elderly in society.

The new models: life-long living and learning centres

If the providers of housing for the elderly are to succeed in the future, they must reinvent themselves out of the past. The college model has some attributes that can be salvaged. The concept of collegiality and "environment matching" is sound. People like to live with people who share their values and ethics. However, most college students spend the majority of their time outside of the dormitory, as opposed to older people, who spend the majority of their time within their private space. Our research shows that (regardless of income) this generation of elders wants larger dwelling units (a one-bedroom apartment with a den is the smallest acceptable unit), more amenities within their units (washer/dryers, microwaves, kitchens, etc.) and less public or communal space. This quest for privacy and individualism will become even more prevalent in succeeding generations.

The most intriguing part of the academic model (and its raison d'être) was originally designed out, and now is being reintroduced. This is the concept of the campus (horizontal or vertical) as a living and learning centres. We have worked with colleges and universities to create life-long learning centres because we have found that many, who are enjoying a longer span of healthy late life, are seeking out opportunities to continue to grow intellectually. Many institutions of higher learning are seeing numbers of non-traditional students flock to their classes. In recognising this trend, and the increasing demand for healthy bodies and healthy minds, we have had the opportunity to design integrated university and retirement campuses. The ancillary services, such as security, maintenance, dietary, transportation, housekeeping, and health care will be amortised over both resident populations. Academic classes and cultural, sporting and social events will be open to all who wish to attend. There will be a symbiotic relationship between the young learner and the mature learner. Some of the academic classrooms will be on the retirement campus, as will dining and hospitality services. The interplay between the two populations will be self-selected, and will not impinge on the privacy of either. It is anticipated that many retired faculty will welcome retirement in this academic setting, as will many who simply seek an intellectually stimulating environment.

Other models have developed retirement communities that are physically close to universities and are intended to attract alumni. Our model has integrated the programmes of the two campuses, and, I think, offers a more innovative opportunity for inter-generational living, within the boundaries of a retirement milieu. It also makes efficient use of human and financial resources, which in turn keeps costs competitive for the consumer.

However, with the advent of the Virtual University and distance learning centres, this model could be initiated in freestanding retirement communities or in the community at large.

Another aspect of college life that is applicable to the future campuses is the interest in healthy bodies. The health club (a variation of the traditional gym) has taken a dominant place in the demands of the older cohort. The health club, in fact, has replaced the health (or nursing) centre in the hierarchy of demands. This is expected to be a professionally staffed, dedicated space that includes a weight and exercise room, an exercise pool and lockers with showers. The focus of these facilities is to improve balance and flexibility, as well as to provide a therapeutic environment and rehabilitation.

Managerial styles are also changing to accommodate these new expectations. With more men surviving to late life and selecting retirement communities, and with more self-assured women with business and professional experience, there are more questions about management direction, and we are seeing resident participation on all levels of decision-making becoming more prevalent. Information is more forthcoming. Schedules are being developed based on the desires of the consumers instead of for the convenience of the staff. Buildings are being remodelled or replaced, and programmes are being redesigned. Residents are "ageing in place" in their apartments, and services are coming to them instead of them moving to the services. The desire to die at home includes a home in a retirement facility.

The health care continuum
These shifts in service delivery are beginning to play havoc with other levels of care. Assisted living has become the nursing home of the pre-Medicare past. Nursing centres only care for those who are terminally ill, medically needy or in a rehabilitative regimen, or in late stages of severe chronic disease or dementia. But even in the health care continuum there are increased demands for consumer autonomy and self-determination.

Celebration City in Orlando, Florida, a Disney Community, has developed an innovative model with the Adventist Health System, which may well be the precursor of the future. It is called HealthCompass, which is a personal health management tool that allows consumers to develop a longitudinal lifelong health record for themselves and their family members on the internet. The consumer remains in control of the record at all times, and can add to the documentation as well as allowing access to other providers.

Another dramatic example of this new concept in care provision is at the Kameda Medical Center in Japan. John Wocher, Executive Vice President of the organisation, has instituted a technological system that has created a film-less, paper-less hospital, that is patient-focused and patient care-centred. Each patient has a bedside computer terminal, which provides patient and family access to all records, notes, etc. on the patient's history, as well as documenting patient preferences for the care staff. The patient may add to the files. The record goes with the patient upon discharge, and also becomes a part of a permanent longitudinal record of the individual's health history.

Unique populations
Developing retirement options for people of modest means has been a creative challenge. We have worked on a number of innovative, adaptive reuse projects, which utilise existing structures and infrastructures to minimise capital costs. We have also developed operational programme models that integrate a brokered "care management" package for the residents into the existing community network of services, thereby reducing redundancies in service provision and personnel. It also provides an integrated, cohesive package of services at a reasonable cost. A concierge (not a social worker) accesses the system for the residents, or they can do it themselves through a personal or community-based computer. Technology has been a vital component in making this an efficient and responsive management system. Some of the adaptive reuse projects have included decommissioned military bases, mills from the days of the industrial revolution, schools, convents and hotels.

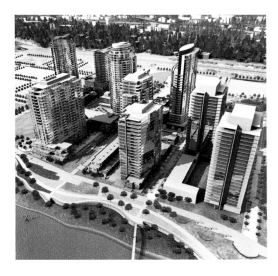
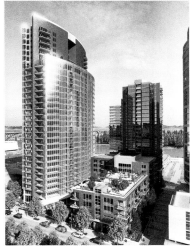
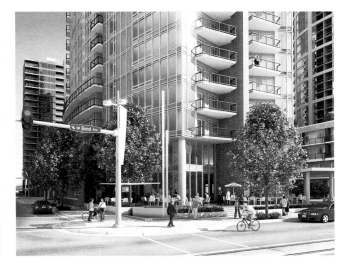
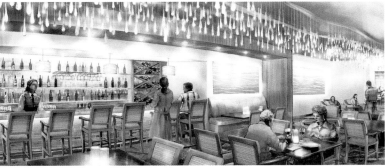
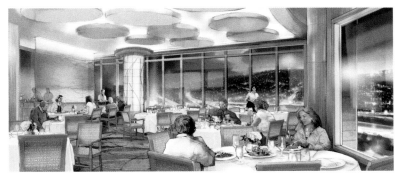

Mirabella
Located in a new urbanism development on the Willamette River in Portland, Oregon, the Mirabella will take every advantage of the neighbourhood's extensive amenities, while also pro-viding robust services for its residents. It is affiliated with the prestigious Oregon Health and Science University, and is situated directly on the light rail line.

Conclusion

The evolution in the United States from a post-industrial, post-technological society into the information age is having a profound effect on how we meet the demands of the elderly. Simultaneously, we are experiencing the influences of the largest, most highly educated, geographically mobile, affluent cohort of older people that we have ever had in our society. The traditional ways are falling aside, and new models are rising. But the gap between rich and poor continues to grow. There are also many new ethnically and culturally diverse populations within our urban and rural communities, and many have immigrated with their elderly. They, like many of their counterparts in their homelands, and their age peers here, are finding that the demands of this new society are breaking down the old order, and the traditional family responsibilities are no longer possible to undertake.

There are lessons to be learned from our evolution. Often wisdom comes from understanding mistakes or misdirections. Moments in history, political decisions, well-meaning attitudes, lack of knowledge: all have created the complex tapestry of the past. As other cultures and countries make this transition from industrial or agriculturally based societies, they too will experience the pain of change but, hopefully, they will avoid some of our missteps, and will learn from our collective pasts. We have an awesome challenge before us as a global community.

Dementia as a mode of being: the living environment and everyday competency

JOHANNA MYLLYMÄKI-NEUHOFF

Dementia affects every fourth person over 65 years of age and the average duration of the illness is around ten years. In some cases the illness can continue for twice as long. During this period around two thirds of all dementia sufferers live at home, nursed and cared for by relatives.

From a medical point of view, the clinical picture of dementia is quickly described. For an unknown reason, protein deposits, so-called "plaques", develop in the brain and disrupt the transmission of information between brain nerve cells, causing them to successively die. The illness generally progresses through several stages and eventually leads to helplessness and hospitalisation. People with dementia first begin to suffer memory loss, then become disorientated and unable to recognise things; in later stages the illness can lead to a loss of identity and social isolation.

For several years, teams of scientists around the world have conducted intensive research into the key causes of this illness. According to the current level of knowledge, the assumption is that the development of the plaques is accompanied by inflammatory processes. At present there is no known medical remedy. Generally recognised therapies include treatments aimed at delaying the onset of dementia with the help of pharmacological and cognitive therapies and endeavouring to improve the quality of life of dementia sufferers.

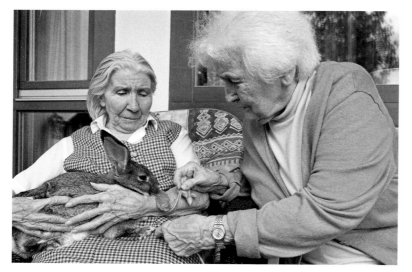 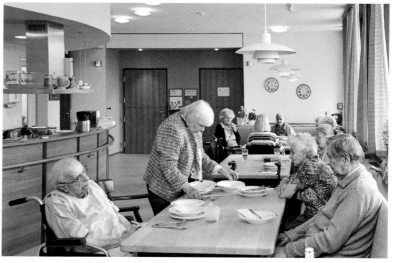

Competence Centre for People with Dementia, Nuremberg; contact with animals and taking part in everyday activities has a therapeutic effect

More recently, a new tendency has emerged in research in which dementia is considered as a psychological development process and not exclusively in terms of coping with an illness. This allows one to develop positive approaches to dealing with the different individual modes of being of dementia rather than focussing entirely on the cognitive deficits of the sufferer.

The sufferer is aware of the developing onset of the illness from an early stage, particularly as their interactions with their surroundings change. Everyone has a specific relationship to their immediate environment which is influenced by the congruence or fit between one's personal wishes and needs and the conditions and demands of the environment.[1] A key criteria for this fit is one's ability to feel competent and therefore independent and safe. Even persons with mild cognitive impairments (so-called MCI patients) exhibit changes in their interactions with their environment. These cognitive impairments lead to errors in one's memory of places and a reduced ability to spontaneously adapt to new spaces and unknown situations. As sufferers begin to realise these changes, they may feel a sense of shame and inadequacy caused by emotional borderline situations resulting from difficulties in knowing where they are, finding their way or performing normal daily routines.

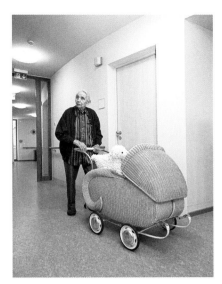
People with dementia often live in a world of their own

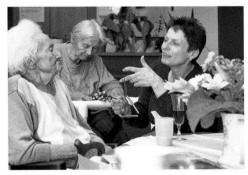
Individual communication and stimulation

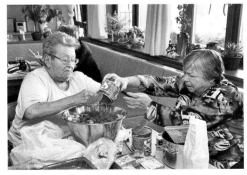
Catering for the needs of the residents

The home and immediate surroundings of a dementia sufferer may on the one hand become a corset, and on the other provide compensatory elements as, according to ecological psychology, people are influenced in their experiences, thoughts and actions by their environment and where they live.[2] This means that people and their actions are inseparably and mutually linked with their immediate surroundings, a fact that applies to people who are healthy or impaired alike. In order to better understand the behaviour of dementia sufferers and to adapt their living environment better to their needs with a view to enabling them to live independently, we need as much knowledge as possible about the effect of spaces and environments on their complex experiences and actions. At present we are still in the starting blocks. The little we are able to learn at present is limited to eco-gerontological knowledge about appropriate environments for old people and what relatives and carers observe about the sufferer's interactions with specific environments. Practicable instruments with which to assess the dementia sufferer's own subjective interaction with different spatial structures and their assessment of the qualities of their environment are still lacking.

Memory loss as a threat to identity and everyday life

In the first years of dementia, memory loss and a loss of orientation are the primary symptoms. More complex challenges in everyday life such as making financial arrangements, staying organised and keeping appointments, finding new places and coping with road traffic are the first things to become a problem. Sufferers are generally quite aware of their situation and attempt by avoiding such situations to disguise their first cognitive impairments behind an intact façade so as not to make a bad impression. The topic of dementia is often taboo for the sufferer and possible interventions are met with vigorous denial and stubborn adherence to how things are. They do not regard themselves as ill and believe they can still solve their problems on their own. Over time, however, situations start to arise where sufferers experience difficulties in dealing with everyday actions, creating uncertainty and worry. Uncertainty leads in turn to a loss of confidence and vitality and can eventually cause the person to withdraw into himself and from interactions with others. These deficiencies make it ever more difficult for the sufferer to come to terms with everyday life. Social contacts with friends and acquaintances become suddenly less pleasurable, and communications and reciprocal interactions with their different environments begin to dwindle and are later avoided entirely. The overall pattern is one of increasing withdrawal caused by a subjective feeling of inadequacy. Little by little they begin to lose control of their own lives.

In many cases people with cognitive impairments lose interest in activities and hobbies that were previously important to them and gradually withdraw from actively and emotionally shaping their direct surroundings. To cite a concept by Albert Bandura, the everyday world of people in the early stages of dementia is characterised by a loss of confidence in their own self-efficacy.[3] They lose confidence in their own competence and ability to deal with things as a result of the difficulties they experience, which to them seem uncontrollable. The doubts in their own self-efficacy allow stress and worry to become overpowering. Their own environment is experienced less and less subjectively as being meaningful. This loss of self-confidence and the increasing inability to master everyday activities is usually closely linked to the person's progressive withdrawal. In such situations changes to the person's everyday life and environment feel most threatening. The feeling of helplessness is exacerbated and with it the problem of self-identity: am I still the person I once was, what can I still do, what comes next?

Bidding farewell to the familiar

The sufferer's interactions with their environment are dominated more and more by stressful situations. In everyday activities they begin to increasingly reach the limits of their physical abilities and find it steadily more difficult to keep a grip on their environment as complex thought processes become more difficult to follow. The repeated occurrence of irresolvable everyday problems results in emotional stress reactions, which do not go unnoticed by their surroundings. These subjective responses to the symptoms of the illness often cause conflicts with loved ones, partners, family and relatives. Because the sufferer's actions are rarely understood by the people around them, their social context has a particularly significant influence on their self-esteem. It is as if an irresolvable vacuum stands between the sufferer's intentions and the observed behaviour. Relatives need a great deal of background knowledge of the illness and practical help in order to better understand and communicate with the sufferer. During this phase it is particularly difficult for the family to come to terms with the inner world and helplessness of the sufferer, particularly as their behaviour follows no logical pattern. It is difficult for them to accept and understand the mistrust, aggression and anxiety that they may be confronted with. For the relatives it inevitably reaches a point where they will have to bid farewell to the familiar behavioural patterns of the person as the key characteristics of their personality gradually recede. Friends and relatives will need to learn to tolerate often strange and unusual behaviour.

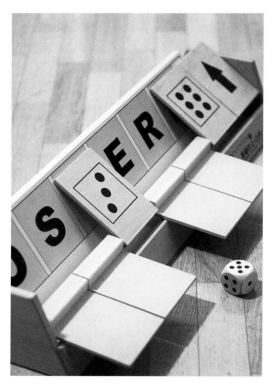

Games can help improve cognitive skills

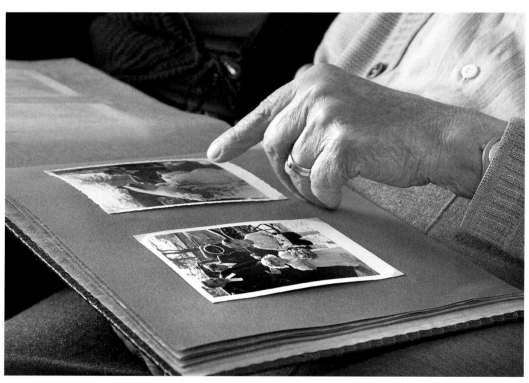

Regular reminding of one's own biography can slow the process of loss of personality structures

Acceptance

The once active and self-driven relationship with personal contexts, spaces or relationships and the continuation of hobbies such as working in the garden become increasingly impossible as the illness progresses. Paradoxically, the more a person begins to lose their sense of identity and will to actively control and shape their environment, the more important their environment becomes for them as a stable and comprehensible background. The constancy of their physical surroundings gives dementia sufferers a feeling of stability and security. In this phase, the long-term memory begins to take over comprehension of surroundings while the "consciously and actively planned present" recedes. The focus shifts from actively adapting to surroundings to tolerating and accepting them.

This viewpoint has in the meantime been taken up in discourse on the professional care of dementia sufferers and the building of appropriate facilities. After a controversial exchange of opinions in the past, professionals have since reached agreement on what characteristics are important for facilities for dementia sufferers. Institutions appropriate for dementia sufferers should take into account and offer three components: the optimal built elements of the facility and ward, the psychosocial milieu and the organisation of nursing and of how people live together. In professional circles, milieu therapy models are currently much discussed as a way of designing an environment that is "appropriate" and "tolerable" for the sufferers.[4]

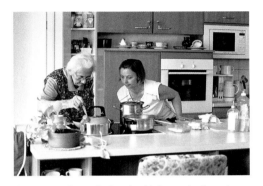

Competence Centre for People with Dementia, Nuremberg; life in an environment designed for people with dementia can help residents regain a sense of everyday competency

The environment should adapt, not the sufferer

Dementia limits the degree of independence, self-control and ability to cope with one's surroundings. Providing appropriate living quarters is difficult when perception, cognition and orientation are so impaired that the entire person-environment congruence has shifted out of balance.

The close relationship between a person and their environment has become so far removed from its previous form as a result of the illness that previously active mechanisms for coming to terms with one's environment give way to coping mechanisms such as avoidance and acceptance. Dementia sufferers are no longer able to react flexibly and appropriately to situations in their surroundings and to engage with reality. They can only react intuitively and emotionally to situations around them. Without any form of selfcontrol it would seem that the sufferer is entirely helpless. The built environment therefore presents a constant challenge for dementia sufferers, its level of intensity affecting their well-being and perception of stress. Their sense of well-being is best when the stimulus provided by the active and compensatory aspects of the surroundings is perceived by the sufferer as consistent and they are subject to neither an excess nor a lack of stimulation. As the illness progresses, even once familiar surroundings can suddenly be perceived differently and even mutate to nightmarish scenarios.

From a neurobiological point of view, this change in perception can be explained by the fact that our direct perception is not solely a real-time response but is also informed by long-term interpretative patterns from the past. Dementia sufferers may therefore experience a dislocated perception of the present situation produced by the "disjointed" brain. Our experience of the world is scenic and that of dementia sufferers is too. The loss of short-term memory means that they are not able to adapt and compensate in the same way as they used to. In situations of unease, patients may fall back on behavioural patterns, such as searching for something, that are rooted in an attempt to escape from momentary feelings. This behaviour is often described as a tendency to "wander away", with the patient acting unsettled and roaming around. The desire to "go home" can be interpreted as a signal that the person feels lost at that moment and seeks a place of comfort and security.

The guiding principle for the creation of environments appropriate for dementia sufferers is to focus on the everyday needs of the patients and to precisely observe the continual changes in their living environments. This point of view opens up new perspectives for the care and housing of dementia sufferers as it allows one to observe the complex emotional and social needs more clearly, and consequently to create more positive everyday experiences and environments for the patients. In a more coherent and predictable environment, dementia sufferers can expect to feel more competent in what they do and as a result the avoidance mechanisms they have developed and negative expectations of their self-efficacy may gradually recede.[5]

Notes

1 R. Lazarus, R. Launier, "Stressbezogene Transaktionen zwischen Person und Umwelt", in J. Nitsch (ed.), *Stress. Theorien, Untersuchungen, Maßnahmen*, Bern: Huber, 1981. R. Lazarus, *Stress and Emotion – A New Synthesis*. New York: Free Association Books, 1999.

2 H.-J. Harloff, "Grundlegung der Wohnpsychologie. Zuhause/Heim als transaktionales Konzept", in *Report Psychologie*, 1989, pp. 10-15.

3 A. Bandura A., "Self-efficacy: Toward a Unifying Theory of Behavioral Change", in *Psychological Review*, Vol. 84, No. 3, 191-215. A. Bandura: "Self-efficacy mechanism in psychobiological functioning", in R. Schwarzer (ed.), *Self-efficacy: Thought Control of Action*, New York: Hemisphere, 1992, pp. 355-394.

4 Ch. Held, D. Ermini-Fünfschilling, *Das demenzgerechte Heim*, Freiburg: Karger, 2nd edition 2006.

5 The expectation of self-efficacy is one of the key aspects of cognitive theories that explain human behaviour.

STEFAN DRESSKE

Living and dying in a hospice

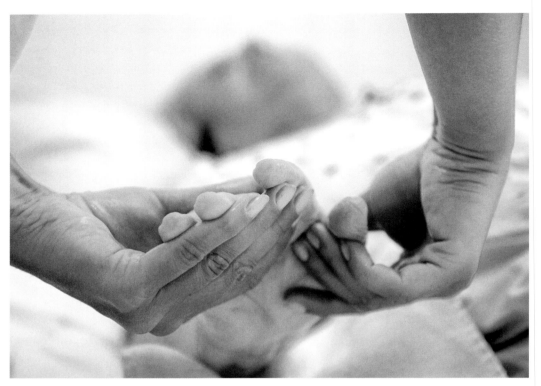

A hand massage as an additional care practice that helps reinforce the patient's sense of identity

In so-called Western societies people are dying at a much older age than ever before. Most people die of chronic degenerative diseases, illnesses that at an advanced stage can no longer be cured and often require ongoing nursing care. Nevertheless many medical options are still available to delay the progress of such illnesses and relieve suffering. The period of time in care and of dying grows increasingly longer and with it the uncertain goal of remedial-medical care. Approaches to medical treatment veer between the opposite extremes of "fighting a battle against death" on the one hand and "allowing the person to die" on the other.[1] In the meantime, independent techniques of palliative medicine have been established that aim primarily to relieve symptoms and provide psychosocial care to improve conditions for the dying person. This new special discipline brings together the fields of medicine, nursing care, social work, theology and voluntary activities built around the concept of a hospice. Hospices can provide both outpatient and inpatient care and were conceived with the aim of helping people face death as positively as possible.

This shift in the form of care provision for the dying and in attitude in general did not materialise out of nowhere. Up until the mid-1980s the topic of death was still generally taboo and fraught with inhibitions. Today, the topic of care for the dying is discussed increasingly openly – although too often in connection with legal regulations or the scandalised reporting of euthanasia or neglect in old age. However, whenever the topic is raised, the mention of hospices as institutions synonymous with dying with dignity follows soon after.

That hospices offer the best possible institutionalised care in the last phase of life is no longer called into question, neither by representatives of charities and the church, who up until the 1980s were concerned that hospices may turn into "ghettos for the dying", nor by doctors who feared their patients would be "abandoned". In fact quite the contrary: hospices are both open and public places, as I was able to verify repeatedly in an empirical study conducted in 2001 and 2002.[2] Nevertheless, most people have little idea about what is involved in providing care for the dying. An example from my observation studies illustrates how hospices work, what patients can expect and what kind of difficulties and problems commonly need to be overcome.

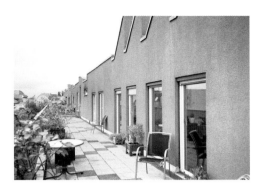

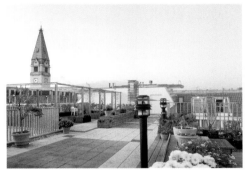

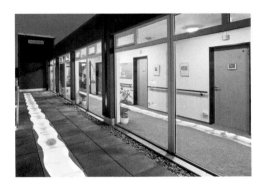

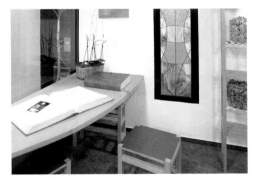

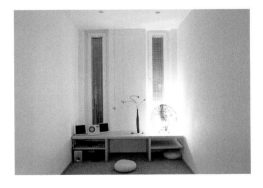

A good death – an example

Our example concerns Mr Bauer, a 95-year-old leukaemia patient. As Mr Bauer is admitted to the hospice, his condition is relatively good: he is without pain and can move around the hospice on his own. His main problem lies elsewhere: originally his daughter was supposed to take care of him in return for him financing the building of her house. However, when the time came, his daughter changed her mind. As a result, Mr Bauer is forced to live in the hospice and is accordingly aggrieved. There is nothing the nursing staff can do to appease him. He complains to the doctor treating him, makes the staff explain his medication time and again and obstinately asserts his independence. Nevertheless, the sisters and staff patiently fulfil his "special requests" and discover that he is, in their own words, a "fascinating person". While talking to him they discover that Mr Bauer was a "talented dancer" and passionate chess player and soon afterwards they initiate a game of chess with him. A few days later, Mr Bauer is so "uncooperative, stubborn and difficult" that his carer loses patience and reprimands the patient. The next day Mr Bauer does not feel well, complaining of sharp pain, dizziness and nausea. He is generally disorientated and miserable. At the end of the shift, his carer reports that "he now no longer refuses to be helped". And, as the carers later note, Mr Bauer "wept bitterly". His condition worsens and he no longer gets out of bed. The hospice calls his daughter, who until now had stayed out of things. To begin with she watches the carers do their business and sits in silence for a while with her father. The next day one of the nurses asks her to help hold her father while he is being washed. At the end of the shift the nurse describes this as a kind of embrace, which the father also reciprocates, an act that can be understood as an unspoken "reconciliation". The daughter now spends more time with her father and they even talk to one another. In the following night, three weeks after entering the hospice, Mr Bauer dies peacefully in the arms of a carer.

Supporting the identity of the dying person

From the viewpoint of the hospice, Mr Bauer's story can be regarded as a successful example of the care they provide. But what does successful mean in this context and how is this achieved? As in many other institutions, hospices also employ a systematic programme of techniques. Specifically, this includes biographical work with the patient whereby the staff constantly seek to learn more about the patient's sense of identity by watching out for references to his or her past. This is particularly effective for patients who have spent long stretches in hospital with various illnesses or who previously lived alone at home. Communication also encourages patients to express their wishes, with particular emphasis on their immediate well-being and on pleasurable experiences that the patient can enjoy then and there. Expressing one's wishes, even small wishes such as playing chess, becomes an act of self-affirmation. Such encouragement is not only expressed verbally but also through the practice of caring, which generally goes far beyond the necessities of hygiene. These "wellness" offerings in the broader sense include morning care programmes, massages with aromatic oils, bathing, accompanied walks around the hospice, joint meals etc. The care practices themselves are aimed at reinforcing the identity of the patient; the emotional care and attention provided by the staff has to do with more than just cleanliness, it is valuable in itself. Care and treatments that are stigmatising are avoided where possible, and when they are necessary, for example the use of a feeding cup or incontinence nappies, then with as little distress to the patient's personality as possible. Having to be nursed reminds patients enough of their frailty and of the fact that they are dying. The staff themselves rarely address the topic of the patient's death openly and directly, although when patients are admitted the doctor will have spoken to them about the incurability of their illness and the time they can expect to live. The doctor's explanation is, however, generally speaking a rational-cognitive process that is often not emotionally "absorbed". Many patients still harbour hopes of recovery and occasionally have quite unrealistic expectations. As Cicely Saunders (1918-2005), founder of the modern hospice movement, always said, the aim of a hospice is "not to prolong the days of your life but to improve your quality of life for the days that remain".

"Controlling the process of dying"

The physical treatments undertaken in hospices can be regarded primarily as a concerted programme of socialisation. This kind of care is supported by and indeed made possible by the programme of medical ther-

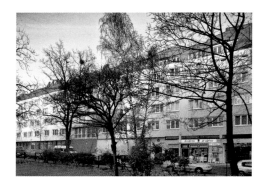

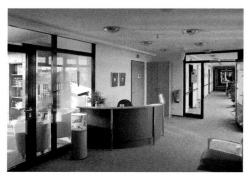

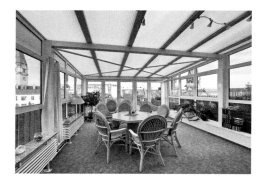

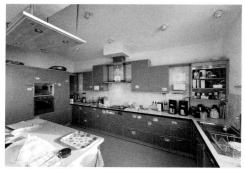

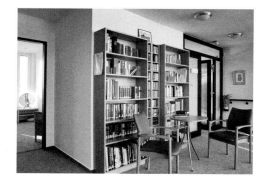

apy, as can be seen in our example too. Before the patient was admitted to the hospice, he had received a blood transfusion. The hospice doctor was somewhat sceptical, citing that although patients feel better immediately after such treatment, they feel that much worse a few days later. And indeed, Mr Bauer did not feel so well three days after being admitted, a fact which the staff attributed to the effects of the transfusion subsiding. The hospice does not try to counter or even fight the deterioration of the patient but rather to make the downward trend as bearable and smooth as possible. The practice of achieving "highs" at the cost of sudden "lows" is avoided. The aim is to anticipate and minimise the suddenness of downturns, all the while weighing up the current well-being of the patient against the prognosis of deterioration. Care provisions, medical interventions and communication with the patient aim to synchronise the mental condition of the patient with their progressive physical deterioration. When the time comes, the patient dies peacefully. This controlled process of deterioration is in some cases thwarted, for example when patients are confused and bewildered or suffer from dementia or as a result of non-treatable pain or through the outward spread of metastases. Here the nursing and care staff can only try and master the uncertain process of deterioration, and sometimes the only consolation is the knowledge that one has done the best one could. Two key dimensions determine the nature of a hospice: the focus on biographical identity and the attempt to control the course of dying as a peaceful and pain-free process.

The design of the living environment

As with any health care and social welfare institution, a hospice needs to outwardly represent its function while at the same time be a private retreat for patients and their relatives. Its architectural design can contribute to reconciling these opposing functions. For acceptance by the general public, it is important that the hospice is embedded in its immediate urban and historical context. If built as part of a hospital complex it can refer to the historical dimension of medical and health care. If extensively-glazed it can symbolise openness towards its surroundings. Openness is also an important criteria for the patients in order not to feel excluded. This can be achieved by providing ample glazing, conservatories, sheltered interior courtyards and terraces and floor-to-ceiling windows that allow bedridden patients a view of their surroundings. A further dimension of openness is the use of spaces within the hospice for exhibitions, small concerts, readings and so on. Foyers, corridors, common rooms, kitchens, "living rooms" and team rooms can be designed as a hierarchy of spaces that become progressively more private. More intimate spaces still need to be created that, while not entirely enclosed, provide patients and relatives with a spot to retreat to and be undisturbed. As places for leading one's everyday life, hospices should fulfil normal expectations with regard to domestic privacy.

The process of dying is accompanied by a simultaneity of quite different emotions. Joy, sadness, reflection and sincerity must all be accounted for in the design of the spaces so that there is place for them as everyday means of communication. Open living areas, kitchens or kitchen-living areas and clearly defined sitting areas in corridors, on terraces or in the garden offer opportunities for patients, relatives and staff to come together. Typical communal activities such as mealtimes, watching television, reading and resting should take place in semi-private, sheltered environments. In addition to facilitating everyday communication, the hospice also contains memento mori, symbolic representations of death reminding people of their own mortality and referring to the purpose of the hospice. Although not continually verbalised, death is ever present and there are sufficient opportunities for reflection and contemplation.

The patient's room is the core of the private sphere and should only be interrupted by nursing care and treatments. In addition to its functional requirements the room should provide opportunities for the patient to personalise the space. Furniture, including cupboards, should be movable and where possible there should be enough room for patients to bring smaller items of their own furniture with them. Sideboards should be visible and reachable from the bed. Family photographs, keepsakes and personal items provide points of contact and make it easier for staff to relate to the patient and make suggestions accordingly.

The overall design of the hospice should be able to accommodate entirely different personal projections – for some it is a home, for others a hospital or care home, for others a hotel. In most cases, however, patients know that they are in an institution with its own set of rules and regulations, even when these are more oriented towards their needs. It is also important to remember that most patients do not stay for very long in a hospice. Almost 70% of patients die within three weeks.[3]

Perspective on other types of care facilities

The question arises as to whether the model of care provision and ideology behind the hospice can also be of relevance to other institutions where people die. In a hospice, all the institutional provisions are directed without exception and for all patients towards accompanying the process of dying, even when the day-to-day work concentrates on upholding the identity of the person and improving their well-being. The fundamental premise is that all attempts to cure an illness are discontinued in favour of measures that alleviate its effects; in a hospice all patients are therefore dying persons. Although mortality rates in old people's homes and nursing homes are increasing, these institutions are not primarily oriented around the process of dying to the same degree as a hospice is. Individual aspects of the care provided in a hospice – symptom-oriented medical care, attentive care and support, communicative orientation, symbolism in the interiors – can most certainly be transferred to other institutions. Nevertheless, a key difference remains: the ideological position of a hospice is unequivocal, and both patients and professional staff share an awareness of the central aim of being able to die with dignity. This commitment is not as clear-cut in other kinds of institutions. In a nursing home a member of staff may need to leave their watch over a dying person in order to deal with an emergency with another patient. Here other necessities – not least to save lives – take precedence over the provision of care for the dying. However, there is one key aspect of the hospice ideology that can without doubt be transferred to other realms: the demonstration of solidarity with and affection towards the critically ill.

Notes

1 U. Streckeisen, *Die Medizin und der Tod*, Opladen: Leske & Budrich, 2001.

2 S. Dreßke, *Sterben im Hospiz. Der Alltag in einer alternativen Pflegeeinrichtung*, Frankfurt a.M.: Campus, 2005.

3 Ch. Pfeffer, „Statistik der Bundesarbeitsgemeinschaft Hospiz für das Jahr 2004", accessed on 4th June 2008: www.hospiz.net/themen/statistik.html#Hospizstatistik_2008.

Page 35, from top to bottom
Ricam Hospice, Berlin-Neukölln; rooftop addition with full-height windows and roof garden | Planted roof garden overlooking the roofscape of the surrounding neighbourhood | An artwork symbolising the flow of life | Room for remembrance of the dead | Room for peace and meditation

Page 36, from top to bottom
Ricam Hospice, Berlin-Neukölln; the hospice embedded in its urban context | Entrance area with reception and office | Seating in the conservatory | Open kitchen in which meals can be prepared according the patients' wishes | Small library in the corridor

On the essence of living:
safety – security – orientation

INSA LÜDTKE

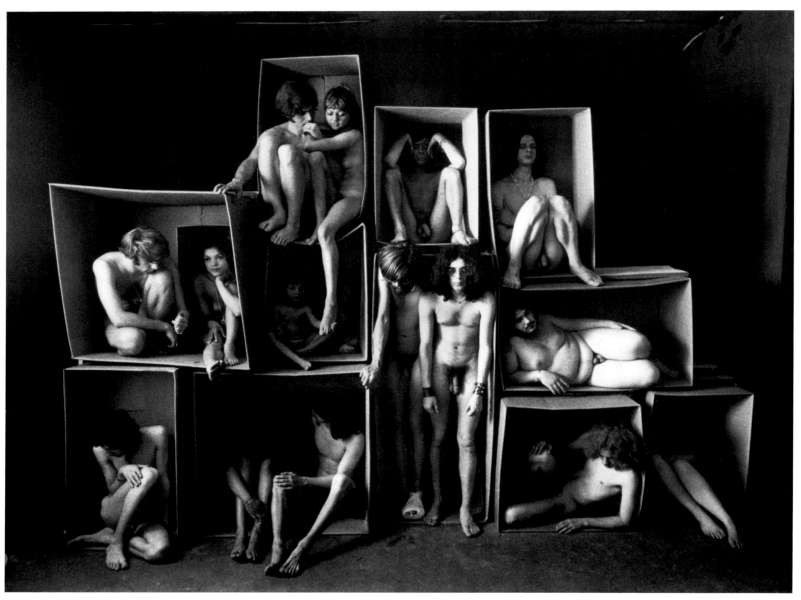

Actors of the musical "Hair"; photograph by Will McBride

"He who is unhappy with his existence will have difficulties fully living."
Immanuel Kant[1]

The catchy and provocative slogan "Still dwelling or already living?" ("Wohnst Du noch oder lebst Du schon?") is for German consumers synonymous with an international furniture retailer. Making skilful use of the stylistic device of semantic friction, it sets up a rivalry between the verbs "wohnen" (living as in dwelling) and "leben" (living as in being), and implies, through its use of "still" and "already", an evaluative opposition not present in everyday usage. The English language is by comparison not as discriminating, using the verb "to live" to denote both meanings.

The message behind the slogan implies the promise of a more dynamic, more intensely lived domestic experience.[2] Whether this can be attributed to the then (mid-20th-century) revolutionary, low-cost concept of a Swedish furniture retailer where the customer becomes part of the production process and assembles the furniture himself is doubtful. A contradiction in terms therefore remains; after all dwelling is by definition inherently linked to the notion of settlement. So where does the supposed opposition between "dwelling" and "living" come from? Without wanting to give the game away: the "essence of living" is always characterised by a degree of ambivalence.

Strictly speaking, to live, although an active verb, is not an activity in itself. It would seem ridiculous to say "Right at this moment, I'm living" while standing in one's home. People usually talk about how they live when they are outside of their own four walls: "I live on the edge of a wood ... on the third floor ... have lived alone for twenty years ... in lodgings..."[3] So although not a distinct activity in itself, the act of living can be regarded as a succession of many individual actions. These are by no means trivial things: a large part of our lives consist of ritualised activities, for example cooking, eating, washing, sleeping and clearing up. Through their regular repetition, consistent pattern and our own recurring gestures, we internalise them physically until they happen "of their own accord" without us having to think about them. The repetition and regularity with which we do things becomes habit and creates a feeling of dependability and security and not least relieves us of the need to continually make new decisions.[4]

For this reason, "to live" can mean to have found one's place. The notion of living derives from the root of the verb "to gain" and "to wander", "to roam", "to search for something". In the history of mankind, living is a comparatively recent manifestation. The primeval cave, hut or tent has little in common with our contemporary understanding of living. It was not until the Middle Ages that the notion of residing in one place, "to remain", "to stay", "to become accustomed to" became anchored in the Old Saxon verb "wonen", which in turn was derived from the Germanic root "wunian" meaning "Wonne" (delight), "well-being", "to strive for something", "to enjoy", "to be satisfied" and not least "to be enclosed" or to be physically protected.

"To stay" (indoors, in a building), however, does not fully render the contemporary understanding of living. If I stay with a friend, this does not mean that I live there. One's home represents much more: it is one's "third skin", a place of one's own, a place that encompasses the self. As such, living belongs unequivocally in the category "modern identity",[5] as echoed by the saying: "Show me where you live and I'll tell you who you are."

The ongoing process of habituation results in a growing sense of familiarity with our surroundings that we can call living in a both narrower and broader sense. Through habit we impart a sense of familiarity on a strange environment and begin to live our own lives. Thus living signifies how intricately habit and home are interwoven. It is this interlacement that turns a place where we live into our home. The turbulences associated with moving house have much more to do with breaking with old patterns and developing new habits than with adjusting to a different spatial configuration.[6] We only need think back to the first days and weeks after moving into a new home to know how powerful the force of habit can be.

An inevitable habitual activity that is quite possibly inherent to living is the gesture of opening and closing. Entering and leaving a room is framed by this twin gesture.[7] The door, its frame and the threshold beneath our feet represent a transitional space that we experience physically, whether it leads from one room to the next or from the apartment into the outside world. We also open and close curtains and blinds, cupboards and drawers, a jewel box or a laptop. Superficially, this act describes how we enter or leave a room or our home, how we regulate how much light enters the room or put away our belongings, but at a deeper level it is about experiencing spatial boundaries between "the world" and our own private realm.[8]

Conversely, opening up our private space to strangers means that we reveal information about ourselves and the conditions in which we live; the latter is a more meaningful indicator of ourselves than other supposedly intimate personal details we might volunteer such as "I am vegetarian". How we choose to live is an expression of our inner selves, externalised outwardly in the form of furnishings as well as the kind of flat or house we live in (period building or new building, terraced house or penthouse). Living is an interactive process between the inhabitant(s) and the room. This interdependency is indissoluble; as I shape the space I live in, so too do I form myself, and vice versa. For the German philosopher Martin Heidegger, being and the built are entwined at a level far greater than "one's own four walls". For him "bauen" (to build) as it was originally spoken, "buan, bhu, beo", is directly related to "bin" (to be). Here the notion of dwelling, and with it the radius of one's being, is extended far beyond the boundaries of a single enclosed space: "To be a human being means to be on the earth as a mortal. It means to dwell."[9]

Designing how we live

As intimated at the outset, living can only be superficially shoehorned into "two rooms, kitchen and bathroom". How and where we live is both trivial as well as deeply existential. For each of us, home is where our own private lives begin, that which makes up who we are.[10] That said, contradictory characteristics arise as soon as the question shifts to qualitative issues such as what form the place where we live should take. On the one hand people suppose that they will find utter bliss in their dream home, on the other "an apartment can kill a man just as easily as an axe!"[11] Accordingly, the question of what an "ideal floor plan" should look like has preoccupied generations of architects for years.

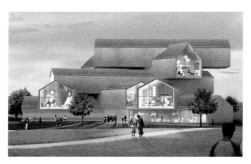

Herzog & de Meuron: "VitraHaus" on the Vitra Campus in Weil am Rhein, project design 2006

One possible approach, as proposed by the mathematician and architect Christopher Alexander, may lie in distinctly smaller spatial elements or configurations. Alexander strives for a more humane architecture oriented around basic human needs and advocates the dissolution of customary architectonic structures in favour of needs-oriented elements. Rather than placing one room next to the other, in 1977 he proposed a series of basic (relational) patterns which can serve as a basis for the design. According to the architectural theorist, the 253 patterns contained in his book "A Pattern Language" form a structure much like words in a sentence, which can be assembled without having to concern oneself with the actual architectonic appearance. Here Alexander is much more interested in archetypal spatial qualities and elements that apply across cultural boundaries, for example "a bench in front of the house".[12]

Another building that eschews traditional architectural plans is the so-called "Future Evolution House" being built in Vienna at the time of writing. As its name suggests, the architectural concept of the building not only picks up on Alexander's ideas but also takes into account the factors of time and evolution. Appropriately, the building will be the home and work space of the future consultant Matthias Horx and his family. The building plan has straightforward labels such as "Love" for where he and his wife will spend time together and "Guests" for the children's room. The latter may seem shocking for those with a more traditional notion of the family, but as Horx explains, "such thinking supposes that their children will never grow up and leave of their own accord [...]. Most people who build a house claim that they are building it for their children. That is utter rubbish." A house, according to Horx, should not constrain but provide orientation; it should be a hub from where the inhabitants can move around.[13]

Ever since the terrorist attacks on 11th September 2001, sociologists and trend researchers report an increasing tendency towards introversion and staying at home. Professionals use the term "cocooning", conjuring up images of the caterpillar spinning a cocoon around itself. This withdrawal into the protective sphere of one's own four walls is posited as an expression of our basic need for safety and security. This return to domesticity is not entirely new. The pioneering American trend researcher Faith Popcorn claims to have "discovered" this tendency as far back as the beginning of the 1980s. At that time cocooning was a synonym for cosiness. The futurologist Horst W. Opaschowski explains the new-found enthusiasm for the home as follows: "The desire to come to rest, to be left in peace and to take things easy points to a shift of consciousness in which the home and home environment play a more important role in one's quality of life."[14]

Living in the future

But what is new about the way we live? Our notion of the home is indeed a phenomenon of the modern age and is in the first instance a most personal affair. At the same time it has also become a collective experience. Notions of contemporary living are always an expression of the respective conditions in society and are as such constantly changing. This is particularly evident in the increase in floor area per person, which according to the German Federal Statistical Office has risen sharply over the last few decades: between 1968 and 2002 the average floor area per person has risen by nearly 70% to over 40 m². The trend researcher Harry Gatterer predicts that "the trend towards large living quarters will continue in the future".[15] At the same time there will be a shift in the way living quarters are arranged: in future, living quarters will be divided into wellness, entertainment and "work@home" zones, according to a study by the Zukunftsinstitut.[16]

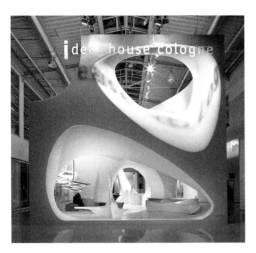

Zaha Hadid: "Ideal House Cologne", presented at the furniture fair "Imm Cologne", Cologne 2007

Notes

1 After: V. L. Nicolic, *Hausleeren*, Tübingen, Berlin: Wasmuth, 1998, p. 125.

2 R. Krause, "Lebst du schon?", in: *TAZ-MAG*, 3rd May 2003.

3 V. Kern, "Was ist Wohnen? Fünf logische Antworten", in: *TAZ-MAG*, 3rd May 2003.

4 W. Schmid, *Philosophie der Lebenskunst*, Frankfurt am Main: Suhrkamp, 2001.

5 V. Kern, ibid.

6 W. Schmid, ibid.

7 G. Selle, "Öffnen und Schließen – Über alte und neue Bezüge zum Raum", in: *Gebaute Räume – Zur kulturellen Formung von Architektur und Stadt*, 9th year, No. 1, November, Munich 2004.

8 G. Bachelard, *The Poetics of Space*, translated by Maria Jolas, Beacon Press, Boston, USA, 1969.

9 "Building, Dwelling, Thinking" (Lecture held in Darmstadt, 1951), in: *Poetry, Language, Thought*, translated by Albert Hofstadter, Harper Colophon Books, New York, 1971.

10 H. Hilger, "Die dritte Haut des Menschen", in: *Monumente*, 07/ 2006.

11 H. Zille, quoted in J. Reulecke (ed.), *Geschichte des Wohnens*, vol. 3, Stuttgart: DVA, 1997.

12 Chr. Alexander, *A Pattern Language. Towns, Buildings, Construction. New York: Oxford University Press, 1977*.

13 W. Letter, "Der Aufbruch", in: *Brand Eins*, No. 07/2008.

14 J. Bölsche, "Wohnen statt Leben", in: *Spiegel Special*, No. 05/ 1997, p. 16.

15 H. Gatterer, C. Truckenbrodt, study "Living in the future", Kelkheim: Zukunftsinstitut 2005.

16 Ibid.

17 S. Berg, "Schöner Wohnen", in: *Arch⁺ Zeitschrift für Architektur und Städtebau*, 38th year No. 176/177/ May: "Wohnen", pp. 40-41, Aachen 2006.

"The conventional separation into three or four rooms will disappear," explains Gatterer, "what was once home sweet home" will in future have to fulfil a whole variety of different requirements and needs. The home will serve simultaneously as a place of retreat, of self-fulfilment and as a platform for outward display. One's living quarters become an expression of one's personality.

The role of the kitchen in the future will likewise change: living and cooking areas are already fusing optically into a single room with an increased emphasis on comfort and leisure. Friends and family now meet around the kitchen counter. As the social role of the kitchen increases, even those with little interest in cooking are investing in more expensive kitchen fittings. The bathroom, which is already experiencing a shift from washroom to wellness oasis, will be just one of a series of further places for relaxation and contemplation. For example, a private garden, balcony or loggia becomes a place to allow one's creativity free reign in the outdoors.

The dedicated study or workroom has seen its day. Wireless communications allow one to work with the laptop on the terrace or at the kitchen table. In addition, the "Smart Home" of tomorrow will be equipped with in-built sensors for a more personal ambience and greater security. For example, one will be able to switch between different lighting scenarios via a touch screen, and a fingerprint scanner would obviate the need for door keys.

The desire for greater security is already affecting the structure of cities and neighbourhoods. People with similar cultures and financial backgrounds will congregate in certain neighbourhoods. According to the experts, Gated communities for senior citizens of the like seen in the USA are unlikely to gain ground in Germany; new forms of living for the elderly will, however, certainly become more popular. Most old people today want to live their own lives in a manner they are accustomed to rather than living in an old people's home.

Whether in old age or as a family, urban living looks set to become a model for the future. In addition to the dense network of services and range of cultural activities that make city life attractive, this tendency could also help improve the environment. Short distances and public transport obviate the need to drive. In addition to reducing petrol consumption, considerable resources can also be saved by building new housing using sustainable building materials and designing them to require less heating.

Such is the opinion of the experts. But are we not all experts in living trends? After all, from childhood to old age we oscillate back and forth between continuity and change and – sooner or later – settle into one or the other semi-permanent makeshift solution. The Swiss author Sibylle Berg finds this reassuring, arguing that "living honed to perfection is a little like being dead".[17]

Floor plan design – providing for the changing needs of the elderly

DIETMAR EBERLE

Compared with their contemporaries in the past, today's architects face a far more complex task in the design of housing for people as they grow older. In the age of modernism, the principle of functional separation extended even to people themselves: elderly citizens simply "moved into" a nursing home. Old age was regarded as a static phenomenon, a special case, while the actual process of growing old was largely ignored. Today, longer life expectancy together with a greater personal awareness of one's needs and development and a greater overall politico-economic appreciation of the "human factor" has opened up a much broader and considerably more interesting spectrum of opportunities for architects than ever before.

In the present discourse, what has perhaps been given too little attention is the level at which interactions between old people, the client and architects take place during the decision-making process. Today the users, "those affected by the planning process" as Ottokar Uhl once provocatively termed them, have found their own voice as active participants in the market economy and are giving greater consideration to their own living situation. Increasingly, they are making their own provisions for old age rather than relying on public welfare provisions. While the familiar surroundings of the home remain the most favoured form of living, people are also learning to proactively take their lives into their own hands. Rather than waiting until they become dependent on help, they look ahead, actively seeking ways of living that are more appropriate to their needs as they grow older than their own four walls. And that is good – for everyone involved in the building process.

The market players are now showing interest in the niche of housing for the elderly and are introducing products whose economic concepts and social orientation differ from those of typical housing concepts. "Thematic living" on the one hand, cooperative "social contracts" on the other – the diversity of concepts responds to the heterogeneity of society, and also provides empirical values for comparing different models. A key basis for such comparisons remains age itself. Which phases can we identify, what kind of activity can we expect from people of different ages? In his illuminating essay "The Adventure of Growing Old: On Growing Old and Staying Young" Herrad Schenk[1] identifies three transitional phases of old age: the Go-gos (55/60 – 70/75 years), the Slow-gos (70/75 – 80/85 years) and the No-gos (80/85+). This differentiation happens to coincide – perhaps by chance, perhaps because it accurately portrays current society? – with three groups of people for whom our architectural office has designed projects. These residential projects for the elderly – the Attemsgasse in Vienna, a housing complex in Zurich-Affoltern and the Diakonie (Christian social service institution) in Düsseldorf – were undertaken for three clients, all from central Europe, with a view to accommodating overlapping phases of life. Although they share a common cultural background, the spatial concepts employed vary considerably.

The buildings in the Attemsgasse in Vienna, built for the Austrian Housing Association (ÖSW), follow the principle of inter-generational dialogue and were designed by Baumschlager Eberle in collaboration with the architect Elsa Prochazka. One of the two buildings is conceived especially for "senior citizens" aged 50+, the other for the increasing number of "young urban professionals" who also work from home. In the design of the apartments, the team avoided rigidly defined functions (dining room, bedroom etc.), instead striving to create flexible floor plans that can be adapted to individual needs. For example, the generous two-room apartments in the building for the over 50s can be divided – should the need ever arise – to provide space for a carer. The prospective residents are therefore making provisions for their own future through their choice of apartment. An essential aspect for the planning team was the configuration of functionally neutral areas which can be used for different purposes or changed as needed to ensure their long-term usability. Given that older people spend a larger amount of their time within their own four walls, the integration of loggias into the living area is of particular importance: the transition between indoors and outside is fluid without thresholds so that residents can enjoy being outdoors while retaining privacy. Similarly, all apartments are barrier-free. Appropriately dimensioned lifts provide access to all floors, the corridors are wide enough to turn around in with a wheelchair and any steps – including those between the apartment and terrace – do not exceed a height of 3 cm. In the configuration of the floor plans as well as the

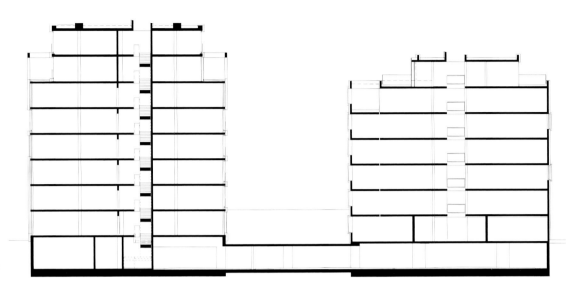

Housing in the Attemsgasse, Vienna; section

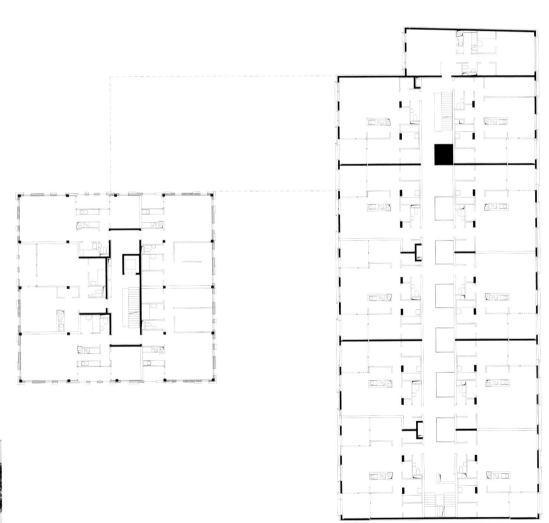

Typical floor plan

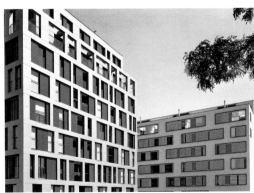

Façade design

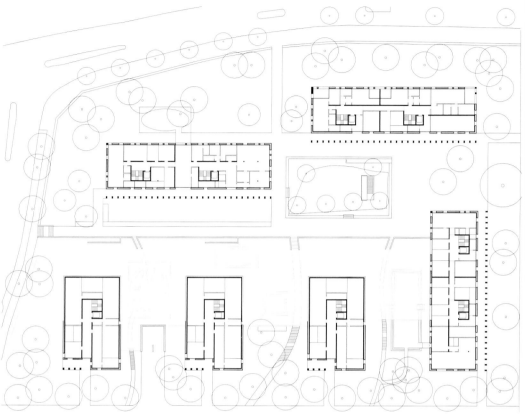

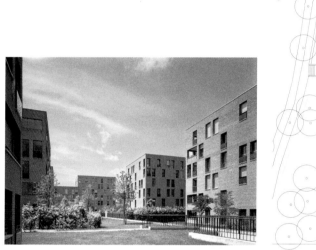

Ruggächern Quarter, Zurich

Ground floor plan

ergonomics of the details, the apartments have been conceived to cater for the needs of older residents and the changing of these needs as old age progresses. The demand for such apartments could not be greater: all apartments had been rented before completion of the project in April 2008.

The second project, the Ruggächern Quarter in Zurich-Affoltern, has a different proportion of private and public areas: built for the Zurich General Building Cooperative (ABZ), the complex features a building specially reserved for people aged 55 plus (the Swiss, it seems, begin to age later than the Austrians!). Fifty residents were selected by the ABZ and view themselves as a "community" and as members of a cooperative with certain obligations within the neighbourhood. The social integration of the elderly citizens is greater than in Vienna, and the spatial concept correspondingly different. Given the "community" concept of the scheme, the ground floor contains rooms that can be used by all the residents. This includes a library, fitness room and therapy room, so that private life and communal life take place within one building. The floor plans of the two to three-room apartments are likewise functionally neutral to ensure their long-term usability as needs change.

Both of the above models for living in old age offer a limited degree of provision for the "worst case scenario" where residents need ongoing nursing care, either through the provision of appropriate rooms or the ability to combine spaces as required. The nursing home for the Diakonie in Düsseldorf is, by contrast, conceived for the intensive care of elderly people. Here it is immediately apparent that much more is needed to offer residents a dignified and adequate living environment. The planning of the building attempts to break down the impression of an "institution" and the concomitant associations of barracks and mass housing. Accordingly, the 90 individual rooms have been arranged in a U-shaped building on three floors. Each "arm" accommodates 15 rooms with care facilities in the connecting section between the two. This results in a

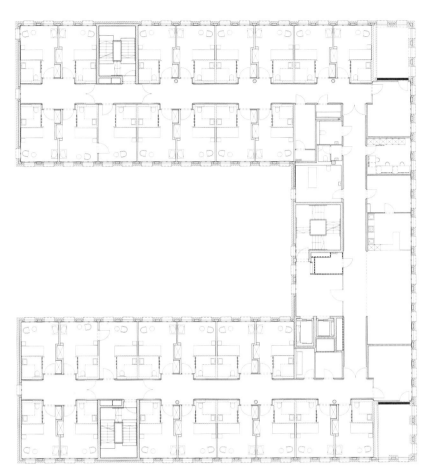

Nursing home for the Diakonie in Düsseldorf; typical floor plan

series of small groups of rooms, each with their own kitchen and communal living room. An additional advantage is that nursing care can be provided with relatively few staff, and that care staff are never far away. Here too, even when mentally or physically impaired, residents in the Diakonie can decide for themselves the degree to which they would like to take part in communal life or be on their own.

The three examples show how with each successive stage of growing older, one's demands on one's living environment change. As externally determined rhythms of everyday (working) life disappear, so too do opportunities for social contact, likewise as physical mobility decreases. For older people it is therefore important that their living environment offers a platform for communication and recreation, just as the so-called "city of short walks", which has so often been proclaimed, is of elementary importance to them. The examples described above help intensify in one way or another the ability to develop a familar, a "habitual" environment in both senses of the word. Sustainable apartments are those that are functionally neutral and can adapt to changing life situations, that are equipped with ergonomic surfaces and furnished with materials that residents find comfortable. Why then, one might reasonably ask, are not all apartments built this way? In fact, studies in Switzerland have shown that this could be achieved with an average additional investment of only 2%! The advantages are clear: the added value for the state as well as for investors is incomparably higher. Such apartments allow residents to remain in their own living accommodation for much longer with a lower risk of accidents, in turn reducing the investment required for associated infrastructure.

Note
1 H. Schenk, "The Adventure of Growing Old: On Growing Old and Staying Young", in A. Huber (ed.), *New Approaches to Housing for the Second Half of Life*, Basel, Boston, Berlin, Birkhäuser, 2008, pp. 15-26.

Interior architecture and product design

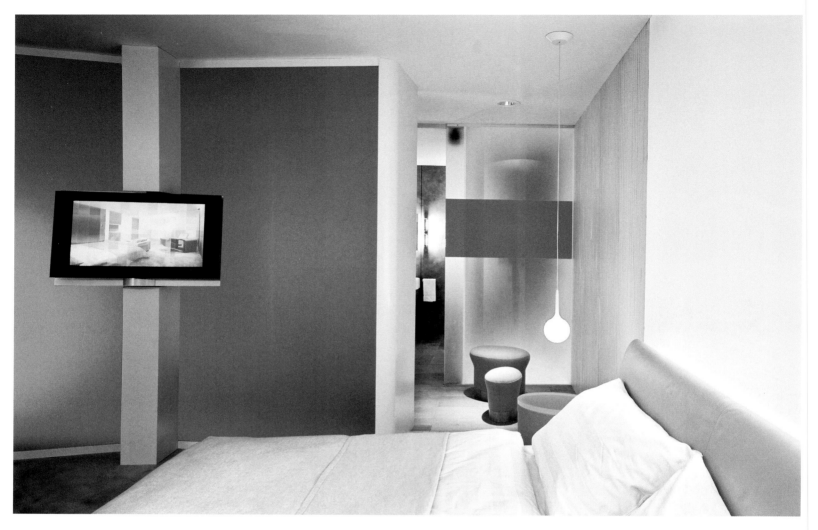

5+ Sensotel, Willisau; double room designed to stimulate the senses

One aim in the design of housing for the elderly is to compensate for physical deficiencies as agreeably as possible. While the impairments associated with old age do not equate to those of a disability, both present similar design problems. The following example, which details our search to find the best possible comfort for elderly and disabled people in the design for a hotel, can therefore also serve as an example of design for the elderly. In previous centuries wealthy senior citizens often took to living in hotels, and although this was a luxury it reveals a fundamental principle: a hotel should, like housing for the elderly, create a world that is distinctive and individual and is both functional as well as aesthetic. Its design should not be lacking in any aspects that correspond to the culture and respective standard of living of its residents. Above all, it should fulfil the needs of the people who live in it.

In 2001 in Rheinsberg, in beautiful surroundings not far from Berlin, the author designed the world's first design hotel for the physically disabled. Since then the building has been awarded four international design awards, not only for its aesthetic qualities but also due to its popularity among its residents, 80% of whom are regulars, and its economic success. The design aims to create a warm and Mediterranean atmosphere that is appropriate to its lakeside location and that is consistent with a holiday and recreational destination rather than a city hotel. The design, for example, refrains from using stainless steel and other metal surfaces to avoid associations with wheelchairs, medical instruments or hospitals. Similarly, the reception is both functional as well as inviting, with a slightly lower counter for guests in wheelchairs alongside a standard-height counter for non-disabled visitors. The reception area opens directly onto the restaurant with a large backlit cupboard in the centre where wheelchairs can be stored out of view. The interior design of fittings and furnishings avoids using specially conceived furniture or products for the disabled as these are rarely aesthetically pleasing and, on the contrary, often disrupt an otherwise pleasant environment. Instead the design employs other means, for example the baths have slanted terrazzo surfaces rounded off towards the bottom, preventing one from bumping into them with a wheelchair. This also made it possible to integrate aesthetically attractive washbasins.

It is through light that colours and materials come alive. Surfaces and surface structures become interesting with the help of light, a principle that applies regardless of the target group one is designing for. However, the quality of light should not be too uniform as this creates a flat, monotonous impression, straining the eyes and causing tiredness. Instead, one should strive to achieve changes of light and shadow where transitions between darker and lighter rooms are clearly evident, creating a sense of homeliness. Furthermore, as can be seen in the example, distinctive colours can be used to mark locations, creating a form of wayfinding system for people with impaired vision.

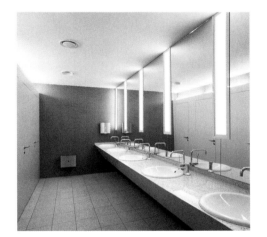

Haus Rheinsberg Hotel am See, Rheinsberg;
low-level washbasins for wheelchair access

In addition to the widespread use of solid wood, for example as protection strips along the walls that prevent users from bumping into them, a special Italian paint has been used that contains crystals. The paint has a uniform colour and can be used on wood to protect against scratching – even deliberate scratching with a key leaves no trace. This has been used for doors as well as other surfaces particularly prone to wear and tear.

A central consideration in the design of the hotel was to help residents wherever possible to be and feel independent. For example, in the hotel rooms, the clothes rails in the cupboards can be electrically lowered so that elderly or disabled visitors can hang up their clothes themselves. After all, one need not be dependent on help for every little task. The pools in the spa and the pool areas offer same-level entry surfaces, and guests can also use a ramp to enter the water. These are just some alternatives to the more conventional means used in most homes for the elderly.

The question of how to deal with the spaces which are to serve old people as a new home is primarily one of creating an appropriate atmosphere; an atmosphere that should be distinctive and communicate a feeling of having come home. Where hotels in the 1980s often had a somewhat impersonal character, many hotels today offer an atmospheric potential that would also be appropriate for living environments for the elderly. This applies equally to senior residences – where one would expect to find a welcoming atmosphere much like in a hotel where one feels well looked after – as it does to rented or purchased flats or apartments for the elderly. In the apartments themselves one should feel free to be able to personalise the space, to shape one's surroundings, while the public areas should, even in rented accommodation, have a hotel-like character. A number of well-designed hotels that have been realised as low-budget projects demonstrate that this is also possible without excessive financial outlay. While the materials used may be less expensive, it is always possible to make skilful use of colour and light without incurring great expense.

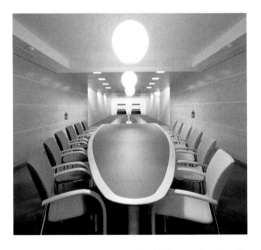

Haus Rheinsberg Hotel am See; disabled access bowling alley

Living spaces for old people must always take into account the needs of the residents for warmth and security and a sense of homeliness and identification. The task is to create a readily identifiable structure with spacious rooms that are clearly arranged and transparent so that all parts of a building are visible and there are no dark corners. Light and colour again play a crucial rule, for example in lessening the intimidating qualities of corridors and stairs as well as ancillary areas, particularly for people with impaired sight or mobility. Signage and directions should be well-illuminated with a light that is warm rather than cool.

Heating and air conditioning represent a further fundamental aspect of the planning of living environments for the elderly, as older people generally prefer higher room temperatures. To enable residents to adjust these to suit their changing comfort needs, easy-to-use touch-sensitive panels can be used. These should always be marked with clear symbols rather than small, hard-to-read labels.

Design is also stimulating. It would be wrong to assume that elderly people only need peace and quiet, meditative spaces and dining and communal areas. It has become increasingly important to create spaces for old people to be active, creative and interact with other people or seek inspiration. For another project, the 5+ Sensotel in Willisau in Switzerland, in which I was able to experiment extensively, the five senses inform the basic principle of the design. As many studies show, sensory stimulus benefits old people greatly, encouraging cerebral activity in general, and the experiences gained in this respect could therefore be applicable to the design of living environments for the elderly. In this sector, feelings and sensations are as a rule particularly important in order to create a general sense of contentment and warmth. This has as much to do with light, colour and materials as it does with the question of how things feel, the haptic qualities materials have, whether they are pleasant to touch. In an exhibition in Los Angeles, I used ten different interior designs to demonstrate how light, colour and form alone influence the atmosphere of a space, ranging from happy to depressed.

One of the strongest senses, which can also be influenced using technical means, is the sense of smell. As certain smells are able to trigger particular memories and pleasant experiences, this possibility is increasingly used to promote a sense of general well-being. Aroma machines are also installed to dispel unpleasant odours. Together with experts in the field I have developed a gadget that can be installed in the wall or in switches or used in an electrical socket. The aromas, which are interchangeable, are anti-allergic and were developed at the New York laboratories of a renowned parfumier. All the fragrances are discreet and, unlike most aromatic fragrances, not oil-based.

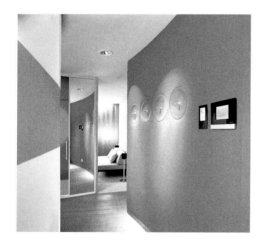

5+ Sensotel; light, colours and materials influence the mood of the resident

Although in every project functional requirements must be fulfilled, functionality should never displace emotional language. We know today that our brains are influenced far more by emotional experience than rational cognition, and the strict dictate of "form follows function" should be reconsidered in light of this. There is much to be said for integrating both approaches; the generation of a form from its function should go hand in hand with emotional aspects of a design.

A further essential aspect of the planning of hotels as well as homes for the elderly is hygiene. All areas must be easy to clean, water should not accumulate and the choice of materials must take into account hygiene considerations. The latter is fortunately comparatively straightforward as many attractive materials are now available on the market that fulfil the requirements and almost radiate a sense of hygiene. Given the increasing cost constraints in the housing as well as care provision sectors, one should ascertain the budget distribution from an early stage as interior design and outfitting is all too often placed at the end of the chain. Cost savings in the interior design of housing for the elderly are ill-advised as old people spend more time at home than younger generations. Where budget constraints are tight, one should focus on accentuating individual areas, deciding carefully where high-quality materials are absolutely necessary and which areas can be given a simpler treatment.

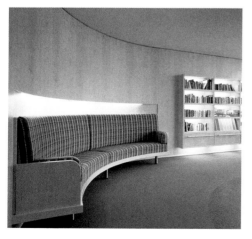

Haus Rheinsberg Hotel am See; seating niche in the fireplace room

The insight that sustainability and ecological principles are also highly important in interior design and particularly in the choice of materials is nothing new. It seems, however, that demand from the general public and the long overdue realisation that our environmental resources are limited were necessary before international action was taken. Many of the ecologically-friendly materials which I have researched for more than ten years are still very expensive due to low demand, comparable with the first organic produce which was far more expensive than it is today now that demand has risen enormously. In the medium term we can expect to see the same pattern for the availability of ecological materials which are fully biodegradable. Interestingly, ever more synthetic materials are being developed that behave in the same way as natural materials.

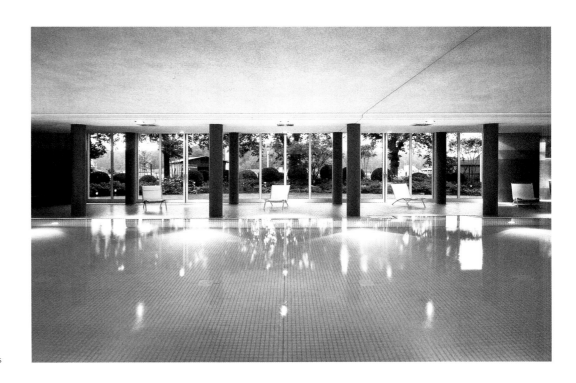

Haus Rheinsberg Hotel am See;
pool with same-level entry surfaces

The principles of "universal design" and "design for all" are widely understood in the realm of design for the elderly. Their implementation in the design of architecture and urban environments are without doubt welcome. In the realm of interior design and product design I would argue that such principles should be applied with care and measure and that they should be considered in the larger context. Even in housing for the elderly it is not necessary to equip all bathrooms with the whole range of fittings, grips, handles and supports from the outset. Instead, the planning should take these into account – in the sense of "pre-procrastination" – for possible integration at a later date where necessary. In fact, interior designers should as a rule ensure that their designs and plans can accommodate several phases of a life cycle so that, for example, a living room can be adapted with little effort to serve the changing needs of its residents as they grow older.

Gardens for senior citizens – a framework for the design of outdoor spaces

HARMS WULF

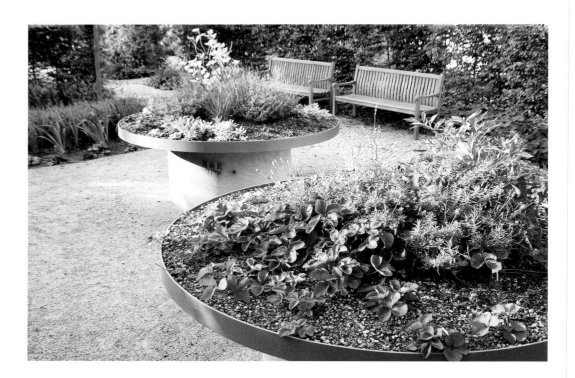

Home for the Elderly, Berlin-Prenzlauer Berg; raised planting beds allow wheelchair users direct sensory contact to plants

People need to be active to regain their health as well as to remain healthy. This credo applies to all stages of life, including for the age group of senior citizens. For a long time, this fundamental need seems to have been neglected, whether for economic reasons or lack of awareness. That the design of outdoor spaces should take into account the needs of older people is therefore a relatively recent realisation, and one that has been rapidly fuelled by the increasing number of senior citizens and the accompanying debate on a better quality of life in old age.

As mobility and responsiveness begin to deteriorate and hearing and sight become impaired, the relevance of the quality of one's living environment, of which outdoor spaces are undoubtedly a part, increases accordingly. The spatial and structural qualities of one's local surroundings are crucial factors in our ability to lead independent lives in old age. Personal mobility and social participation are important conditions for the well-being of all people, old people included. Despite the fact that the need for ongoing care increases with age, the greater majority of elderly people would prefer to live in their home environment. The design of residential environments appropriate to the needs of the elderly therefore requires adequate solutions that address these needs and enable old people to live independent lives on their own terms.

It is generally agreed that the availability and quality of outdoor activities has a determining effect on the behaviour of old people. Where elderly people suffer from cognitive restrictions and a reduced ability to establish social contacts with other people, these deficits will be exacerbated by an unfavourable design of outdoor spaces. Instead, better local conditions can stimulate greater activity and contribute to the physical and mental constitution of old people. In the USA in particular, the therapeutic effect of green spaces has been researched and documented. A growing number of older people with a reduced radius of activity make use of public gardens and green areas in their immediate locality to benefit their health. Outside of one's own living space, gardens are by far the most popular place to be.

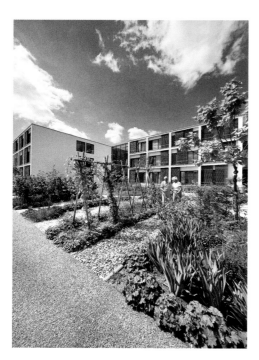

Competence Centre for People with Dementia, Nuremberg; therapeutic garden with traditional fruits and vegetables

Carefully planned gardens and recreation areas can significantly influence people's choices for a particular housing complex or care facility. Moving into a nursing home, for example, is almost always associated with a loss of one's private sphere and sadness at leaving behind one's familiar environment. Attractive green amenities can help divert people's attention from the sadness and pain that accompanies the period of settling-in to a new environment, and in some cases compensate for this entirely.

Clear functionality, a humane scale, a rich variety of activities and a stimulating selection of colours are guiding principles in the design of outdoor spaces, with the overall aim of creating an uplifting and enlivening environment for the visitor. A key aspect is not so much the size of a green area – whether a balcony, private garden, courtyard garden or park – as the variety of experiences it offers. This can be achieved through the provision of spaces of differing qualities and their respective design. Independent of the size of the site, the green area should provide a variety of spatial experiences. Expansive views of open spaces are complemented by protective enclosures. References to individual typical aspects of the landscape, such as the edge of woodlands, meadows or expanses of water create a richness of atmosphere and awaken associations.

It is not by chance that going for walks is one of the most popular outdoor activities among older people. Movement promotes mobility and a sense of well-being. Outdoor spaces for the elderly should consist of a large contiguous open space made accessible via pathways or promenades in the form of a closed network of paths. As the degree of mobility among old people can vary greatly, tangents allow people to take longer or shorter routes. Seating areas arranged within sight of each other offer people with restricted mobility a series of safe havens. Views into the distance, over a clearing or across lawns should also be complemented by more secluded areas. Accordingly, gardens should provide small private zones, niches in the shade with a bench, gazebos or pavilions, places for contemplation or peaceful observation. Sitting and watching from a protected corner is for older people often an important manner of participating in public life and offers an opportunity to come into contact with others.

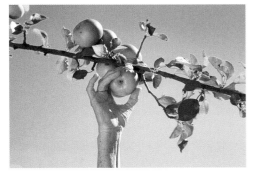

Fruit trees provide sensory as well as biographic stimulation

Outdoor spaces are particularly attractive for older people when they are easy to reach and offer plenty of orientation. Views from indoors onto outdoor spaces serve as enticements, tempting one to go outside and enjoy the garden. Seating areas that are visible from afar, for example arranged around a water feature or embedded amid colourful decorative plants, serve as a welcome invitation. Furthermore, green spaces are especially well-loved when they are always there, changing with the seasons and times of day.

From the point of view of planning and construction, the first thing to avoid is steps or thresholds that inhibit or even prevent old people from getting around. Additionally, people of all ages appreciate being able to use gardens without fear of being accosted, bothered or having an accident. Such worries can act as invisible barriers that prevent people from visiting gardens. Views onto surrounding buildings or bustling activity nearby can help create a sense of security. It is also advisable to mark the boundaries of a garden with some form of spatial closure. This can be achieved by natural means, for example planting and shrubbery, or with taller and more explicit elements such as hedges or fences. Close proximity to a toilet is a further aspect that alleviates worries about going outside, not just for old people. A further factor that contributes to a sense of security is sufficient public lighting, in particular when public gardens are crossed late in the evening or at night.

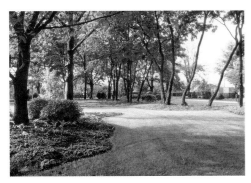

Park-Klinik Weißensee, Berlin-Weißensee; clusters of trees create a variety of different outdoor spaces

Garden users with a greater need for security are in general more dependent on clear signals that aid orientation. A uniform surfacing for the main pathways – for example a gravelled asphalt surface – can help lend people a sense of certainty in finding their way around the park by providing a visual as well as a tactile response. Likewise, unhindered views of a landmark of some kind on the site can help provide orientation, whether it is a characteristic group of trees, a work of art or a distinctive element of a building. Such items serves as signals and can help reassure people, particularly those with perceptive deficiencies, that they have not lost their way.

Our senses serve as our bridge to the world. Older people generally have plenty of time to explore the subtleties of perception or to rediscover these: observing, listening, smelling, tasting – and remembering. The importance of engaging the senses in the design of outdoor spaces for the elderly cannot be emphasised enough. As people grow older, many lose some of their sensory faculties. Hearing and vision are often the first to suffer, later sometimes the sense of smell and acuteness of taste. Similarly, the spectrum of our per-

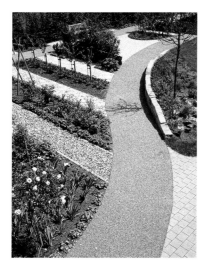
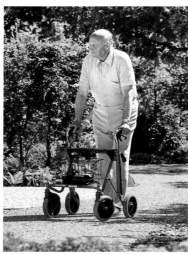
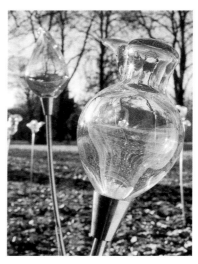
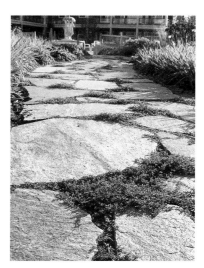

Competence Centre for People with Dementia; circular path with uniform surface treatment for better orientation | Level surfacing suitable for use with wheeled walking aids

Park-Klinik Weißensee; an artwork with aromatic glass 'umbels' by Renate Wiedemann provides additional sensory stimulation | Ida Wolff Geriatric Centre, Berlin-Neukölln; paved stone path with joints planted with thyme

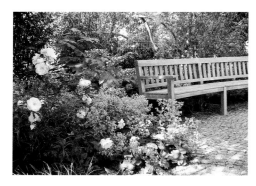

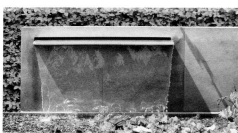

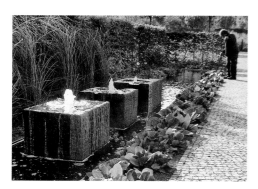

"Gerontogarten", a stimulating garden for seniors, Berlin-Prenzlauer Berg; plants create a pleasant environment for a bench niche | Competence Centre for People with Dementia; the soothing sound of flowing water | Home for the Elderly, Berlin-Prenzlauer Berg; bubbling water fountains create attractive stimulation

ception can shift: colours such as yellow and red generally remain as strong as ever but others may lose some of their brilliance. Here, the provision of a broad palette of sensory stimulants can help compensate for individual sensory deficiencies. The targeted use of planting offers one of the best means of achieving this. Design elements made of wood, water and stone also contribute to the sensory diversity of green outdoor spaces.

The closer one comes to plants, the more they stimulate the senses. When plants can be reached and touched, even older people with restricted mobility or sight can be encouraged to undertake gardening. Raised planting areas, such as table-height planting, planted wall copings, raised beds and planting boxes allow people to come into direct contact with natural plants, lending a garden an additional therapeutic quality. Even greater gardening comfort is afforded by raised beds which are open underneath for wheelchair access.

The element of water enriches any garden. Fountains or water features are a popular attraction for eyes as well as ears. The sound of burbling water can mask out other less desirable sounds in the wider surroundings and has a calming effect, as does watching the movement of water.

The design of gardens for people suffering from dementia is a particular challenge, as it involves more than just compensating for limited perception or mobility. The primary symptoms of the illness include a loss of memory, disorientation and a state of confusion. These can be accompanied by restlessness, depression, aggression, hyperactivity or anxiety. The design of gardens for use by dementia sufferers should first and foremost provide a peaceful and protective atmosphere. Dementia sufferers find intrusive environmental conditions of all kinds – noise, cold, heat and glare – harder to deal with and sometimes they are too much to cope with. At the same time, stimulating elements also play an important role.

People with dementia do not necessarily suffer from physical impairments, so it is important that they are able to move around freely as much as possible. Sufficient opportunities to go outside and move around also help maintain the normal rhythm of day and night, which for many dementia sufferers is imbalanced. Special attention should also be paid to the inclination of dementia patients to wander around, the positive effects of which are now well-known: it improves circulation and contributes to reducing stress and to reinforcing a sense of autonomy. For this reason, gardens for dementia sufferers should also offer sufficient possibilities for wandering around in the form of a self-contained system of pathways.

A further challenge is to contain with positive means the tendency of residents to wander off, i.e. without making them feel shut in. Restrictions can quickly lead to frustration and aggression among dementia patients. To avoid this, fencing enclosures should be made as invisible as possible or concealed using natural means such as planting or hedges.

Gardens designed for dementia sufferers should also provide additional stimulus for activities that they can undertake on their own. Many people identify with traditional plants and practical gardening equipment from their active past. These can bring back memories and animate residents to pick up even long forgotten activities in the garden. Caring for plants and harvesting fruit also helps reinforce a sense of identity with their surroundings and, through association with the resident's earlier lifetime, can arouse positive sentiments.

Similarly contact with animals can enrich the lives of dementia patients. While they are often no longer able to care for a pet themselves, they are able to communicate with them emotionally. Such interaction diverts attention from their everyday difficulties and helps them identify with their surroundings. At the same time the proportion of comparatively active senior citizens, for whom sport is an everyday part of life, is increasing in our society. Accordingly, areas for ball games and physical exercise, a swimming pond, table-tennis table or appropriate fitness equipment are ways of catering for the active needs of such "young senior citizens".

Outdoor spaces for older people should not be misunderstood as a solution exclusively for this particular generation. Although the creation of environments tailored to the needs of older people is extremely important for their quality of life, it runs the risk – even when unintentional – of stigmatising and discriminating those it wishes to help. Garden visitors may be made to feel that they are no longer part of the world at large, creating the impression that they have been closed off in comfortable surroundings so as to be out of the way.

Older people seek interaction and contact with each other as well as with younger generations. As with anyone, they also want to feel noticed and respected – and gardens offer perfect opportunities for this. While the design of outdoor spaces for use by the elderly must take into account their specific requirements, this can already be achieved through the implementation of barrier-free design principles. The realisation of the barrier-free design of our living environment can foster an integrative approach that encompasses all generations and with it an awareness that the removal of barriers benefits all members of society. The terms "universal design" or "design for all" have come to represent this approach. The former term is anchored in the United Nations Charter for Human Rights and formulates the right of every individual to have access to an environment of useful, intuitive and safe-to-use things and spaces. The principles of universal design – applied to the design of outdoor spaces – allow all of us, old and young, with and without impairments, comfortable life in our environment on our own terms.

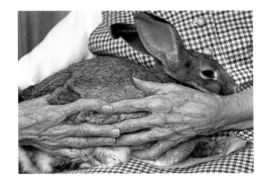

Pets provide a means of non-verbal communication and basic stimulation for people with dementia

The role of the architect in the care provision and housing markets

ECKHARD FEDDERSEN

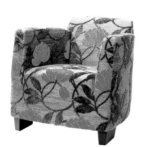

"How well cushioned are you?" asked the exhibition "I'll live until I'm 100. New ways of living for the over 50s", Swiss Federal Institute of Technology Zurich, 2008

In the last 20 years, the fields of activity and with them the role of the architect have shifted considerably. A trend towards greater specialisation, and in this respect professionalisation, through a greater concentration on only specific services is unmistakable. Planning services are increasingly covered by specialised offices: hospital planners, office planners, industrial architects; specialised fields have formed in all sectors creating a barrier for talented young architects entering the field. Selection procedures for competitions, consultancy and job applications follow the same pattern.

Accordingly, what were previously fields of planning are regarded increasingly as sectors in a planning market. Buildings for the elderly fall within a segment of the planning market for social buildings. In order to be able to maintain a high quality of architecture that remains relevant to society's needs in the context of such changes, we will need to develop new patterns of behaviour founded on a fundamental understanding of the changed conditions. These changes in the planning process, in the contributing participants and their respective legal position with regard to one another lead to a redistribution of rights and obligations.

In principle, the new developments represent a fusion of international, and particularly American, planning procedures and prevailing Central European planning methods. Only 20 years ago in Europe, building for the elderly was characterised by a single client who was both owner and operator of the care facilities. In this constellation, which is still a model for charitable associations today, a single owner of a site approached an architect of their choice with a functional idea for a building and pre-arranged funding. State funding in the form of subsidisation of investment costs became available in return for an ability, on the part of the state, to apply conditions to the planning. State intervention was primarily limited to ensuring equality, both with regard to the applicant as well as the later residents. Legislation was introduced to underpin this form of influence.

This approach has remained largely unchanged in all European countries where state subsidisation for the building of housing for the elderly is anchored in legislation. But here too new, less restrictive, market-financed models are surfacing parallel to the old federal culture of state subsidisation, and even gradually replacing it, depending on the country's budgetory constraints. To begin with, this applied only to facilities for the richer classes, projects with a high return on investment, but today projects financed with private capital and bank mortgages dominate the market.

What has long been the case in Anglo-American countries will follow suit in Europe too: the ownership and rental or leasing of a property is becoming increasingly independent of the provision of care services by another company.

As a consequence, the architecture and the architect will need to address two different sets of interests in the planning of a building: on the one hand the design of an attractive property for rental that is highly flexible and has a long lifetime at minimum cost, and for the operator, a high-quality building with low maintenance and operating costs, a strong image and excellent functionality appropriate to its needs. To achieve these aims, both with regard to quality and costs, a project controller is often employed by both of the contractual partners. The banks, who require additional expertise to assess, plan and monitor the financing of such "special properties", also draw on the services of specialist consultants and controllers.

The availability of property independent of an operator leads to its classification as commercial property, with the result that an operator needs to contractually guarantee a minimum of ten to 15 years rent. An obvious response is to pool several properties which are then of interest as an open-end or closed-end fund, rather than as individual properties. This has resulted in a strong tendency towards the unification of care properties on the market, which in turn has lead to a standardisation of the accommodation-related costs on the operator's side and to a greater degree of comparability than has ever been the case in the past.

While the above describes the situation for nursing homes, the range of residential alternatives for the elderly are diversifying ever further. The spectrum ranges from nearly 50 Euros per m² monthly rent to 8 Euros including a fixed price security package. The professional investor market has shown little interest in this market segment due to its lack of clarity and low returns.

For architects this situation means that they are often dealing with highly volatile projects which are dependent on highly diverging investor interests: from a single owner to an owner consortium to closed-end and open-end funds. Similarly, the operator can vary from a small family-run business to a public corporation. Project financing varies from classic private capital to company capital of all kinds to closed-end or open-end funds and leasing systems.

In such cases the architect is often the only one with a non-materialistic interest in achieving a good overall result for all interested parties. Very often the diverging interests of the different parties only become apparent as the planning process progresses. The planning process therefore requires a high degree of coordination and transparency from the very beginning. The architect must know the respective applicable parameters for costs, quality and function inside out and have a broad awareness of the legal position of the other participants.

On the side of the operator, the range of service providers in the elderly care sector can be loosely divided into "inpatient" and "outpatient" sectors. If the market for inpatient care is already difficult to describe, the market for outpatient care defies definition entirely. It ranges from a single district nurse to operators with thousands of care assistants in dozens of cities and rural municipalities. Demand for planning services in the outpatient sector is, however, limited as most such services, with the exception of a few small wards, are housed in existing residential and commercial buildings.

The situation is different in the inpatient care sector. The most obvious and most profitable sector is that of nursing homes, which represents the main form of care service offering aimed at an estimated 5% of over 65-year-olds. Closer inspection shows that current societal demand for available places would be fulfilled when places are available for around 2% of 85-year-olds, a percentage that is expected to rise in future, particularly in view of the fact that the average age at which people enter a nursing home is already 83 years. The average residential period falls as the age of entry rises and is at present approximately 1.5 years. In institutions offering special facilities for people with advanced dementia the average residential period can fall below a year.

Architects working in this sector therefore need to acquire a high degree of knowledge regarding current care service offerings. Areas such as night-time care or special services for people who have suffered a stroke, people with progressive dementia or requiring post-operative care feature more heavily than they did a few years ago, when people without a constant need for nursing care also lived in nursing homes. The architect has to reconcile the medical and hygienic requirements of the nursing care regulations with the homeliness and comfort requirements of the residents in such a way that care provision and living in old age are no longer perceived as contradictory. Cooperation with colour psychologists, interior decorators from good furnishing houses and lighting consultants can be of value here. Similarly, grading systems, much like that of hotel star-ratings, are being developed that combine standards of furnishings and materials with carefully selected design requirements to define different standardised levels of quality. However, in all cases the most important aspect of a design is and remains the desire of the resident to be welcomed by a homely atmosphere in their time of need.

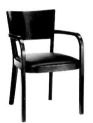

Armchair, chair and stool symbolise the spectrum of financial possibilities

Planning and designing for people with dementia

R. WELTER, M. HÜRLIMANN, K. HÜRLIMANN-SIEBKE

Methodical approaches and design principles for residential care facilities

In recent years there has been a fundamental shift in the awareness of the needs of people suffering from dementia. Where previously care focussed primarily on medical and social factors, today we are aware of the importance of a more holistic approach that upholds the quality of life and dignity of the sufferers. An essential aspect in this respect is the appropriate spatial and organisational design of the sufferers' environment.

From a holistic point of view, the care and support of dementia sufferers should always be an integral part of a communal network of provisions for the elderly. People with dementia are no different to the rest of us. It is just that they have to deal with the challenges of a particular illness. Accordingly, the closer they live to their home environment and the better their care facilities are integrated into the local neighbourhood, the more they can make use of their individual resources and that of their social environment. A variety of living alternatives and care facilities are necessary in order to be able to provide sufficient choice both at a macro-scale (community, neighbourhood, institutions, forms of living and so on) as well as at a micro-scale (spatial arrangement and design).

The planning and building of inpatient care facilities for the elderly, including those suffering from dementia, is particularly challenging. It is generally agreed that the traditional nursing home arrangement is just as unsuitable for dementia sufferers as it is for the elderly in general: very few people wish to enter a nursing home regardless of their illness. As a result, in Switzerland since the 1980s a large number of decentralised residential group care facilities have sprung up. In the meantime many homes for the elderly have expanded to provide similar residential group care which has enabled them to cater for the increasing demand for care provision without incurring excessive investment costs. The positive experience of this form of residential care for the elderly has helped establish it as a model for the care of dementia sufferers: residential care group facilities allow greater flexibility with regard to their architectural design and can accordingly correspond more closely to the residents' familiar patterns of living.

It is well known that people suffering from dementia react more sensitively to their environment as their ability to adapt and compensate deteriorates. Their behaviour, however, can point to general inadequacies in the design and planning of their living environment and as such we can learn from them as 'seismographs' of good or poor environments. Planners and designers need to be good at observing in order to learn what they can from people with dementia about planning and design principles that have the potential to benefit us all.

The following discussion elaborates suggestions for methodical approaches applicable in both the planning as well as the realisation of projects, and points to important decisions at a macro-scale as well as examples of the effects of the design of spaces at a micro-scale. Decisions made at an early stage in the planning process, such as choice of location (regional, community-based, neighbourhood-level), model type (integrated, annexe, semi-autonomous, fully autonomous) and kind of care provision (mixed or specialised), affect the quality of life for the user just as much, for example, as the floor plan arrangement or colour scheme.

People who suffer from dementia have a greater need for clear orientation, security and freedom to move around than most people do. However, it would be short-sighted to assume that this necessitates specialised accommodation and care in special-purpose facilities. Rather, we need to find innovative organisational and architectural solutions that create optimal environmental conditions that allow dementia sufferers to live their lives among us.

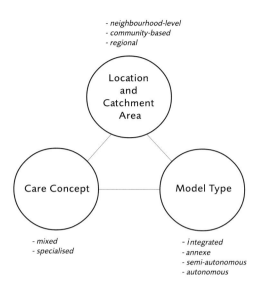

- neighbourhood-level
- community-based
- regional

Location and Catchment Area

Care Concept

Model Type

- mixed
- specialised

- integrated
- annexe
- semi-autonomous
- autonomous

The three planning elements and their relationships
to one another

Fundamental planning decisions (macro level)

Before one can begin with the interior and exterior design of a facility, the planning team first needs to consider several important criteria at a macro level. There are three key elements that need to be decided during the initial planning:

- The choice of the location of a facility;
- The choice of care concept;
- The choice of model type.

All of these aspects concern both the architecture as well as the operating concept and have implications, individually as well as in combination with one another, for the dementia sufferers, their relatives and the care staff. The following diagram illustrates the relationships of these three planning elements to one another and the resulting constellations.

As consultants, the authors often encounter different combinations of these three elements. The following are typical constellations:

Example 1 Regional location: serves a large catchment area. Model type: autonomous – a large dedicated and independently-run facility. Care concept: specialised – catering for dementia sufferers only.

Example 2 Regional location: for example in a rural or alpine catchment area. Model type: integrated – different residential groups are part of a single building.Care concept: mixed – residential groups consist of both dementia sufferers and non-sufferers.

Example 3 Community-based location: the facility is designed to cover the demands of a community.
Model type: integrated – residential groups with dementia sufferers are cared for as part of an existing home. Care concept: specialised.

Example 4 Neighbourhood-level location: the facility as part of an urban quarter or neighbourhood.
Model type: autonomous – the facility is not part of any other institution. Care concept: specialised.

Example 5 Community-based location. Model type: annexe – an existing nursing home provides care for two residential groups of dementia sufferers, for example in a separate villa or an apartment building near to or on the grounds of the home. Care concept: specialised.

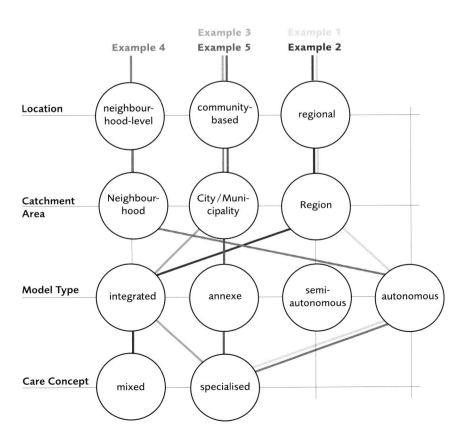

Schematic diagram showing combinations
of planning elements

Planning elements: Location and care concept

The following overview draws on studies and consulting undertaken by the authors and shows examples of the effects of the choice of location and the choice of care concept.

The effect of facility location on...	Local/decentralised facilities	Regional facilities
Elderly persons	• ability to remain in familiar spatial and social surroundings • greater normality	• involves moving away from home • home or hotel-like character • more additional services • more anonymous • greater danger of stigmatisation
Relatives, neighbourhood	• more social contacts • neighbourhood help • greater acceptance	• further away from relatives • greater sense of isolation • risk of greater alienation
Municipality	• small local facilities • municipalities have greater influence on services	• larger facilities with special character • municipalities are partners in a consortium
Financial investment	• smaller facilities, possibly less efficient • lower investment costs • can be converted at a later date	• rational organisational units • greater investment cost
Spatial/organisational	• fewer formal (house) rules • less available space	• explicit house rules • more space • additional services possible
Care provision	• less formal daily routine • lower staff-to-resident ratio • more like everyday life, staff need to be generalists	• stricter daily routine • flexible deployment of staff • specialised care and activities

Selected examples for the effects of the choice of location

The effect of care form on...	Mixed care concept	Specialised care concept
Quality of life for people with dementia	+ mixed group = normality + more extensive social contacts, memory through experience - stress as a result of "misunderstandings"	+ sheltered social environment + specialised care - decision to enter facility may be made by others - stigmatisation - risk of less normality, location can be far from home
Quality of life for other residents	+ greater security of being able to remain even if one's well-being should deteriorate + new tasks in life - stress and disturbances resulting from dementia sufferers	+ no stress and disturbances resulting from dementia sufferers - worries about one's own "deterioration" and the possible need to move at a later date
Activities of care staff	+ emphasis on normality and continuity in day-to-day care - additional mediation role - possibly fewer and less well-qualified staff	+ particular focus on relatively homogenous needs groups + more and better qualified staff - work in a "specialised facility" leads to a greater risk of strain
Spatial and organisational design	+ necessitates careful planning (also for dementia sufferers) +/- residential care group situation necessary - greater investment in facilities and useable floor areas	+ systematic planning and creation of centres of competence +/- residential care group situation necessary - greater investment in facilities and useable floor areas

Selected examples for the effects of the choice of care form

Planning elements: Model type

The following overview of the four aforementioned model types is based on field studies undertaken by the authors and their personal experience. It is intended to encourage planners to consider a variety of options from which to develop their own solutions.

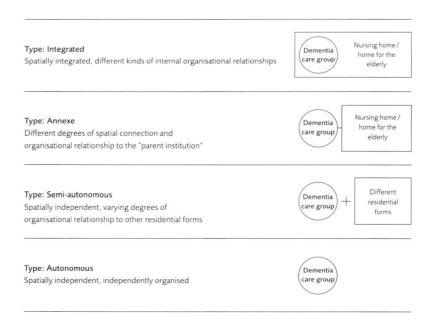

Type: Integrated
Spatially integrated, different kinds of internal organisational relationships

Dementia care group — Nursing home / home for the elderly

Type: Annexe
Different degrees of spatial connection and organisational relationship to the "parent institution"

Dementia care group — Nursing home / home for the elderly

Type: Semi-autonomous
Spatially independent, varying degrees of organisational relationship to other residential forms

Dementia care group + Different residential forms

Type: Autonomous
Spatially independent, independently organised

Dementia care group

An overview of model types according to their spatial and organisational arrangement

The potential and limitations of different model types

Model type: Integrated | Potential

Existing capacities within a pre-existing facility are repurposed, often with minimal built interventions and financial expense, at comparatively short notice for use by dementia sufferers in a residental group.

The residential group of dementia sufferers have access to the staff, infrastructure and service capacities of the "parent institution", particularly in times of extreme stress and tension.

The direct relationship to the "parent institution" offers opportunities for exchanges and synergies.

Model type: Integrated | Limitations

Spatial and architectural design possibilities are limited by the provisions of the existing building, for example with regard to creating a normal living environment, providing sufficient movement and direct outdoor access.

It is difficult to free the new facility from the institutionalised character of the "parent institution".

The larger the institution, the greater the tendency to make use of the resources of the "parent institution" rather than develop operating concepts and care forms that are more appropriate for dementia sufferers.

Model type: Annexe | Potential

A new building or conversion offers a greater chance of improving the architectural quality of a facility, particularly with regard to creating a normal homely environment, the provision of sufficient space to move around and direct outdoor access. The facility loses some of its institutionalised character.

A direct connection to the "parent institution" offers opportunities for exchanges and synergies.

If necessary, sufferers in the later stages of the illness can be transferred to an in-house care wing.

Model type: Annexe | Limitations

This model type takes longer to realise and requires more significant financial investment.

Its larger capacity and corresponding higher concentration of residents means that it serves an extended catchment area (residents are further from home), reducing its semblance of normality.

People with dementia run the risk of being transferred away from their environment and segregated into a special in-house ward once their level of illness becomes sufficiently serious.

Model type: Semi-autonomous | Potential

The creation of a semi-autonomous residential group derives from a conscious decision to implement a particular care concept or cater for a particular group of people with dementia. Typically this will follow a particular model and will accordingly be well-planned.

Semi-autonomous residential groups represent a major step towards living in normal surroundings. They are very often integrated into urban quarters, or at least nearby, and are not overly large.

Typical everyday activities prevail within a friendly and familiar atmosphere. Residents are more actively involved. Depending on the set-up, external services are not used in favour of working together with a neighbouring institution.

Model type: Semi-autonomous | Limitations

A semi-autonomous status generally means that the operator alone is responsible for establishing, financing and operating the facility.

The capacity of smaller independent facilities with regard to staff and infrastructure is more limited than that of the "integrated" or "annexe" model types. This has implications for their cost-effectiveness and flexibility, for example limiting their ability to provide external outpatient and day-care services.

Staff must fulfil several functions. A decentralised structure means that staff must be more flexible and independent.

Model type: Autonomous | Potential

A specially-developed concept and planning allows one to develop tailor-made spatial and architectural solutions.

The use and conversion of existing spaces is flexible and in most cases also reversible at a later date.

A new building or conversion offers a greater chance of improving the architectural quality of a facility, particularly with regard to creating a normal homely environment, the provision of sufficient space to move around and direct outdoor access. The facility loses some of its institutionalised character.

Model type: Autonomous | Limitations

This model type takes longer to realise and requires more significant financial investment.

Depending on the capacity of the facility, people with dementia, once their level of illness becomes sufficiently serious, may have to be transferred out of their everyday environment into a specialised external facility.

In combination with the "specialised" care concept, there is a certain risk of ghettoisation.

Design principles (micro level)

Design principles concern the spatial and design characteristics of an environment. They apply to all the built qualities of a residential facility from the access and floor plan arrangement to infrastructure and equipment as well as materials, fittings and lighting. As part of the environmental conditions they represent important resources for residents and staff alike.

By making specific use of existing resources, it is possible to influence the progression of the illness, lessen the occurrence of symptoms and accordingly improve the quality of life for dementia sufferers. The schematic diagram details, in the context of the individual potential of a person with dementia, the most important available and exploitable resources in their living environment. These represent the sum of all spatial, organisational and therapeutic structures which can help dementia sufferers to actively use their still intact capabilities and retain a sense of independence. In the following section we will focus primarily on physical resources in particular, such as orientation, security and room for movement.

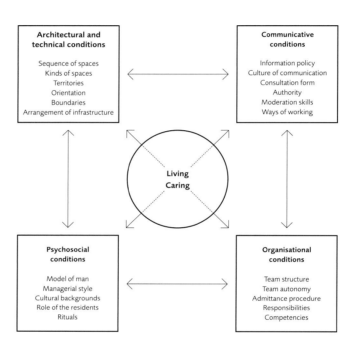

A resource model of the living environment of people suffering from dementia

In professional literature and in our personal experience, there are no indications that the needs of the elderly with regard to their living environment, whether or not they suffer from dementia, are any different to those of other people. The main difference is that older people spend more time at home than people who go to work and younger people. They are also less able to compensate for deficiencies in their environment and so are considerably more dependent on a good-quality living environment.

While the following design recommendations apply particularly to residential care facilities for people who suffer from dementia, that does not mean that they constitute an argument for developing specialised facilities for this group of people. On the contrary, they should be regarded as generally applicable criteria for high-quality living environments. Where such recommendations lead to design concepts that can be realised in general housing, they will improve the quality of life for elderly residents in general as well as dementia sufferers.

The design of spaces creates living environments with a degree of permanence and constancy. It has a direct effect on the well-being of the resident while also supporting the staff in their care and therapies. The design recommendations detailed here are intended as a general indication of concerns that need addressing and not as normative stipulations.

Design recommendations for orientation and wayfinding

Spatial structure: A clear and easy-to-comprehend arrangement of spaces assists orientation greatly. The use of light and a clear contrast between floors and walls can guide movement and help one to find one's way around. Similarly, arrangements that are familiar from normal living environments, such as open kitchen-living rooms, short corridors to individual rooms and toilets that are outside one's bedroom tap into habitual experiences and assist orientation.

Indoors – outdoors: Transitions from outside to inside, such as when entering a residential group (e.g. via a front door) and from there to communal areas should be clearly recognisable.

Paths with places: Situations that act as markers along a path (indoors or outdoors), for example seating niches, a particular piece of furniture or an inspiring view, evoke memories and create places that serve as destinations or places to rest and enjoy.

Kitchens: Open kitchens, with seating arranged so that one can watch or help, reinforce a sense of taking part in everyday activities with their familiar sounds and smells. Alongside the spatial aspect, other characteristics also assist orientation, for example a regular pattern to the day, meals that awake memories of the region of birth and from childhood or familiar music. The day-to-day operation and care provisions therefore also provide orientation.

Design recommendations for security and safety

Security and orientation are closely linked and for the most part complement one another. Nevertheless, certain measures are recommended to ensure the security and safety of the residents and staff.

Stopping residents wandering off: The boundaries of a residential group should in principle always be contained. Indoors, this can be achieved by keeping doors and windows closed or using doors with number codes. More subtle methods include disguising doors using colour or items placed in front of them such as folding screens, furniture or plants. Outdoors, dense planting, stacked piles of wood or raised beds can serves as natural boundaries. New technology also provides more individual means of being able to find people, for example a transponder chip with alarm. However, some very simple measures are often adequate, for example a gong on the door that lets the staff know when it has been opened or a gate with a mechanical latch that dementia sufferers in advanced stages will have difficulty opening.

Safety measures: Indoors, locks on kitchen or bathroom cupboards can ensure that residents cannot access medication or delicate objects. Dark floors and deep niches can be disquieting for dementia sufferers and this phenomenon can be used to discourage access to rooms such as service and heating rooms. Corridors and toilets should have sufficient railings and grips and centralised light switching to avoid people tripping if they unintentionally switch off the light.

Design recommendations for creating space for moving around

People suffering from dementia rarely spend all day in their own room. They prefer places where something is happening, for example the living room or dining area, the kitchen or the garden. Some sufferers will occasionally become restless and be gripped by an urge to move around, which one can understand as a need to sense oneself and one's surroundings in order to maintain contact with one's environment. To cater for such needs, facilities should provide a roughly even proportion of places of calm and places of activity. A connecting corridor is a natural space to move along and can also provide moments of perception by offering views, pictures, changes of colour or particular lighting.

Places of rest and peace and quiet are similarly important both indoors and outdoors. Long corridors and especially large and monotonous circuits can by contrast create a sense of unease. Simple measures can provide a way out of the monotony, such as the provision of seating areas where corridors widen or plants and furniture which one needs to walk around.

A guiding principle that governs all design measures is to create a familiar everyday atmosphere that as far as possible is reminiscent of the residents' previous living environment. Numerous examples as well as our own experiences have shown that the principle of normality, whether achieved through family-house floor plans, participation in day-to-day activities around the house or the presence of one's own furniture, is most beneficial in helping the elderly, including dementia sufferers, to maintain and make use of their own resources.

Towards the development of innovative solutions

The development of – or hindrance of – innovative solutions is dependent to a large degree on the approach taken by the planner. As there is no professional consensus as to what constitutes the "right" solution, it is important to lay open the available options during the planning process. The following section details some examples from our experience as consultants in which planners have adopted an open, non-ideological approach to finding locally appropriate solutions. "Locally appropriate" solutions make use of both pre-existing as well as newly created resources such as communal principles, existing buildings and concepts for caring for dementia sufferers, the attitude and self-conception of staff and the capabilities of the residents and of their relatives.

Thinking in terms of options versus "tunnel vision"

Project teams should examine and discuss the conceivable options on an ongoing basis from project inception and throughout the development of the project. This applies equally to the aforementioned three planning elements as well as the design principles.

It is important to avoid "tunnel vision": exclusively following the first acceptable solution one chances upon or a solution that has worked elsewhere invariably results in the late recognition that other possible solutions would have been more appropriate. In such cases one has little option but to start over or leave as is. Much time and energy is wasted and very often not all team members are willing to start over. Such "tunnel vision" generally results in second-hand copies of previous solutions instead of innovative solutions born of local conditions.

Early clarification of the role and purpose of project groups

Project groups generally consist of an interdisciplinary group of professionals. Team members have different ways of working and bring different knowledge and skills to the group. Likewise they have different expectations with regard to the aims of the project.

It is therefore useful to note down important facts in the form of a project outline (not to be confused with a sketch plan). This should address among other things the following questions:
- What is the starting point for the project development?
- What has the project group been set up to achieve?
- Who are the project participants?
- Will experts be consulted for special advice?
- What rules govern collaboration within the project group?
- How much time will the participants be expected to devote to the project?
- Are all team members able to actively take part in the project development?

A project outline of this kind serves as a framework agreement which all team members can abide by from the project outset onwards.

One's own living requirements are not necessarily applicable for dementia sufferers

Most project participants have themselves not yet reached "old age" and therefore can only try and put themselves in the position of their "target group", and of people who suffer from dementia. The danger is that they pursue their own requirements for their living environment rather than the needs of the future residents.

It is instructive to visit existing facilities in order to experience day-to-day life in residential care facilities and to better understand the importance of the physical and organisational conditions. This makes it far easier to imagine oneself in the position of a resident. It can also be useful to simulate restricted perceptive faculties. It is possible to simulate common deficiencies in our sense of hearing, sight, smell and taste which restrict our degree of orientation using relatively simple methods[1] as well as with the help of special technical aids, such as an Age Explorer.[2]

Methodical principles and further examples of design recommendations can be found in the authors' publication, *Gestaltung von Betreuungseinrichtungen für Menschen mit Demenzerkrankungen* (*The Design of Care Facilities for Sufferers of Dementia*), published in 2006 in Zurich and on the website www.demenzplus.ch.

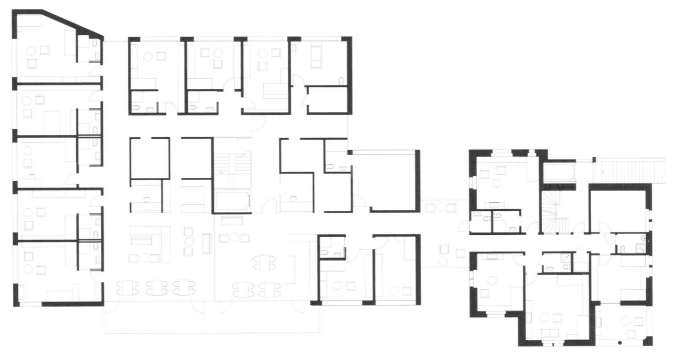

Floor plan of a dementia care group in an urban neighbourhood

Notes

1 See fcs.tamu.edu/families/aging/aging_simulation/index.php and www.allgemein-medizin.med.uni-goettingen.de/literatur/instant+aging-zfa2007.pdf.

2 See www.mhmc.de/HTML/age_explorer.html.

The life cycle and energy balance
of residential buildings

GEORG W. REINBERG

For the environment, only the overall ecology or energy balance is relevant. Accordingly, every planning task must aim to minimise its overall environmental impact. Although a variety of highly sophisticated instruments are available for assessing the environmental impact of a building, these can only be applied once the building has been planned in its entirety. During the design process itself and the conceptual development of complex buildings, such as housing or homes for the elderly, one must instead follow basic principles, which, once the design has been drawn up, can be evaluated and optimised using simulation programmes.

The following section examines how fundamental principles and hierarchical criteria can be employed for the design of residential buildings for the elderly. Special attention is given to "energy consumption" as a key indicator of environmental impact. To determine an ecologically relevant energy balance, the architecture must be considered in its totality: over the entire life cycle of planning and construction, the building's use and operation, and recycling.

A | Planning and construction

The basis of every ecological measure is the planning of the building itself. It is at this stage that environmental pollution and energy consumption can be reduced most at comparatively low cost. This applies to an even greater degree to regional and urban planning. Large-scale regional and urban planning measures, which for example are responsible for regulating transport and the routing of utilities, have a fundamentally greater effect than individual measures at the level of a building. For the elderly, this means that they should be able to live nearby so that they are able to take part in public life. This not only helps prevent the isolation of older, less mobile people but also reduces traffic (and the associated environmental pollution). In this respect, the integration of old people in their traditional environment and their close proximity to friends and relatives can be regarded as an "ecological measure" in itself.

Planning dependencies in the various life phases of a building

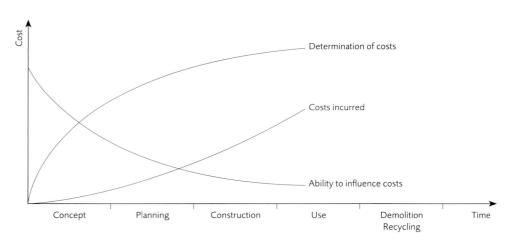

For the building itself, increasingly effective energy-saving measures in the construction of a building ("embodied energy") have resulted in a proportional increase in the relevance of the energy expended for the day-to-day running of buildings. Careful planning offers great potential for implementing effective ecological measures without great expense. A key factor for the ecological balance of the construction is the quality and environmental friendliness of the building materials used as well as their performance in relation to their environmental impact (a particular level of performance, such as structural stability, fire protection or thermal insulation is assessed in relation to its environmental impact and the embodied energy of the respective material). Different models are available for evaluating the ecological quality of materials.

In addition to selecting appropriate building materials, it is also necessary to consider transport and the organisation of the construction. Here too, this should not solely be considered and decided from a technical point of view but be regarded as an aspect of the planning process and design. For example, soil that does not necessarily need to be excavated will not require transportation or result in environmental pollution; lighter materials with more manageable dimensions are easier to transport to the site. As roughly 90% of construction transport requirements result from excavated mass and the building carcass, this is where optimisation will be most effective. Similarly, as almost all environmental pollution resulting from the transportation of building materials is caused by heavy goods vehicles, rail-bound means of transport (trains and trams) represent an attractive alternative that should be considered wherever feasible.

Well-organised building site practices can – when exploited – improve the overall architectural quality, for example when the finished building serves as a "testimony" to its construction and reminds one of its own history. For the construction, building materials should be easy to detach and separate from each other, i.e. through mechanical rather than adhesive fixture. Building elements should be easy to reach and replace where necessary – the "longevity" of a building contributes significantly to its ecological balance – and where possible should consist of recycled or "replenishable" materials (building materials made with renewable resources). Many replenishable building materials are also healthy from a building biology perspective and therefore well-suited for old people.

B | The use and operation of a building

Heating energy consumption is the first area where energy-saving measures should be applied as here the largest and most cost-effective savings are to be made. The energy reforms in recent years have therefore rightly focussed on reducing heating energy requirement. For the elderly, this is all the more relevant as older people generally feel comfortable at higher room temperatures during the heating season. In addition, older and less mobile people spend more time at home than younger people.

In a traditionally insulated house, a temperature rise of 1°C corresponds to a 6% increase in heating energy consumption. Housing for the elderly should therefore be better insulated than standard housing. Note that although in absolute terms, energy consumption in highly-insulated houses increases more slowly with indoor temperature than in poorly-insulated houses, its proportion as a percentage of overall energy consumption rises more quickly.

One can improve the indoor climate of a building by adding energy from outside and/or through its structure and construction. The more sustainable solution is through construction measures aimed at minimising heat loss through the external skin of the building and/or recovering heat loss with the help of technical installations.

Retaining warmth

Building measures aimed at retaining warmth include:

Reducing the external surfaces through which heat is lost, by improving the surface area to volume ratio (less surface area, or a greater volume for the same surface area, equates to less heat loss per heated cubic metre), improving the building's geometry and reducing the external temperature through the addition of buffer spaces (unheated extensions) or by partially burying the building (in winter the ground is warmer than the air).

Improved thermal insulation:

• **Opaque building elements (walls and ceilings)**: A layer of thermal insulation of at least 20 cm (for example cork) for external walls and 30 cm for roofs represents an economically viable level of insulation. From an ecological perspective, even thicker layers would be advantageous but significantly reduce the amount of useable floor space where the building itself cannot be made larger. Vacuum insulation materials are more effective, offering a similar level of insulation at around a tenth of the material thickness compared to conventional insulation materials. At present these materials are, however, very expensive and are not easy to correctly install in practice.

• **Layers of insulation** are generally placed on the external surface of the construction (improved indoor climate, upkeep of the construction). Highly-efficient insulation reduces the level of energy consumption and also provides a more comfortable indoor climate as our subjective sense of well-being indoors is dictated largely by the temperature difference between the surface temperature of walls and the air temperature. Where room temperatures are higher, such as where old people live, this temperature difference becomes particularly important.

• **Transparent building elements (windows)**: Today many improved products are available, such as triple-glazing with dense gas fillings or reflective coatings as well as associated products such as laminated glass inserts and thermally-efficient frames. Because transparent elements generally insulate less well and highly-insulated glass is expensive, it is important to take into account their colder surface temperature, particularly where old people are concerned. A sufficient level of indoor comfort – where the temperature difference between window and air is as low as possible and circulating air does not cool excessively on the inner surface of windows – can be achieved by selecting windows with a "passive house" specification ($U_w < 0.85$ W/m² K).

• **Construction details**: As the thermal efficiency of the aforementioned opaque and transparent materials improves, heat loss through poorly executed details becomes proportionally greater. Likewise, poor detailing can more rapidly lead to building defects.

• **Airtight building envelope**: The loss of (warm) air from the building is closely related to the construction details. The greater the indoor to outdoor temperature difference, the stronger the pressure of air movement from indoors to outdoors. Should warm air penetrate the construction and condense, it can lead to serious building defects. Housing for the elderly should therefore fulfil the airtightness requirements of passive energy standards (measured using a blower door test which creates a 50-pascal pressure difference between indoors and outdoors; the air change rate under these conditions should not exceed 0.6 per hour).

• **Minimisation of ventilation heat loss**: As inhabitants require constant fresh air (approx. 30 m² per person per hour) there is a limit to the amount of heat loss one can prevent via the building's envelope. However, warmth contained in ventilation and flue gases can, to a large extent, be recovered before it leaves the building by passing it through a heat exchanger. Although older people are less active and may therefore require less fresh air, homes for the elderly are often more densely populated. As a result, the need to recover the warmth in the air is more important than it is for general housing. A mechanically-controlled ventilation system fed through a heat exchanger also ensures optimal fresh air quality, which is important for people more susceptible to illnesses; it also efficiently removes odours.

Building measures aimed at retaining warmth ("passive energy house standards") can be an economically viable means of reducing the energy demand to a level of 40 to 50 kWh/m² per annum in regions with a Central European climate. Internal heat sources can provide around a third of the energy demand; the remainder must be covered through other means.

Heat gain

Typically, the largest directly available source of renewable energy is the sun. The sun can be used in architecture in a variety of ways:

Passive solar gain:

The sun has a stimulating, healing and enlivening effect on people and is correspondingly important for old people as well as the frail. Passive solar gain, which admits as much solar energy into a building as possible, is therefore a doubly valuable way of providing warmth in housing for the elderly. In winter, however, the sun shines only part of the time and irregularly, making it difficult to predict the effect of passive solar gain. Because it is influenced by a large number of different factors (level of insulation, room temperature prior to solar irradiation, level of comfort as temperature changes, regulation mechanisms for parallel heating systems, heat flow in the building, user behaviour, thermal absorption capacity of the building construc-

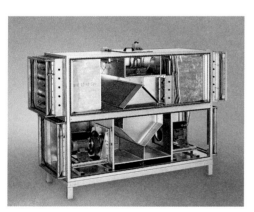

Supply and extract-air unit with cross-flow heat exchanger

tion, furnishings and so on) it is highly complex to calculate and requires computer simulation tools. As a result, planners have often adopted other systems that are easier to manage and predict, and the benefits of sunlight for the residents of low energy buildings have been exploited only rarely. The low popularity of this form of solar gain represents a missed opportunity for elderly residents in regions of Europe that are not particularly sunny.

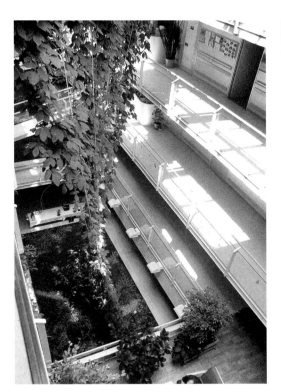

Home for the Elderly, St. Pölten; a glazed roof allows sunlight to flood the atrium

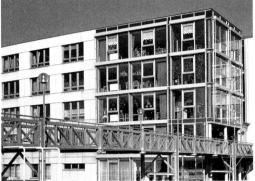

Home for the Elderly, St. Pölten; conservatories as sun verandas

Home for the Elderly, St. Pölten; a conservatory or winter garden provides an ideal way of enjoying the winter sun

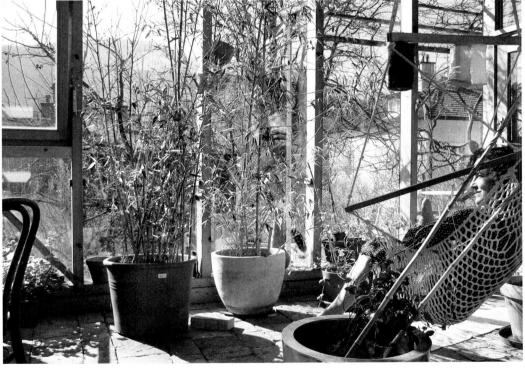

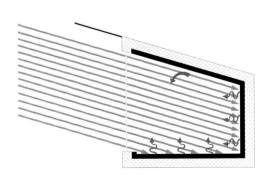

The principle of passive solar gain

A simpler alternative to direct passive solar gain (heat retention directly in the living space) is an "isolated" form of passive solar gain using a winter garden or conservatory. Here greater temperature fluctuations can be tolerated, making it possible to increase the amount of glazing and – despite its comparatively low efficiency in absolute terms – to absorb considerable passive solar energy. The heat gained must first, however, be transferred to the rest of the building, which is most simply achieved by incorporating the winter garden directly in the building's automatic ventilation system. Conservatories also provide an ideal means for elderly people as well as the infirm to enjoy direct sunlight. Here they can experience the healing power of the sun; an old man who was hard of hearing once told me enthusiastically that he could hear better after a few hours in the sun in the conservatory.

Computer simulations have shown that conservatories which are attached to the building's ventilation system provide a heating contribution of around 20%.

Further variants of exploiting passive solar energy include translucent thermal insulation or similar absorptive thermal insulation systems. These kinds of insulation allow sunlight to penetrate into the structure of the insulation, warming either air that is trapped in miniature cavities so that it cannot circulate causing it to act as an insulator, or the material itself. A further kind of solar collectors are windows containing adjustable metal lamella in the cavities between the panes that absorb solar energy and warm the air between the panes to a relatively high degree so that it can be transferred to a thermal mass.

Passive solar energy can be used to cover a further third or half of the heat demand of a building. This leaves only a small remaining amount of heat demand – that cannot economically be reduced any further by ecological means – which can also be covered using energy from the sun (approx. 5-15 kWh/m²a).

Active solar heating:
The term active solar heating was initially used to denote all systems that required some form of technical installation. Today many "passive" solar strategies also employ automatic control and ventilation systems (hybrid systems) and the term active solar heating now refers predominantly to solar water heaters. In addition, there are also solar air heaters, though these are comparatively uncommon.

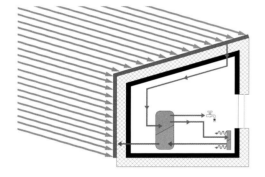

Active solar water heaters are elements that although technically independent should generally be integrated into the building for better performance. The collectors are mounted on the south-facing surfaces of the building, which means that elderly residents cannot benefit from direct sunlight in these areas. Their advantage is that the water in the collectors has good thermal retention properties and is able to store the heat of the sun and provide warmth when the sun does not shine (passive solar gain is by contrast only usable for the duration of each day). The heat generated by the solar water heaters can be used effectively in low-temperature heating systems. Such heating systems require large heat-emitting surfaces and provide primarily radiant heat. This form of heating is known to be physiologically beneficial for older people.

The principle of active solar heating

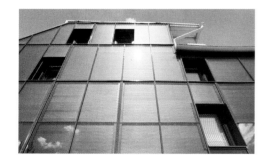

Given the low altitude of the sun in winter, its weaker strength and lower abundance, relatively large collector surfaces and large thermal reservoirs are required to be able to cover the heating requirement (simulations are necessary to calculate its efficiency) and the collectors should be arranged at a steeper incline rather than a low angle (in winter vertically-arranged solar water heaters offer similar performance to 45° inclined collectors, while avoiding overheating in summer). Future technology will further improve the efficiency of these collectors, for example by making better use of lower temperatures using heat exchangers or through the generation of electricity from excess heat using a Stirling engine.

Indirect use of solar gain:
This refers to the use of warmth from the sun stored in the ground or in water: air inlet pipes in the ground or water tubing laid underneath a building serve as earth-air or earth-water heat exchangers. Heat pumps are also effective means of recovering energy from the heat stored in ground water or in deeper underground strata (geothermal energy).

External energy sources:
These should only be used to cover any "residual heat demand". Here too, ecologically-friendly alternatives that make use of renewable energy sources (such as biomass) are preferable to methods that negatively impact the environment (for example large hydroelectric power stations). Non-renewable energy sources should not be used for heating purposes.

Hot water
If measures for retaining heat, as described above, have been implemented and a building fulfils a low-energy or passive-energy standard (heat demand per m² floor area is not more than 15 kWh per annum),

the domestic hot water demand will be equally large or even exceed the heating demand. As elderly people generally require more water for washing clothes and dishes, from an ecological and economical point of view it makes more sense to reduce hot water consumption, for example through savings and the use of more efficient fittings, than to further optimise heating energy demand. The remaining heating energy demand can, for the most part, be covered by solar energy using one of the aforementioned active solar heating systems. These are also well-suited for hot water heating, more so in fact than as an energy source for heating (only larger installations are able to provide more energy than required for hot water provision in the winter months).

As a rule of thumb, 1 m² collector surface area is required per inhabitant for hot water heating, with three to four times as much for additional room heating provision. The necessary heat reservoir should be dimensioned for the respective needs. The location of such reservoirs, which can sometimes be more than a storey high, should be considered in the initial planning phases. Heat pumps can be used to utilise ground water or geothermal energy for hot water heating. Thermal collectors are now available in technologically advanced forms and, given the steadily increasing energy prices, represent an economically viable means of covering around 60% of the hot water demand of elderly people.

Electricity

In traditional housing, electricity consumption represents the smallest part of the overall energy consumption. Following the examples above, ecological measures can here too be economically implemented. A kilowatt-hour of electricity cannot, however, be compared directly with a kilowatt-hour of heating. This higher level of energy requires more primary energy expenditure for its production and compared with thermal energy should be multiplied by a factor of three in order to be comparable from an ecological point of view.

In the past older people traditionally consumed less electricity than younger people as they made less use of technical equipment such as computers. More recently older people have begun to make increasing use of today's modern electronic technology and in future they will use these increasingly to compensate for physical deficiencies. As they require more light as their eyesight deteriorates, it will become increasingly important when building for the elderly to provide ecologically-friendly electricity at a constant and affordable price. Electricity – as a higher order form of energy than heat – will become a particularly sensitive form of energy required for household use.

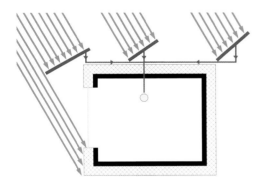

The principle of photovoltaic solar use

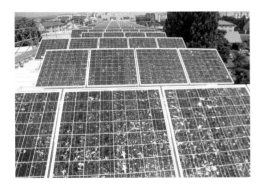

Here too the locally available energy source is once again the sun, which can be converted directly into electricity using photovoltaic collectors. This form of energy extraction is comparatively expensive. In practice only around 10% of the solar irradiation can be converted into electrical energy. By comparison, thermal collectors have a conversion rate of around 50-60%, passive solar gain around 90%. One option is to use photovoltaic solar collectors to serve multiple functions (greater economic feasibility), for example as shading elements for passive solar glazing. Photovoltaic collectors (PV) should be arranged at a shallow angle as the summer sun from above is much stronger than the lower winter sun. They should also be well ventilated as most PV technology becomes less effective at producing electricity as their temperature increases. Photovoltaic should therefore not be integrated into the building but be installed as an additive measure.

Electricity can also be generated using combined heat and power systems (generators which in addition to generating power provide heat as a by-product). One should prevent energy generation methods in the thermal energy sector from incurring energy requirements in the more ecologically-sensitive electricity sector, for example as a result of the need to power pumps and control systems for the aforementioned thermal collector systems. Here the additional electricity demand should as far as possible be covered on site. If there is no possibility or insufficient possibility of generating electricity onsite, one should attempt to derive the remaining power using electricity from alternative power sources such as wind, biomass, small power plants or similar.

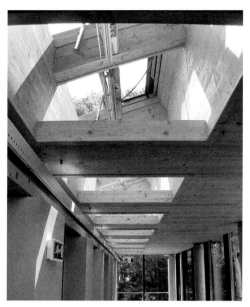

Automatic vents at the highest point of the building for night-time ventilation

Air conditioning in summer

Although old people generally find higher temperatures more comfortable than younger people, the prevention of overheating in summer is just as important for one's quality of life as heating in winter.

In most cases, protection against overheating in summer for all generations in Central European climates can be achieved using appropriate building constructions alone. The most important criteria is sufficient insulation (as it is for warmth in winter), a high thermal mass and the reduction of passive solar gain in summer. A high thermal mass allows the cool night-time temperatures to counteract the heat of the day and avoid temperature extremes (the absorption of warmth reduces temperature fluctuations). All translucent building elements (such as windows) must be well shaded, in particular east and west-facing windows which can lead to overheating. Internal sources of warmth (for example, lighting and technical equipment) should likewise be minimised through the use of low-energy lamps and equipment. Finally, night-time ventilation should be ensured (including adequate protection against rain, burglary and insects) to allow the entire mass of the building to cool down overnight.

In addition to these passive measures, ground water or geothermal cooling can be used to keep building elements cool (water cooling pipes are laid inside massive parts of the building construction) or via an earth-air heat exchanger to pre-cool fresh air as it enters the building. If incoming air is passed over water surfaces, this too can have a cooling effect. Only in special circumstances – and when all other methods have been exhausted – should additional active measures be taken, which will consume energy. In such cases, existing installations should be utilised wherever possible, for example solar water heaters, which in conjunction with new technology can be used at relatively low temperatures (such as those provided by flat panel collectors: under 100°C) for cooling purposes. Similarly, PV collectors can be used to power conventional air conditioning equipment.

The role of the residents

The final most important factor for the efficacy of all the measures described above is the people for whom we undertake such measures: the residents. Passive measures in particular are largely dependent on the behaviour of the inhabitants. Residents should understand, value and experience the benefit of the ecological measures undertaken. The most valuable medium for communicating this is the architecture of the building itself. Its experiential and communicative qualities play a decisive part in creating a sense of well-being for the residents.

Solar architecture in particular offers an opportunity to communicate technology and to turn technical advantages into beneficial qualities for living environments. Old people often suffer from orientation problems or are unable to see as well as they used to. Sunlight (see passive solar utilisation) can be used to guide orientation. Daylight is always better suited to people's needs than artificial light, and people who are bedridden benefit greatly from a view out into the countryside. Lastly, natural building materials are advantageous not only from an ecological point of view but also because they are non-toxic, thereby improving conditions for old people who are generally less resistant to toxic substances than younger people.

Maintenance and modernisation

From an ecological as well as energy balance perspective, maintenance and ongoing modernisation is an equally important factor as the construction and running of housing for the elderly. Flexibility and adaptability are key contributors to sustainability. Buildings for old people should therefore be easily adaptable to changing uses and requirements (which we may not yet be aware of) and easy to repair, for example by separating structure, infrastructure (water, electricity etc.) and furnishings so that these can be repaired or renewed separately according to their different lifetimes. The relevance of maintenance and modernisation is underlined by the fact that over an 80-year period, almost one and a half times as much as the original building costs are expended on the upkeep of a building.

C | Demolition of the building

The demolition of a building can only be undertaken without environmental reservations if a building has been built according to the principles of building biology from the outset. Building biology is a prerequisite for ensuring that the demolition and disposal of a building can be undertaken with minimal energy expenditure – a process that already begins on the construction site (disposal of waste material from the building site). In the planning and realisation of buildings the following hierarchy of priorities applies: avoidance of waste, recycling and utilisation of waste, followed lastly by the ecologically appropriate disposal of waste. Measures include limiting the variety of different materials used, the coordination of the lifetime and usage periods of building elements, the use of recyclable building materials, the avoidance of composite building materials, clear product declarations and so on.

Only when the entire life cycle of a building has (next to) no environmental impact have we managed to successfully balance energy usage, protect the climate and environment and, not least, build sustainably for the elderly.

Reference literature

J. Fechner (ed.), *Altbau-Modernisierung – der praktische Leit-faden*, Berlin, Heidelberg, New York: Springer Verlag, 2002.

M. Hegger, M. Fuchs, T. Stark, M. Zeumer, *Energy Manual: Sustainable Architecture* (Construction Manuals), Basel, Boston, Berlin: Birkhäuser, 2008.

G. W. Reinberg, M. Boeckl (eds.), *Reinberg – Ecological Architecture – Design – Planning – Realization*, Berlin, Heidelberg, New York: Springer Verlag, 2008.

G. W. Reinberg, *Offenes Wohnen im Alter – Pensionisten- und Pflegeheim St. Pölten*, Vienna: Österreichischer Wirtschaftsverlag, 2001.

NIKOLAOS TAVRIDIS

Operators, service providers and clients in the housing and nursing care industries

A new reality for investors and operators

In 1995, the German legislative assembly decided to withdraw all regulatory control from the field of care for the elderly and to allow it be regulated by free-market mechanisms. For the first time, nursing homes no longer needed to fulfil statutory-driven planning requirements and certification conditions, the assumption being that by lowering the market entry threshold this would lead in the long term to a healthy balance of supply and demand. The drawback was that this meant that operators needed to rapidly learn how to live with economic risk. Today, nursing care institutions in Germany are free to determine their own package of care provisions, as long as they fulfil statutory quality requirements, and to offer these on the market. They bear the responsibility as well as the risk – for profits and for losses. At the same time, most federal states in Germany reduced the level of state funding for nursing institutions, on the one hand to avoid skewing the market and on the other due to the fact that state budgets were no longer sufficient to provide such funding.

The free-market regulation of the nursing care industry led to a further change. Property of some form or other is generally the foundation for care for the elderly and this requires sufficient capital. Accordingly, only those with enough capital will therefore be able to offer care for the elderly. The withdrawal of the state as a backer for property acquisitions after 1995 opened up a key role for institutional and private investors. The so-called "institutional investors" – a broad term encompassing financial institutes, banks, funds (closed-end or open-end), pension funds and insurers – are now of particular importance in the nursing care industries. There are many different reasons why institutional investors invest in property or institutions in the care industry,and these motives depend on the readiness, or resistance, to take risks. Institutional investors can differ here quite considerably.

The greater the risk for the investor, the higher the risk premium, i.e. the return on the investment, should be. The expected return on investment for the investors is also influenced by the refinancing conditions as these institutes commonly invest in a combination of own and borrowed capital (pension funds being an exception). If conditions for borrowed capital worsen, the expected return has to rise so that the return on own capital remains constant. Although banks do not differentiate between own and borrowed capital in calculating their return on investment, the refinancing conditions also play an important role for banks as they define the "acquisition costs" of the bank's capital. The higher the interest, the higher the financing conditions for the bank.

In Germany, the branch is relatively new, and more experience with financing and collaboration with institutional investors still needs to be gathered. Since its beginnings in 1995, the nursing care industry has not seen constant development. A phase of initial enthusiasm after the introduction of long-term care insurance was followed by a phase of disillusionment at the end of the 1990s accompanied by a series of spectacular failures and significant bad investments. In the years 2001 to 2005 the market more or less ground to a halt. The institutional investors – despite attractive yield premiums – were no longer willing to invest in the nursing industry as they remembered only too well the losses of the preceding years. By mid-2005, the reticence had evaporated and indeed the reverse situation arose. In 2006 the nursing industry was suddenly awash with a flood of capital provided by domestic as well as foreign institutional investors. The risk premiums shrunk to a hitherto unknown dimension and investments in nursing and nursing care institutions were suddenly the talk of the day.

Following the general liquidity crisis which has gripped the financial markets since mid-2007, investments have since slackened as was to be expected. However, the nursing care industry has been less affected by this than other property classes. The reason for the large-scale investments by foreign institutional investors in particular has less to do with the care industry itself and more with the overall liquidity of the financial markets during this period. The high level of liquidity meant that the profits in primary property classes, such as housing, offices and retail, were very low due to the high flow of capital, and that secondary property classes, such as hotels, logistic property or nursing care facilities were more attractive as the return on in-

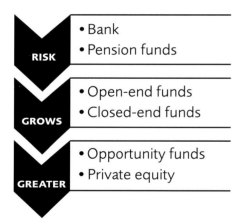

RISK
- Bank
- Pension funds

GROWS
- Open-end funds
- Closed-end funds

GREATER
- Opportunity funds
- Private equity

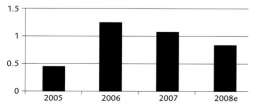

Investments by institutional investors (billion Euros)

vestment was considerably higher. After the flow of capital also began to sink considerably in the secondary property classes – with the exception of the care industry – investors saw an opportunity to increase mean returns by including nursing care facilities as a component of larger mixed property portfolios. Institutional investors still expect investments in the care industry to perform better than other kinds of property and accrue a greater return.

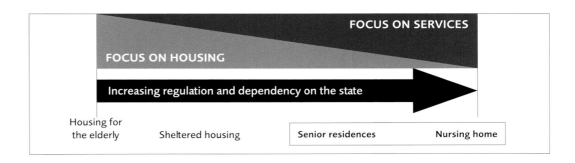

Every investment in a property in the nursing industry has to consider two "layers". The relative weighting of these determines the degree of risk and the overall estimation of the property investment, including expected profits for the investor. At one end of the spectrum, there are investments where physical property is the dominant aspect of the product, for example housing schemes for the elderly. These are in essence very similar to normal housing projects except that they are specially equipped to fulfil the needs of the elderly (according to the German norm DIN 18025). Typically no or only a low level of services are provided. The higher costs are a product of the requirements of the DIN, which results in 10-15% higher rent income. At the other end of the spectrum one finds the typical institutionalised nursing home, in which property features as just one of a series of "hygiene factors". Whether or not the property is of great importance for the product, its primary constituent is the service and with it the operating concept. The larger the role of the services, the more the profits depend on specific "soft" factors such as operator and concept.

Between these extremes there are other forms such as sheltered housing or senior residences whose profitability consists of a combination of property and services in differing proportions. In general one can assume that the greater the focus on services, the older the customer, in this case the resident, is likely to be and therefore the more dependent they will be on these services. Because of the need to protect the interests of the particularly vulnerable residents, these institutions are subject to a greater degree of statutory regulation by state agencies. The long-term care insurance covers a large part of the financial cost of care and accommodation. The regulatory framework of the state and the economic dependency on the state are considerable. Since the introduction of long-term care insurance in Germany, institutional investors have focussed more on fully institutionalised nursing care facilities despite the fact that these are more dependent on monetary support from the state. In fact, this tendency has increased over the past few years. There are a number of reasons for this which reflect the different evaluations of inland and foreign institutional investors.

A widespread opinion is that as a result of state funding this class of property has a firmer footing than other property investments for the elderly lacking such state support. Many investors are also of the opinion that demographic changes point primarily to a greater demand for fully institutionalised care facilities. Although these views are still the subject of much discussion, the advantages of fully institutionalised care facilities (demographic factors, state support and high return on investments) are easily communicated and understood, and many institutional investors are attracted to them as a result. Less interest has been shown in investments for housing for the elderly, for sheltered housing schemes or communal housing.

From the viewpoint of institutional investors, care properties have the following inherent risks:
- Fungibility, i.e. little or almost no possibility of reuse through third parties;
- Limited transparency with regard to the operators;
- Different functional concepts;
- Lack of independent consultants (brokers often call themselves "independent" consultants but have an inherent conflict of interests).

Despite the above risk factors, investments in this branch have developed spectacularly over the last few years. As mentioned earlier, for the institutional investor it is important to achieve a reasonable return on investment where the risks involved are as transparent as possible. As a result, the following key aspects of a care facility play a decisive role in the decision whether or not to invest.

1. Location

After several attempts in the 1990s to build nursing facilities on greenfield sites, investors realised that isolated facilities are rarely successful. Whether the location is urban, at the outskirts or embedded in a residential area depends in part on the clientele it aims to attract. Residential schemes for the elderly or sheltered housing for clients (residents) who are still sprightly and relatively active will need to provide a greater variety of recreational activities than a nursing home whose residents are generally no longer as mobile. For old people's homes, locations in residential areas can be advantageous in order to be near to one's relatives. Connections to other health care institutions such as hospitals, rehabilitation clinics or medical care centres are favourable. It is essential to ascertain the realistic demand for the planned location. In recent years opinion has changed. Up until 2005, institutional investors assumed that net demand was the most important determining value for the choice of macro location. Since then, a more aggressive competitive approach has proven that it can also be successful.

2. The operator

The spectrum of operators on the German market is very fragmented. The largest segment, representing nearly 55% of the market, are independent non-profit organisations, while private operators currently make up around 37% and rising. The remainder of the market is shared among municipal operators who are increasingly being forced out of the market. This fragmentation at the level of the operator means that very few operators are able to entirely safeguard against failure, either through their financial standing or as a result of the size of their organisation. An investor will need to examine how competent the operator is and assess their professionalism. A number of factors are relevant including the quality of the management, links to the local market, particular strengths, a convincing operator concept and not least previous track record.

3. Lease agreement

The lease is in a manner of speaking the clasp that binds together property and operator. It has to clearly and transparently regulate the distribution of rights and obligations for both parties. The lease must also take into account that for operator-managed facilities a large part of the value of the property lies with the operator itself. Given the high degree of fragmentation in the market for operators, the lease must regulate what happens should the operator fail, in order to ensure that the value of the property is affected as little as possible or ideally not at all. The lease must reflect the investor's need for security.

At present, institutional investors tend to prefer small facilities with a minimum size of 60 to 80 beds. Larger institutions with 150 or more beds have become much less attractive in recent years. Investors are most interested in facilities with a high proportion of single rooms, with 60% being the lower limit. The size of the individual units should likewise not be too small. The average expectation is at least 40 m² net floor area per apartment or suite. With regard to the risk of an operator going out of business, a shift has become apparent over the last two years. From 1996 to 2005, institutional investors clearly preferred working with the few big players on the market. Today, investors are also willing to work with smaller operators who run between three and five facilities. A reason for this is that in their endeavours to net the "scarce" larger operators, the investors often had to accept a painful cut in profits and less favourable lease terms. Higher profits and more favourable lease terms can be agreed with smaller operators. Most investors have since realised that they can compensate for the risk of a possible operator failure with the higher returns possible with smaller operators.

4. The development of profits

After the introduction of long-term care insurance in Germany from January 1995 to the end of 2004, the returns on investment for nursing care facilities were surprisingly homogenous and robust. The average return on investment during this period lay by 8% for contracts where the tenant bore all costs except for maintenance to the roof and external surfaces. As a result of the massive flow of capital, the situation changed dramatically from the end of 2005 onwards. Almost overnight the return on investment sank to between 6 and 7% and more or less regardless of the quality of the property concerned. From mid-2007 onwards the situation readjusted somewhat and by autumn 2008 the return on investment lay by on average 7.5%. From the viewpoint of the seller of such properties, it is a problem that the realisable return on investment is not affected greatly by the quality of the investment. According to our calculations, the difference in return on investment between a good and a poor object on the market lay by less than 0.75%, a value that is extremely small in comparison to all other classes of property (in housing the difference can be as much as 4 to 5%). The reason for this low differentiation between good and poor properties with regard to return on investment is the investors' comparatively homogenous opinion of care facilities coupled with their unwillingness to accept a low return on investment given that any involvement in this market bears a higher risk.

Outlook

The professionalisation of investments in care facilities has led to a considerable flow of capital on the one hand but also made the nursing industry more dependent on the general cycles of the financial markets. This has become ever more apparent since the third quarter in 2007. The key new features of the long-term care insurance scheme (introduced with the Pflegeweiterentwicklungsgesetz in 2008) have yet to impact noticeably on the disposition of the investors. In fact, the increasing investment in the nursing care industry has led to greater competition in many locations, which in turn exacerbates the risk of operators going out of business. Investors must examine the core business of the operators in greater detail and the investment product itself is becoming ever more complicated. Future investment activities will also depend on how the returns on investment in other alternative property classes change, which for most investors are easier markets to access than care facilities. One can expect investments in the care sector to be accordingly volatile.

The reticence among investors to invest in housing or sheltered housing schemes for the elderly could disappear as soon as suitable investment products appear on the market. A prerequisite for this is that such products should hold their value and that investors can readily see this without the need for excessive analysis, which at present is not the case. As a result of the proposed shift in emphasis towards outpatient care, as heralded by recent legislation, the demand for such products is likely to rise dramatically, representing a chance for investors too. It is, however, down to project developers and operators to devise concepts that are oriented towards the needs of the investors.

BERNHARD HEIMING

Project controlling and cost management of housing projects for the elderly

In the property market, housing projects for the elderly are no longer a niche segment. By the year 2020 almost a quarter of all German residents will be older than 65 years of age. The number of people interested in forms of housing appropriate for the elderly is increasing rapidly and a consumer group is growing whose needs the property market will have to cater for in the coming years. This trend began three to four years ago with a sharp uptake in the number of nursing home projects and is currently expanding to address a variety of different forms of housing for the elderly.

In recent years, it has become increasingly clear that project controllers are being involved in building projects at an ever earlier stage. In many cases there is no longer a single client but rather a consortium of financial investors and project developers. In the case of housing projects for the elderly, they are often joined by the operating agency during the initial phase who, although not actually the client, plays a major role in defining the planning and building parameters. This constellation makes it absolutely necessary to obtain professional advice on costs, time schedules and risk assessment in advance of going ahead with a project in order to determine the basis for a collaboration between investor and developer, and in this special case also the operator. Although this initial involvement on the part of the project controller is very often not remunerated – many regard this as part of acquisition – it nevertheless requires special care as the parameters laid down in this preparatory phase are very difficult to change once the project is under way.

The proactive project manager

In the past project controllers were regarded much as "building accountants" or as "protocol clerks", and the German guidelines for planning services (HOAI §31) underlined this with their heavily simplified, formalised definitions. Modern project controlling is, by contrast, an active management task with the project controller situated between investor, developer, planning team, building contractor and the final user. The aspects discussed below apply in general, not just to the specifics of managing projects for the elderly, and are important for an overall understanding.

Of the tasks a project controller undertakes, cost management is one of the most extensive, and is especially important not least because the effects of time scheduling and quality control can have implications for the cost. Cost management is divided into three sections:
• Cost planning: determining the budget on the basis of a cost estimate;
• Cost control (planning phase): monitoring adherence to the budget as the planning progresses and in the awarding of contracts;
• Cost control (construction phase): anticipation and assessment of cost risks, intervention where costs are likely to be exceeded and the arrangement of corrective measures.

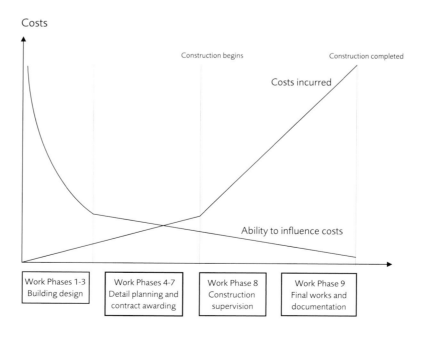

Costs incurred and potential influence on costs over the duration of a project.

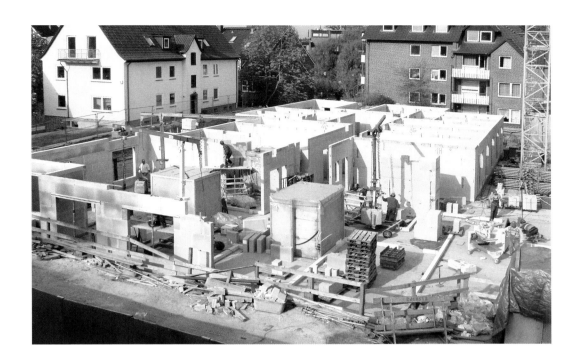

Sunrise Reinbek (April 2004); the installation of prefabricated bathroom cells

As the diagram shows, the ability to influence the project costs reduces significantly as the project progresses, meaning that cost management plays a particularly important role during the early phases of a project. It is therefore necessary to recognise potential risks that may affect costs as early as possible and to implement appropriate measures to stay within the projected costs. Typical risks include:

Deadlines – delays in the time schedule can quickly lead to high additional costs, potentially endangering the budget. This risk can be reduced through:
• Professional project coordination, clear organisational structure and operating schedule and the choice of appropriately experienced project partners.
• Regular communications with all project partners;

Stipulations of the planning permission require:
• Early communications with all relevant authorities involved in assessing planning permission;
• Proactive and clear elaboration of all aspects that deviate from the building regulations or require exceptional consent or permission; where necessary obtain advance clarification via a preliminary building permit.

Increasing construction costs – this risk is difficult to avoid but can nevertheless be minimised through the following:
• Invite tenders of all major building works and trades in advance of construction. Typically the building structure, façades and technical installations already cover between 65 and 70% of the overall costs.
• Obtain recommended prices during the planning phase for all special materials and construction techniques where insufficient prior knowledge is available.
• Determine alternative choices for materials and planning variants.

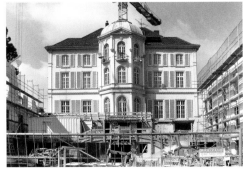

Sunrise Villa Camphausen, Bonn; rearward extension

Contractor's risks – most notably the issue of adequate capacity and the risk of bankruptcy which one must attempt to minimise as follows:
• Obtain information about the size of the company, number of staff and reference projects and talk to the company's other clients.
• Obtain economic data on the tendering companies, such as legal form, annual turnover, capital resources, stakeholders and annual accounts. For very large contracts it can make sense to draw up a "business rating" method based on this information.

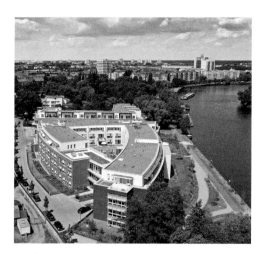

HavelGarten Residences, Berlin-Spandau; aerial view

In addition to these general risks, specific projects may exhibit special risks which one should try to anticipate and ascertain early on as they can result in unexpected costs. These include, for example:

Building site risks: Prior research into the site's history can determine whether the soil is polluted (from a previous use) or whether munitions or ground monuments are likely to exist. A soil investigation is always advisable to ascertain the load-bearing capacity of the site and to determine the ground water level.

Connections to utilities: In some cases it is not possible, or expensive, to connect a site to the necessary utilities. It may not be possible to channel rainwater into a canal, making it necessary to construct a soakaway. The water supply pressure may be insufficient, necessitating a pressure booster station. A transformer station may be necessary to ensure a constant electricity supply.

Neighbours: In a number of cases, permission will be required from the neighbours without which planning permission cannot be obtained or building works may not commence. By way of example these can include insufficient distance to neighbouring buildings and underpinning works or the anchoring of foundation revetments on the neighbouring plot. It is much easier to reach an agreement early on than when under pressure to commence building works.

For the investor, or for the client, it is crucial that the project controller reports back in regular intervals with a compact, understandable and concise overview of the essential facts, project data and progress. Such data needs to be condensed to a level sufficient to provide an at-a-glance overview of the salient points. An overview of the budget, for example, is mandatory, as is a register of possible risks and a diagrammatic time schedule. The report should contain all details necessary for the client to make informed decisions and to fulfil his or her obligation to banks, lenders, partners, supervisory boards and so on.

Requirements specific to projects for the elderly

A number of additional factors apply to projects designed for use by the elderly, which in many cases can only be mastered by a project controller with extensive knowledge of this particular field.

Accessibility: In comparison to normal housing projects, additional costs can arise from:
- Larger bathrooms (transit areas according to DIN) with floor-level shower and additional grip rails
- Handrails in all public areas, corridors etc.
- Motorised door openers on main entrances
- Larger lifts
- Even thresholds between rooms and onto balconies and terraces
- In many cases larger balconies (sufficient room for manoeuvring)
- Emergency call and alarm systems
- Non-slip floor surfaces

Care home regulations: If a project is for use by the elderly and is subject to care home regulations, for example for use as a nursing home, it differs fundamentally from normal projects in that it must conform to a series of stipulations. For example, nursing homes and old people's homes must offer a certain level of staffing, offer particular facilities and technical installations, fulfil hygiene guidelines and organisational structures. As properties run by an operator, they are monitored by the supervising authority. The planning of a nursing home must be carefully negotiated with all relevant authorities as not only planning permission is required but also a permit for running a care home. This form will only be chosen where health and nursing care is envisaged. This can be a sticking point for sheltered housing or assisted living projects. In Germany, for instance, responsibility for nursing home regulations was transferred to the individual federal states in 2006, with the result that each state has its own regulations. The point at which a project is subject to these regulations differs sometimes considerably. In some cases, the level and kind of services offered determines

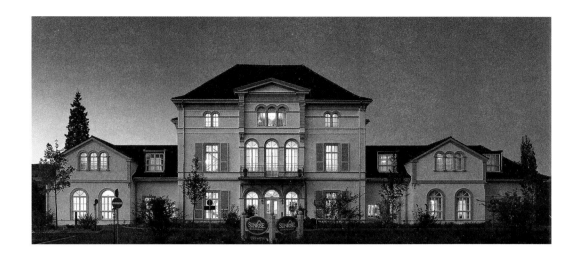

Sunrise Villa Camphausen, Bonn;
street elevation at dusk

whether or not the regulations apply, even when these services are not directly related to nursing care. For assisted living and sheltered housing schemes, it is important to establish that nursing home regulations do not apply and where necessary to consult the relevant authorities in order to avoid that a scheme is barred from operating because it does not fulfil regulations for which it was not built, effectively endangering the entire investment.

Fire safety: Nursing homes are subject to special fire safety requirements. While the guidelines are now no longer as strict as for hospitals, the necessary fire safety requirements are still determined by certain evacuation scenarios in combination with alarm systems and the like. As there are no universal rules and regulations, this needs to be discussed and agreed for each individual project. Conflicts can arise, and may have to be reconciled, between more modern home concepts with airy, open common areas and the level of fire safety measures the authorities would ideally like to see. Sheltered housing schemes differ only slightly from normal residential schemes and for the most part are not subject to extra fire safety requirements. More stringent regulations can apply, however, for communal forms of living where living quarters are shared, for example with regard to fire alarm systems and fire-protection ratings for walls and doors between the individual living quarters. Again, here too there are no universally applicable regulations, necessitating prior negotiation with the fire safety authorities in order to ensure that the planning process can proceed without unforeseen problems.

Parking provisions: In most cases car parking provisions for residential schemes for the elderly are much lower and savings can be made through the reduced number of car parking spaces, which in turn can be offset against greater expenses in other areas.

Early recognition aids problem solving

To conclude, it is important to realise that project controlling involves not only the smooth running of processes and the protocolling and documentation of results but also the anticipation and early recognition of possible general and specific project-related risks, along with the steps necessary to resolve them so that their implications can be assessed, particularly with regard to costs. The earlier one is aware of these, the easier it is to make adjustments to compensate for them. It is important that the client is given all information necessary to make clear and informed decisions before it is too late, even when in isolated cases this could mean abandoning the project. More typically this will involve adjusting the planning, construction or time schedule to stay within the boundaries and framework of the project. One way or the other, the earlier one is aware of problems the better.

HELMUT BRAUN

Quality management
and user satisfaction surveys

Focussing on the resident

Until well into the 1970s, the dominant form of institutionalised care for the elderly in Germany was a tripartite facility, the so-called three-stage home. Regarded at the time as modern, it comprised a combination of residences for the elderly, an old people's home and a nursing home in a single facility and necessitated that residents move as their health deteriorated and care needs increased. The principle of ensuring that whenever possible people could remain in their own homes, a long-standing socio-political fundamental, was therefore compromised not just once but repeatedly.

In history, the building of almshouses for the elderly, usually through the initiatives of local communities or groups of citizens, shows that this did not have to be the case, and their organisational concept and physical structure offer lessons that still have potential today. Instead of rooms with a washbasin, there were apartments with a bathroom, a room for living and sleeping in, a kitchen and a cellar. Help, support and nursing care were provided there where the old people lived. Although, then as now, living and nursing areas were separate from one another, it was up to the resident to decide if and when they needed extra care as they became more infirm.

Since then, progressive housing concepts for old people with and without the need for care and assistance have successively eroded the distinction between outpatient and institutionalised care, offering serviced apartments in combination with reliable nursing care. Over 89% of residents in sheltered housing and applicants awaiting a place cite the ability to receive nursing and health care in one's own home even when frail as a key factor in their choice of this type of housing for the elderly.[1]

Three significant changes in the demographic structure have had a major effect on the market for "housing for the elderly", both conceptually as well as in terms of built form:
- more people live to an advanced old age
- there is a greater proportion of elderly women
- a greater proportion of elderly people live on their own

People of an advanced old age are more prone to negative side-effects brought on by ageing, such as isolation, increased susceptibility to illness or the need for constant care. The increasing number of people over 80 accordingly places greater demands on housing and accompanying services for the elderly. The proportion of elderly women to men in residential and nursing homes is currently approximately 80%. Future planning proposals need to take such structural demographic changes into account.

Preferred residential forms

In every survey conducted, people's first choice of where they would prefer to live in old age is always the same: the familiar surroundings of their own home. Serviced or assisted residential housing occupies second place, followed thereafter by a conversion of their own home. Purpose-built residential alternatives such as retirement homes do not rate as highly. Similarly a flat in or adjoining the children's home is not the most popular choice. Other alternatives such as communal flats or co-housing are only gradually entering the scene while the traditional old people's home is now generally regarded as undesirable. Given that most old people would prefer to live in the familiarity of their own home, this should serve as a guiding principle for future residential and special-purpose residential forms for the elderly.

Qualitative criteria

The single most important reason why old people move into residential housing is to feel safer, both in terms of receiving adequate care and assistance as well as with regard to personal safety. Furthermore, the average senior citizen today wishes to remain self-sufficient and independent, to live in pleasant surroundings, to avoid daily stress, to maintain social contacts and interaction, partake of health offerings, enjoy good food and to be guaranteed value for money for the services they receive.

Facilities and fittings

Surveys also show that residents wish their living surroundings to be as normal as possible, whether or not they live in an old people's residence or nursing home.

This means each apartment should have:
- Its own doorbell
- Its own letterbox
- Its own storage
- Been planned in accordance with relevant DIN norms
- A bath suitable for old people
- An emergency call system
- Its own kitchen
- Special safety measures

Buildings should have:
- Gardens or a park
- A common room
- Washing and drying facilities
- Small common rooms
- A restaurant/dining room
- Gymnastic and fitness facilities
- Where possible a swimming pool
- Where possible a wellness area

The surveys also indicate that demand for single-room flats has all but disappeared and that flats with at least another small room, better two good-sized rooms, are preferred.

Services

What range of services and provisions are potential residents looking for?
• Help in planning their move
• A reception that is manned day and night
• Qualified personnel on all floors and in management
• A safety concept
• Lunch or evening meal
• Weekly cleaning of the apartment
• Emergency call button linked to the reception
• Valet parking
• Cultural and recreational activities
• Arrangement of supplementary services
• Special care for acute illnesses
• Additional domestic services
• Caretaker services

Health care and nursing

Outpatient services must be able to provide reliable and dependable help and care in the resident's home. Residents of all disability levels can be cared for in their own apartment: experience has shown that with careful planning and good organisation this is possible. Transfer to a nursing home or care facility need only be undertaken if the resident so wishes.

For residents requiring psychological support, the complex can provide a form of day-care facility where qualified personnel can provide the necessary care and support.

Residential living and nursing care are no longer mutually exclusive concepts, blurring the boundary between outpatient and inpatient care. Services are becoming increasingly tailored to the needs of the individual, allowing the recipients greater freedom to choose what they need. Greater flexibility can and must be provided at different levels regardless of whether elderly people choose to live in a private household or a nursing home. The strict division between housing and nursing care must give way to more flexible forms of living and health care. The historical example of the almshouses shows that this is possible, and this could once again serve as a model for future developments.

Future perspectives

The immediate and distant future of housing for the elderly will be dominated by three market segments:
• Private households supported by outpatient health care services,
• Institutionalised nursing care whose services and standards are generally determined by the provider (insurance scheme, social security provider), a sector that will increasingly need to upgrade its concept and quality standards
• A broad spectrum of residential forms of living, that draw on and pay for services as and when required.

The residents and tenants in each of these three segments have one thing in common: they want to be able to live safely, self-sufficiently and independently, retaining control over their own lives, even as their nursing care and support needs increase. This necessitates that all professionals involved – architects, service providers, insurers, the housing industry as well as policy makers – work towards developing networked solutions oriented around the needs and wishes of the elderly themselves. Building projects and operating concepts that do not sufficiently take this into account are destined to fail, as several short-sighted projects have shown in the past. Only when the needs and aspirations of the target group are considered in the planning stage and realised in the operating concept will the various users be suitably satisfied.

The coming generation of senior citizens is used to clearly articulating its needs and will without doubt place greater demands on their living environment and care facilities. The ensuing demand in the marketplace has implications for both existing as well as new projects, and poor-quality concepts will need to respond rapidly in order to survive. And, last but not least, all those involved in the planning and conception process should not forget: everything we build now, we are also building for ourselves.

Note

1 For a comparison with the situation in the USA, see a study on user satisfaction in approximately 40 residential facilities published in the *Design for Aging Review* by the AIA: American Institute of Architects Design for Aging Center, *Design for Aging Post Occupancy Evaluations* (Wiley series in healthcare and senior living design), Hoboken: Wiley, 2007.

In response to the socio-demographic, cultural and organisational transformations described in the first section of this book, the spectrum of approaches to living for the elderly has broadened and diversified considerably over the last ten years. Never before have so many people been able to look forward to 15 to 30 years of active and self-determined life after retirement – the time span of an entire generation. The ongoing trend towards individual and diverse lifestyles is also continuing on into old age. Both the housing and the care provision sectors have become more and more aware of the potential of this market segment and are responding to the growing demand for diversity with a variety of different operating concepts.

As a result, the previously separate realms of housing and care concepts are beginning to mesh with one another in a variety of different constellations. The grouping of the projects shown in the following section reflects different variants of such hybrid concepts.

In the following we have identified six key thematic groups, all of which have their own particular formal and design considerations but are nevertheless related to one another: **inter-generational living, assisted living and serviced apartments, living concepts for specific user groups, living concepts for people with dementia, residential and nursing homes** as well as **integrated housing** and **neighbourhood concepts.**

Where ten years ago it was difficult to clearly differentiate between an old people's home and a nursing home, in recent years a series of new terms such as residential care, serviced apartments, residential care groups, co-housing and others show clearly how the spectrum of care provision has broadened. This new diversity is also reflected in its architectural expression, while at the same time lending new momentum to the cultural exploration of the public face of the elderly in town planning and the city.

Statements such as "old age is colourful and varied" are commonly cited, often with the implication that buildings should also be – but is this necessarily the case? Where existing buildings are adapted to accommodate the needs of the elderly, the focus as a rule will be on urban integration and offering something familiar. But what about a new building in a clearly defined urban environment – should it assert itself or blend as far as possible into the surroundings? Examples from recent years show a much greater tendency towards individual expression than only two decades ago. As long as the architectural quality is coherent and consistent, anything is possible, from a neo-classicist adaptation to a radically modern building; the choice depends only on the client and their budget.

While a more conservative tendency is inherent in old age and in the aesthetic expression of old age, it is by far not the only way. Examples from Switzerland demonstrate in their aesthetic diversity that housing for the elderly has likewise remained open to local as well as international architecture and that appropriate options are available to fit every taste. National typologies such as large-scale residential projects in Holland

Living for the elderly
Typologies and projects

or the Swiss condominium concept are also to be found. By way of a counter-example, the difficulties experienced by Sunrise after opening senior residences in Germany show that it may not be sufficient to transplant American ways of living and "Laura Ashley style" into a new context, primarily because it neglects to take into account the biographical background. The careful study and adaptation of a region's architectural language could be a possible way of providing people in old age with an attractive living environment.

The most interesting initiatives of building for the elderly emerge in integrated concepts. Do these projects resist the tendency towards individualisation? Homes for the elderly, regardless of whether they are rich or poor, should no longer be – and often no longer want to be – solitary buildings, but arise in all kinds of urban and functional mixtures: with children's nurseries, next to schools, sharing buildings with shopping centres, adjacent to swimming pools or health centres. More design possibilities emerge – and while it is up to the designers and decision-maker to opt for more urban unity or for greater variety, it is precisely this approach that in one way or another strengthens the sense of neighbourhood that, in design terms as well, we need to foster in our society. The spectrum ranges from the return to small-scale town life to large expressive and sculptural forms that avoid a tired repetition of standard solutions on the one hand and wilful otherness on the other.

Local small-scale solutions are still the most successful examples: Béguinages, neighbourhoods with a dense pattern of street frontages and private courtyards to the rear, or the European turn-of-the-century type of buildings with shops on the ground floor and living on the upper storeys. In the European city, which typologically may be of interest to other continents, it is not always essential to have a car, an advantage for older people who may no longer feel able to drive. It is along those lines that we should re-examine what has proven itself over thousands of years. Let us use these elements as building blocks to reformulate in architectural terms a new diversity in housing for the elderly.

Inter-generational living

Many older people would like to live near to their children and grandchildren or among young or younger people – close by but with their own space. Whether in the oldest form of cohabitation, the traditional family unit, or embedded in the context of an extended family – one's own or, as is becoming increasingly common, one's family of choice – inter-generational living has the potential to accommodate diverse housing needs and wishes.

Inter-generational concepts offer a variety of flexible housing provisions that allow different generations to live together in different ways and can respond to changing demands as residents grow older. The success of such concepts is, however, very much dependent on the personal commitment of the residents and their degree of interaction.

In addition to providing a range of different sizes and types of residential units as well as flexible floor plan arrangements, such concepts also need to offer opportunities for the residents to come together, for example communal spaces for meetings and festivities, sports, a children's nursery etc., according to the respective concept.

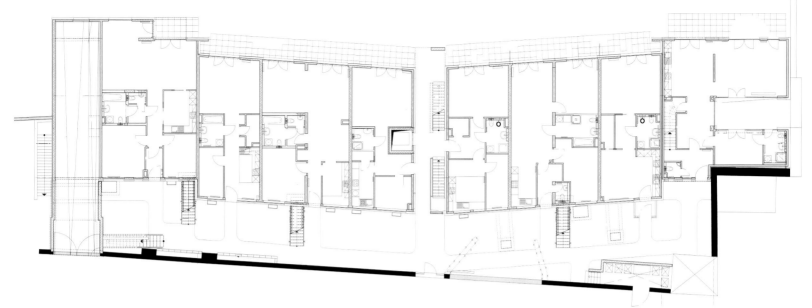

Ground floor plan, apartment building

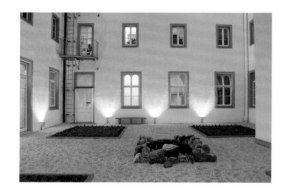

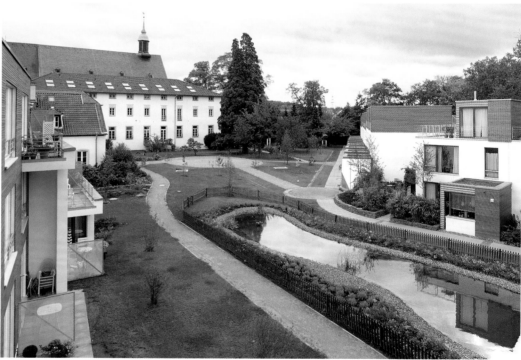

Courtyard in the existing monastery | View of the complex from the north

Carmelite Monastery

Bonn-Pützchen, Germany

Architect	Fischer – von Kietzell – Architekten BDA Partnerschaftsgesellschaft
Client	gwk neubau gmbh
Completion	2000 existing building / 2003 new buildings
Useable floor area	6,864 m²
Units / Capacity	existing building: 31 apartments new building: 16 terraced houses apartment building: 21 apartments

Communal living is the central principle at the heart of the entire scheme for the former Carmelite monastery which is now an inter-generational housing project. This sense of fellowship continues a long-standing tradition of communal living in monasteries as well as in "village communities". The monastery, which dates back to 1706, is surrounded by 6,000 m² of gardens. Together with the neighbouring site belonging to the Order of the Sacré Cœur, it constitutes a green "oasis" of almost 15 hectares on a site that has a rich tradition as a pilgrimage destination.

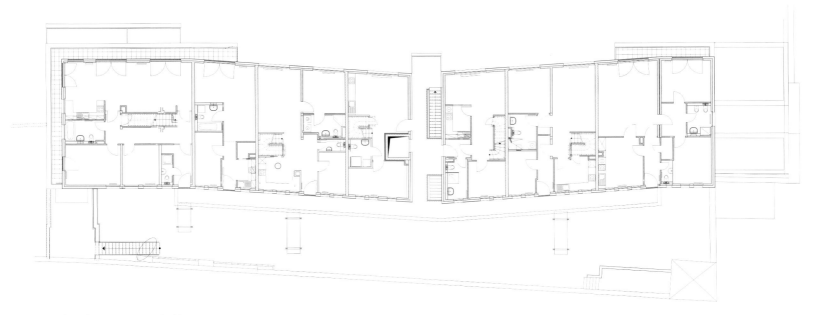

Roof level plan, apartment building

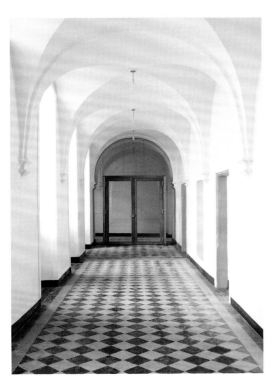
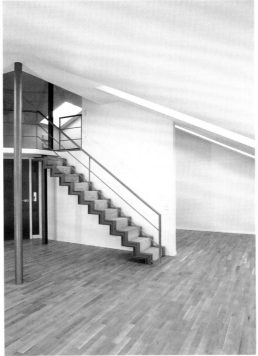
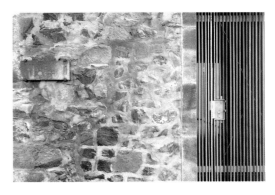

Fully preserved cloister hallway | Apartment in the attic |
Modern entrance gateway in a historical wall

The renovation and conversion of the former Carmelite monastery – a listed building with fully intact cloister – resulted in the creation of 31 privately-owned apartments with floor areas ranging from 50 to 98 m². In addition, a row of 16 two-and-a-half-storey terraced houses ranging from 134 to 148 m², each with a 30 m² outdoor courtyard, was erected parallel to the monastery's boundary wall. These private areas are supplemented by roof terraces. Embedded between the monastery garden and the boundary wall, the clear rectangular forms of the building have a distinctive quality. Both the new houses as well as the monastery are occupied predomi-

nantly by childless couples, single-parent families or singles.

The long three-and-a-half-storey building opposite the terraced houses that forms the east edge of the monastery garden is an apartment building with 21 apartments. Most of the apartments are occupied by families with one or two children. The floor plans as well as the sizes of the apartments vary considerably, from 58 to 134 m². The variety of apartment types reflects the fact that young and old people have different living requirements. Maisonette apartments with roof gardens, single-level apartments, multi-storey

apartments with a central atrium and apartments for families with their own entrance stair are all integrated into the homogenous form of the building. Individual elements, such as a separate entrance, help residents develop a sense of identification with their own home. An underground garage beneath the monastery garden with 69 parking spaces for the residents keeps the complex almost entirely free of cars.

The single-level apartments in the monastery and in the new buildings are almost all suitable for barrier-free access and all the remaining apartments also cater for the needs of elderly resid-

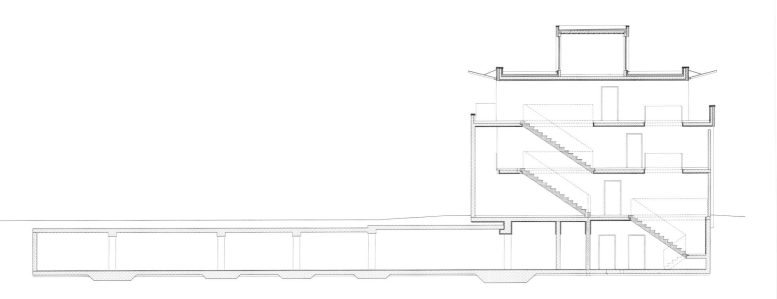

Section through apartment building with underground parking

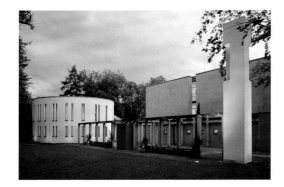

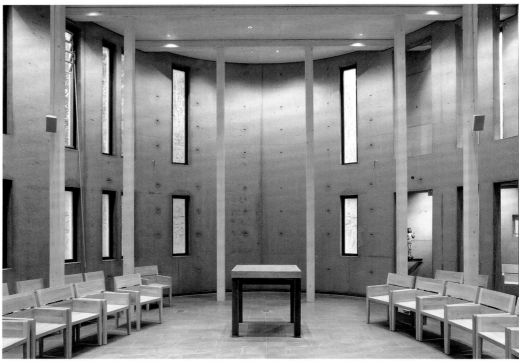

Chapel at the end of the apartment building | Interior of the chapel looking north-east | Rectangular forms of the terraced houses, facing west | Semi-private entrance areas

ents. The close proximity to a home for the elderly means that older residents can draw on additional help as required.

The idea and intention of the housing project is based around communal living for young and old. Facilities such as the residents' association, the communal rooms, a guest room and the café, as well as the communally maintained gardens, together form a "village community" within the local district of Bonn-Pützchen. They also attract outside interest, stimulating interaction with the local neighbourhood and district. These are supplemented by semi-professional recreational activities, arranged by the residents for the community and the neighbourhood.

The monastery garden is divided into different areas to cater for the differing needs of the residents and for different activities. The gardens consist of a landscaped park with pond, a playground with play house and open areas around the terraced houses and the apartment building. In addition, the private courtyards and roof terraces, as well as semi-private niches in the transitional area between public and private, offer differing degrees of outdoor usage.

All of the new buildings have been sensitively inserted into the grounds of the monastery, keeping a respectful distance to the monastery itself. Existing views of the monastery and of the park were carefully considered during the planning. The apartment building picks up the building line of the monastery along the street, while the rearward terraced housing lies parallel to the boundary wall of the monastery garden.

Through the provision of a variety of different flat types, sizes and fittings, the complex has attracted residents from different age groups. The integration of different generations has therefore

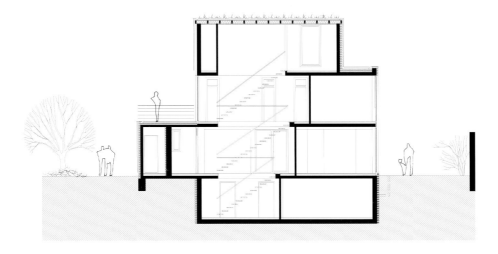

Section through terraced house

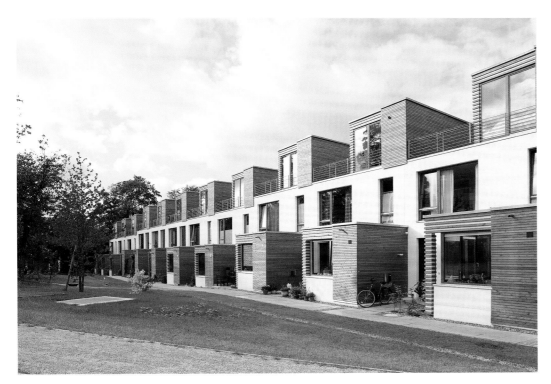
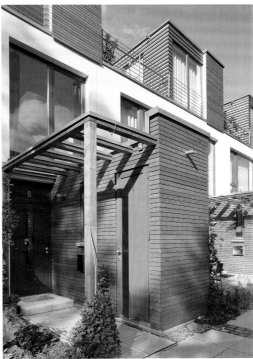

been made possible and is encouraged through the design of the buildings. The successful conversion of the existing building and the compact additions in the gardens form an ensemble of parts that relate to one another in their arrangement and architecture. The complex demonstrates impressively that existing historic building substance can be combined with modern architecture and that old buildings are equally able to accommodate modern living demands.

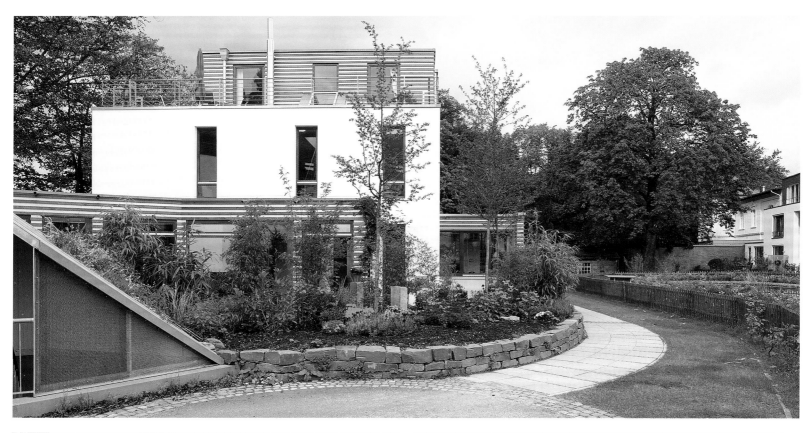

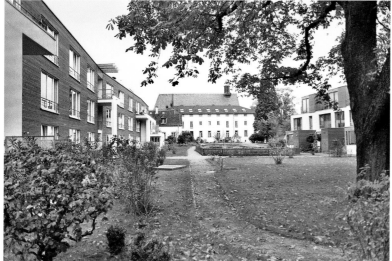

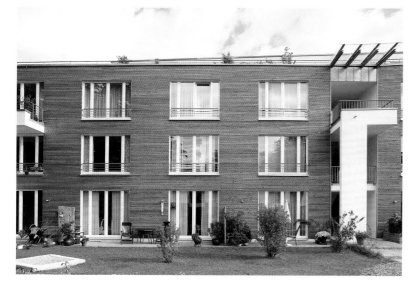

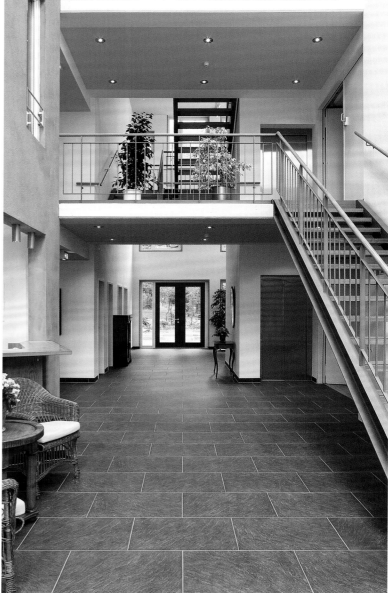

Northwest end of the terraced houses | The new buildings are embedded in the existing gardens | Façade and outdoor entrance courtyard, apartment building | Entrance lobby and circulation space, apartment building

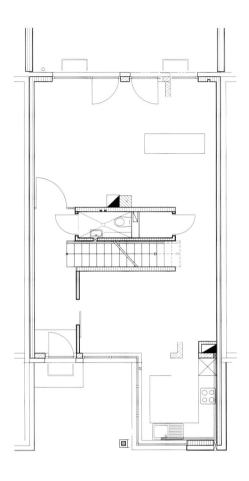

Ground floor plan

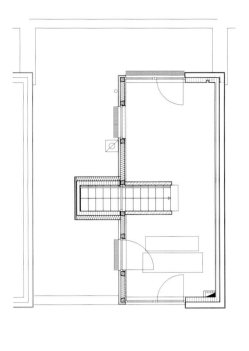

Upper half-storey plan

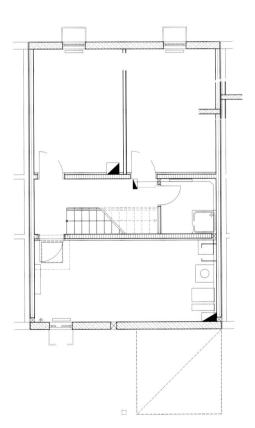

Lower level plan

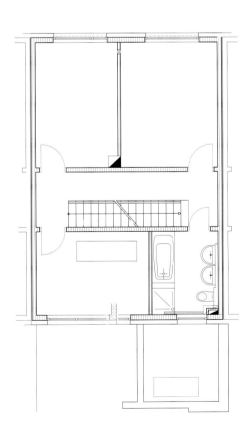

Upper level plan

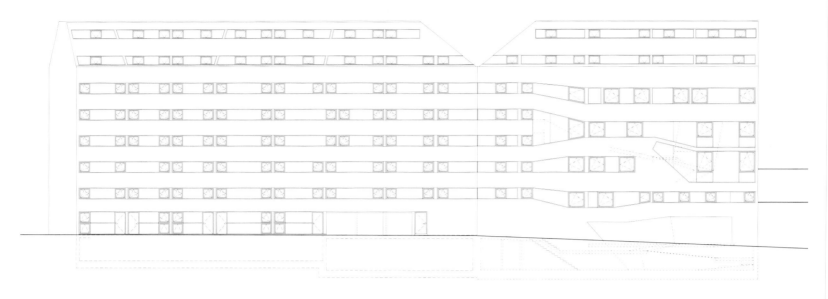

North elevation

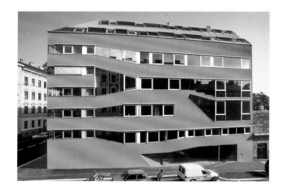

A compact building with irregular fenestration | Location on
the Missindorfstraße

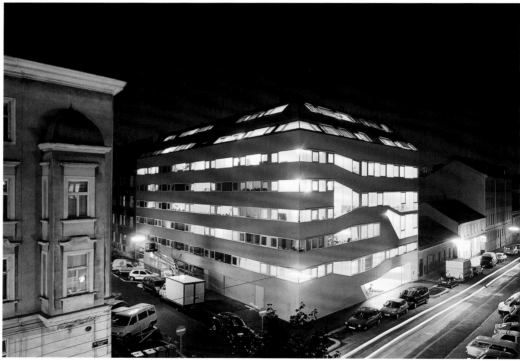

"Miss Sargfabrik"

Vienna, Austria

Architect	MISSARGE / BKK-3 / BK
Client/Operator	Verein für integrative Lebensgestaltung
Completion	2000
Useable floor area	2,820 m²
Units/Capacity	39 apartments

The orange-coloured building in the Penzing district of Vienna owes its strange and somewhat provocative name to its location in the Missindorfstraße and its relationship to the existing housing project, the "Sargfabrik" (coffin factory). Miss Sargfabrik is the younger offshoot of probably the largest self-initiated and self-run housing, cultural and integration project in Austria.

The new building, designed by the architects BKK-3, is a continuation of the planning philosophy and functional mix previously realised in the earlier Sargfabrik project, opened in 1996, which is designed to accommodate social diversity. In

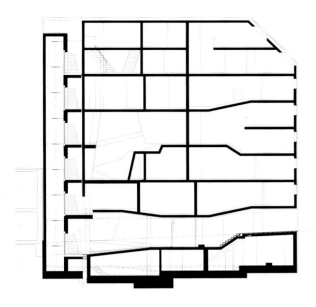

Section

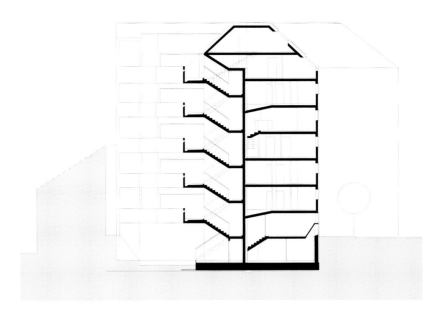

Section

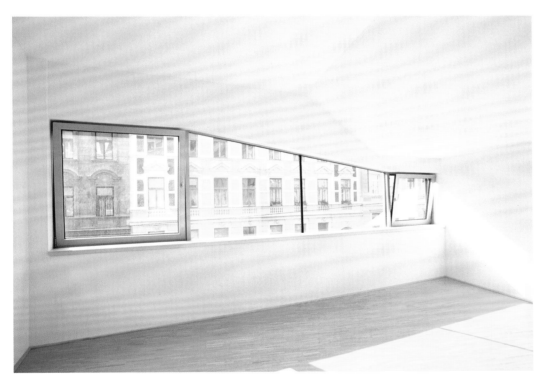

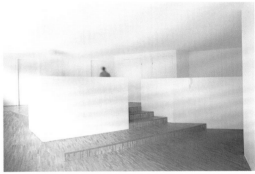

Interiors of the apartments on the third floor and ground floor

this respect, the building is a living environment and meeting place for people of different ages, lifestyles and cultures and is equally open to children, young adults, pensioners, refugees or disabled people, whether men or women. All key decisions affecting the project as a whole are made by a general assembly of the Association for Integrative Lifestyles, who serve as the legal owners of the complex. As such, as far as the residents of both buildings are concerned, the complex and its facilities belong to no-one and to everyone.

Compact and solid-looking on the outside, the building on the corner of the street contains an

impressive array of flat types which the planners have stacked and nested around one another to create a "landscape within the house". The use of an overly rigid grid has been deliberately subverted through the bending and folding of walls, the switching of floor plans and changes in room heights, sometimes with fluid transitions from 2.26 to 3.12 m. On the ground floor the two, sometimes three-storey atelier-like units are up to 4.10 m high. With their own direct entrances from the street, these can be used as a sort of home office. The average size of a flat in the "Miss", given a predominance of small units, is 50 m², though the often diverse needs of the resi-

dents have been taken into account. Accordingly, there are "open" flat types with large window frontages as well as spaces with fewer windows and more wall surfaces. All the apartments are accessed via open galleries with up to 3 m-wide "terraces" and a weather-protected staircase at each end.

The residential functions are complemented by diverse communicative spaces for communal use: a club room (especially for young people), a library, reading and media room that resembles a walk-in spatial installation as well as a joint kitchen with dining area and a washroom. The residents

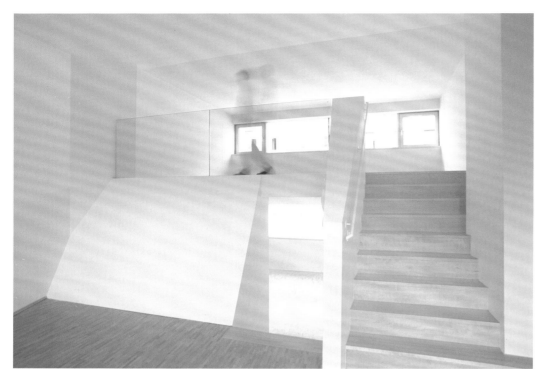

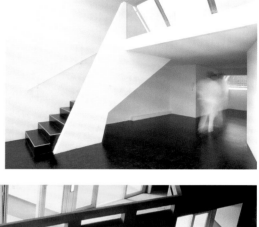

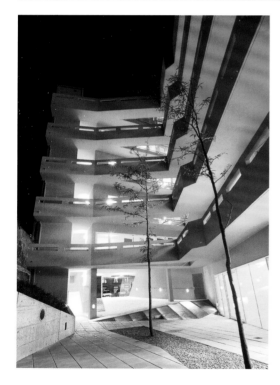

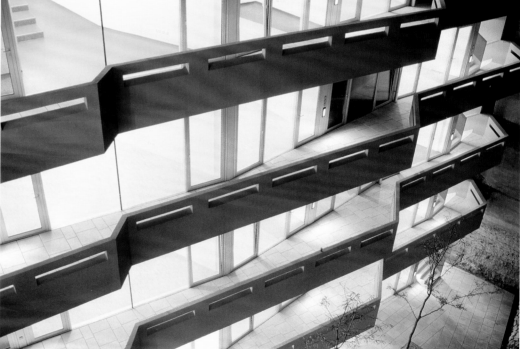

can also use the communal facilities in the neighbouring Sargfabrik such as the children's nursery, swimming pool, seminar rooms, event room, café-restaurant and guest apartment. In addition, residents can use the neighbouring outdoor amenities such as the roof garden with sun terrace, barbecue area, stone garden, vegetable patches, berry bushes and fruit trees, children's play area, green courtyards and last but not least the large pond.

The realisation of the Miss as well as the Sargfabrik integrates numerous ecological principles, both with regard to the building as well as life-style. The external insulation employs a homogeneous non-vapour-retarding system (rockwool and thick mineral render) and the careful detailing of walls and glass surfaces ensure good thermal efficiency and comfort levels indoors. Only ecologically certified and non-hazardous materials have been used in the interior fittings. The use of PVC was avoided wherever possible, even for drainage pipes, where composite laminated piping or welded polypropylene/polyethylene piping was used.

Since its completion in 2000, the affectionately known "orange hut" has, after initial scepticism, proven itself and has earned a reputation far beyond Vienna for a high standard of living. Originally born out of political and social initiatives in the 1980s, the association has remained true to its roots and continues to recruit, in a most professional manner, young people to ensure the ongoing success of the project for coming generations.

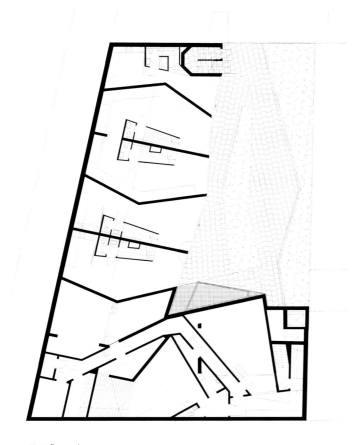

First floor plan

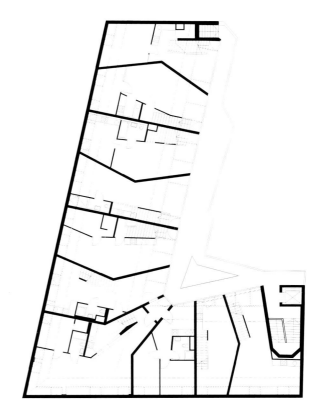

Seventh floor plan

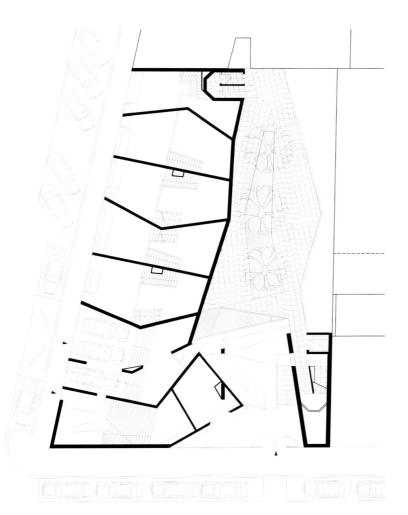

Ground floor plan

Fourth floor plan

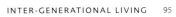

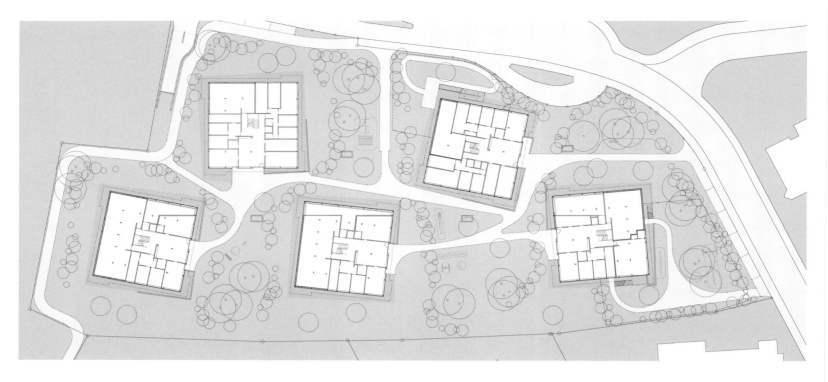

Site plan

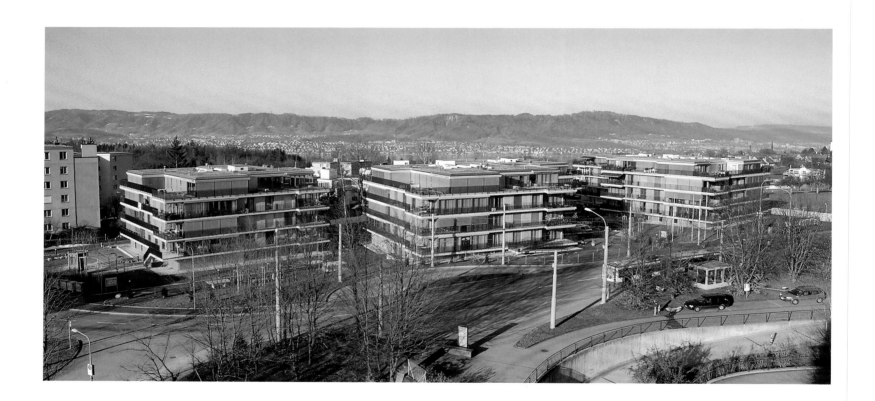

Steinacker
Residential Complex

Zurich-Witikon, Switzerland

Architect	Hasler Schlatter Partner Architekten AG
Client/Operator	ASIG Baugenossenschaft, Wohn- und Siedlungsgenossenschaft Zürich
Completion	2004
Useable floor area	8,754 m²
Units/Capacity	73 apartments, 1 group care apartment, children's nursery with two groups

In the year 2000 the City of Zurich, in its position as landowner, initiated an architectural competition on behalf of a cooperative interested in utilising the site. The aim was to develop a 1.15 hectare-large site on the edge of the city overlooking Lake Zurich with high-quality housing and external landscaping that takes into account the changing structure of society. Furthermore, maximum use of the site was to be made in order to meet the demands of economic viability of the project.

The winning design proposed five freestanding buildings in the form of modern urban villas. The five-storey buildings with full-height glazing

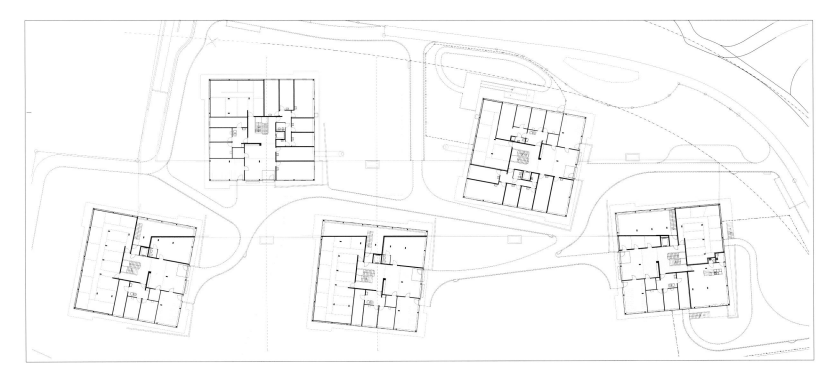

Ground floor plans

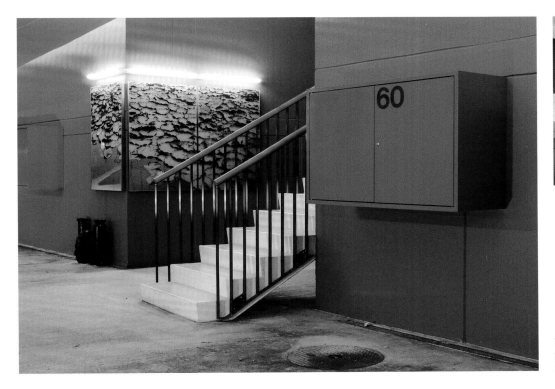

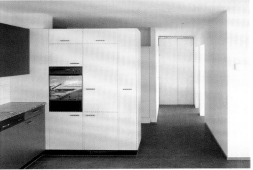

View of the complex of five square buildings from the south-west | Entrance, storage boxes, washroom and hobby rooms on the ground floor | Kitchen design and fittings

bands are placed on the site in such a way that a multiplicity of views and spatial connections result, both between the buildings as well as between indoors and outdoors. The design of the load-bearing structure with cantilevered floor slabs and balcony balustrading on all sides lends the quadratic buildings a dynamic quality. The buildings appear to float above the terrain, an effect that is heightened further by the cladding of the opaque plinth with fixed double-wall glazing elements.

On a typical floor, four apartments are arranged around a central staircase. The rooms follow the arrangement of the column grid and face outwards

with full-height glazed frontages. The bathrooms are arranged in a linear fashion around the central staircase. A larger room is located on each corner so that depending on arrangement, each of the 73 three-and-a-half and five-and-a-half-room apartments can be given a different orientation.

The arrangement of the floor plans and the rooms according to the column grid of the load-bearing structure allow the plans to be adapted in various ways to the needs of the individual residents. Depending on the situation, two apartments can also be combined at a later date to form large apartments.

The housing complex can therefore cater for an entire life cycle: families with children, couples, singles and the elderly. All flats have barrier-free access without thresholds and the entire route from underground car park to the top storey is suitable for wheelchairs. A lift in each building provides direct access to every floor of the building and the lift buttons are arranged lower than normal so that they can be operated easily from a wheelchair or by children. The entrances, equipped with doors that open electrically and at a width of one metre, are wide enough for wheelchair users or people with wheeled walking aids.

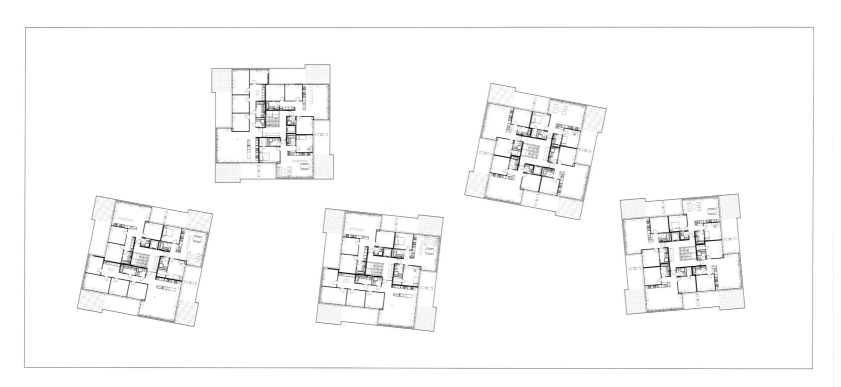

Roof level plans

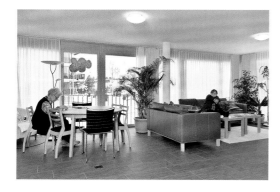

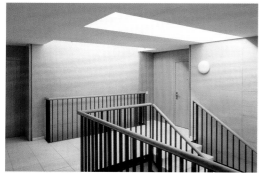

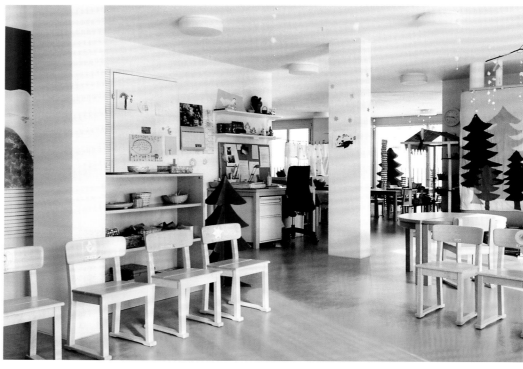

Despite these particular facilities, the apartments are not specially designed for the elderly but are simply spacious and light apartments which are designed so that the needs of old people are not excluded. Old people would like to live for as long as possible in their familiar surroundings and the design of the Steinacker housing complex caters for this need. In the rental of the apartments, special attention was given to achieving a mix of generations.

Barrier-free architecture is also beneficial for parents with prams, and each house has a special area for parking prams. One of the buildings contains a children's nursery that caters for two groups and there is plenty of space for playing outdoors. Another of the five buildings houses a residential care group for up to six older people who are in need of ongoing nursing care. Each resident has their own room within the group and there is a large communal room and spacious kitchen, which is used on a day-to-day basis by the residents and the care staff to cook, sing and for handicrafts.

The Steinacker housing complex was awarded the "Age Award 2005" by the Swiss Age Foundation. The Age Award is presented to innovative projects which are then publicised widely. The aim is, through exemplary projects, to stimulate other new projects and developments. The inter-generational concept of "housing for the entire lifecycle", which informs the design of the Steinacker concept, captured the imagination of the jury.

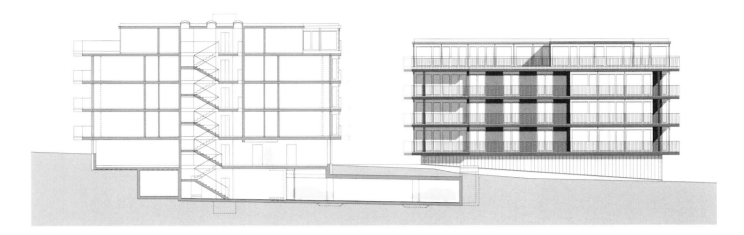

Section and elevation

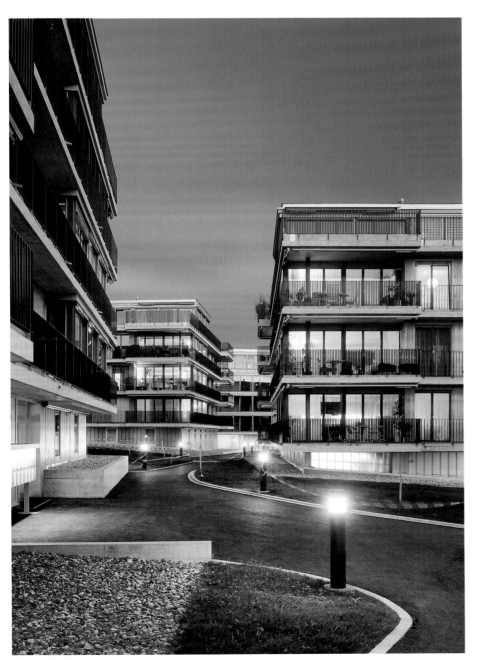

Communal living room in the residential care group | Rooflights in the corridors provide natural light | Children's nursery | Barrier-free apartments and entrances create an environment suitable for young families and the elderly alike

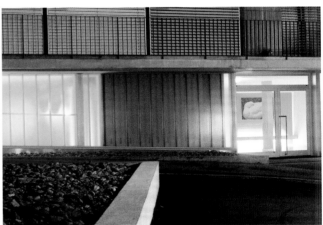

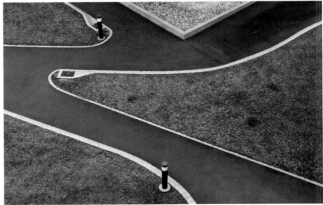

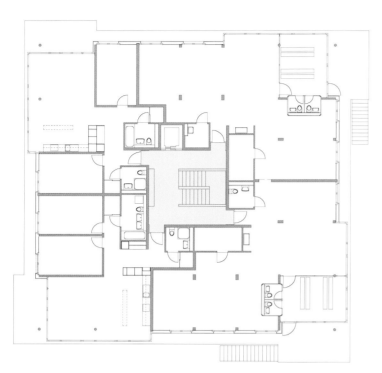

First floor plan, house 1 with children's nursery

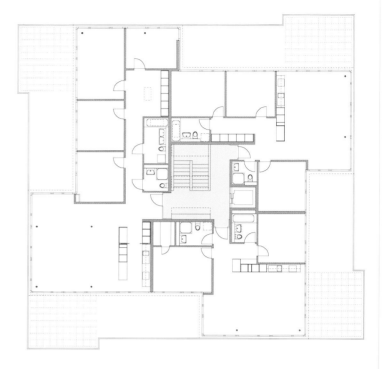

Top floor plan, house 4

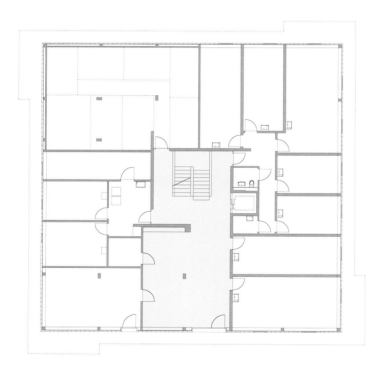

Ground floor plan, house 4

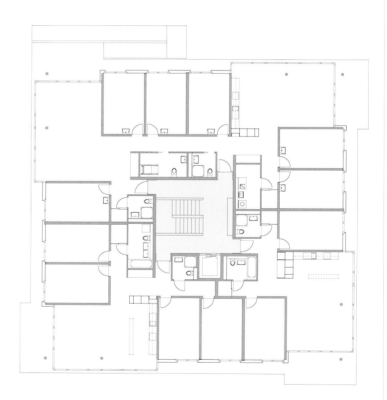

First floor plan, house 2 with residential care group

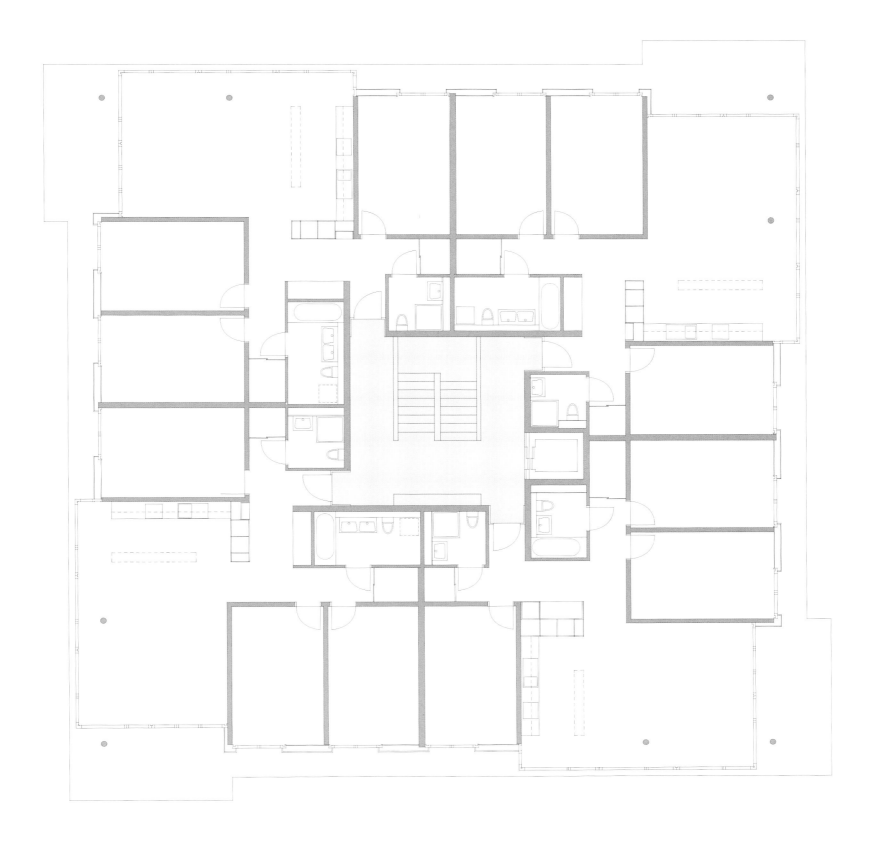

First floor plan, house 4

Assisted living – Serviced apartments

Residents in assisted living schemes and serviced apartments enjoy a way of living that in some ways resembles living in a hotel, with the associated security and comfort it provides at extra cost. This concept comprises a wide range of housing for the elderly with the provision of care services. Typically, a resident will rent an apartment appropriately equipped for the barrier-free needs of the elderly, usually in a special residential complex. The residents subscribe to a series of basic services, for which they pay a flat monthly fee. Basic services typically include consultation and information services and emergency call cover. Residents sign a combined rent and care provision agreement and can purchase additional services such as meals, cleaning and nursing care as required at an additional charge. This form of living for the elderly is not subject to the same regulations as homes and is sometimes also known under other names such as serviced residences and sheltered housing.

Comfort is quite clearly a central aspect of this typology, supplemented by individual personal and health services as required. The notion of aesthetic biography is central to this particular form of living: a concept that describes people's desire to have continued access to that which they have enjoyed throughout their lifetime. This includes interiors that relate to their familiar locality as well as fellow residents of a similar social class or intellectual milieu.

Following the pattern of a hotel, most projects in this typology also offer communal areas and facilities such as a foyer with concierge, a café and restaurant, meeting and club rooms (for example library, games room), wellness facilities with physiotherapy or a hairdresser and cosmetic salon – the size and standard varying according to the class of the establishment.

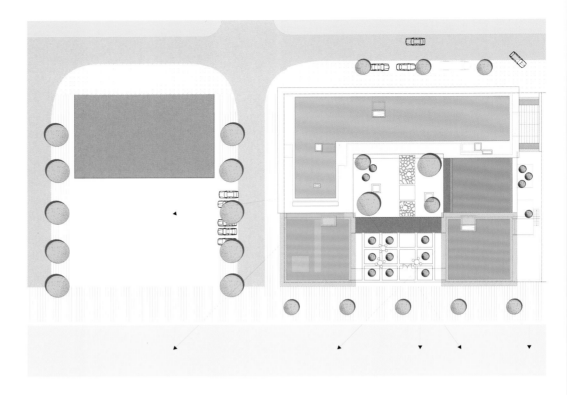

Site plan

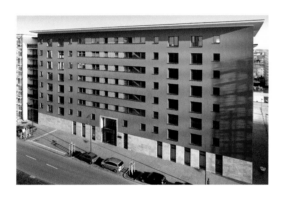

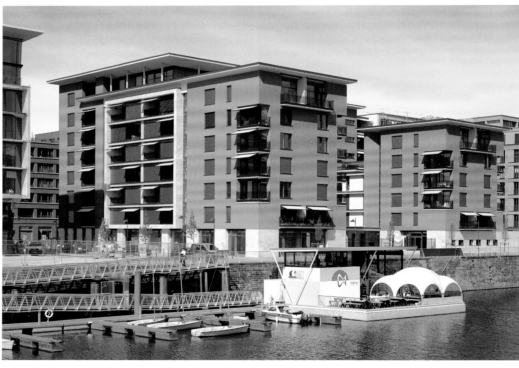

South elevation | East-west orientation of the building between the harbour and Speicherstraße | Central entrance hallway in the ground floor plinth level | Event room on the ground floor

Cronstetten House

Frankfurt am Main, Germany

Architect	Frick.Reichert Architekten
Client /Operator	Cronstett- und Hynspergische Evgl. Stiftung
Completion	2006
Useable floor area	8,289 m² (main useable floor area)
Units /Capacity	75 apartments

The Cronstetten House, designed by Frick.Reichert Architekten, was completed in 2006 and is conceived especially for the 60 plus generation. The name of the building derives from that of the client and operator, a protestant charitable foundation that has existed in Frankfurt am Main since 1753. The site lies directly alongside a harbour separated from the River Main by a pier and is part of a larger project to redevelop the derelict site of Frankfurt's former trading port from the 19th century into a modern urban quarter with offices, apartments, shops and restaurants.

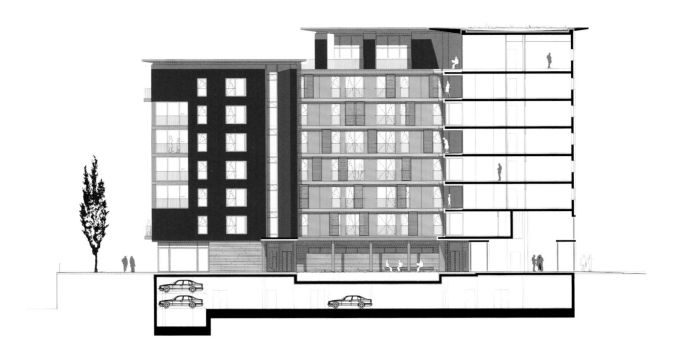

Sectional elevation through section A of the building looking eastwards from the courtyard

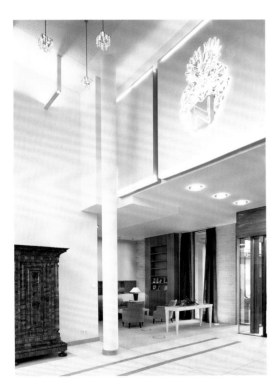

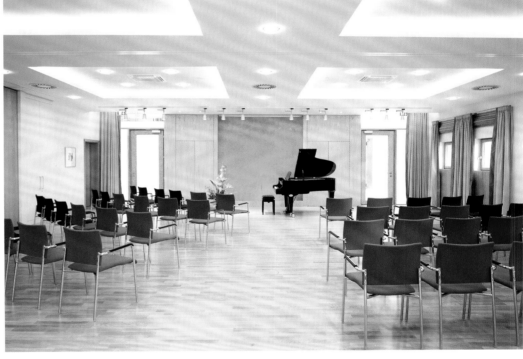

The building extends in an east-west direction between the Ufer-Promenaden-Weg along the banks of the harbour basin and the Speicherstraße behind. The building picks up the height of the urban surroundings and with its 7 to 8-storey-high section along the Speicherstraße forms a clearly defined wall to the "Central Square" on the west side. Towards the harbour basin, the building steps downwards, in the process separating out into a series of individual 'houses' along the harbour promenade. The boundary to the neighbours on the east is formed by a special "filler building" that forms a definite junction between the two. With its set-back façade and

continuous balconies it differentiates itself from the remainder of the complex, emphasising its independence.

The U-shaped floor plan of the building is divided into five sections (A – E), each with their own access stair and lift. This forms a smaller-scale structure which makes it possible to design a more flexible arrangement of different apartment types. From a common entrance on the Speicherstraße on the north side, residents and visitors pass through a lobby into the central entrance hall where they are greeted by a concierge service. From here one can reach the apart-

ments in section C. The entrance hall adjoins an open arcade that runs around the perimeter of the interior courtyard garden. In front of this is a small square that opens southwards via a gate onto the harbour promenade. The arcade leads to four further staircases which provide access to the apartments in sections, A, B, D and E. Each of the staircases is naturally lit and is equipped with a lift so that residents with walking aids or in wheelchairs can easily reach the apartments on the upper storeys.

The ground floor, which is acts as a plinth on which the building sits, contains a variety of

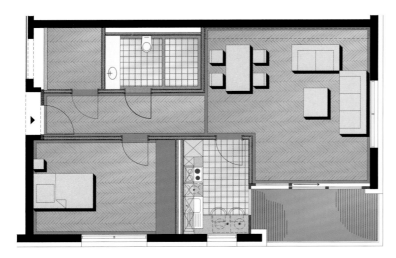

Floor plan of two-room apartment

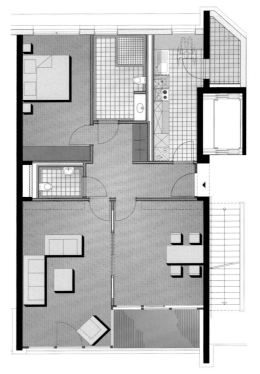

Floor plan of three-room apartment

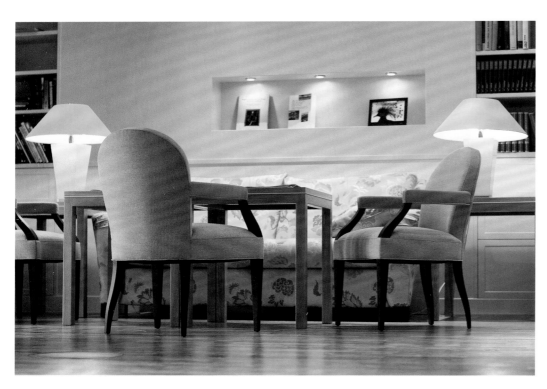

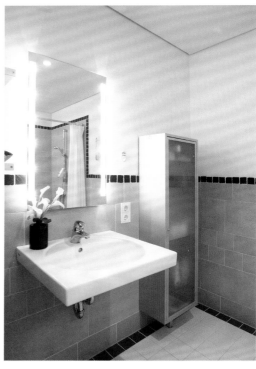

semi-public functions. All the public-facing surfaces on the ground floor are clad in a light-coloured natural stone made of Thuringian travertine, while in the arcade the travertine facing is interspersed with naturally split stone segments. Alongside the entrance hall and the concierge lie the director's offices and administration, a care station and other communal amenities such as a room for events, an art room, a gym with changing rooms and a club room. The latter face onto the arcaded courtyard as the "centre" of the building. It serves as a meeting point and hub of the complex, promoting social contact, conversation and communication between the residents.

The courtyard garden can be crossed and is designed to be an attractive place to spend time. The public facilities such as restaurant, shops and other rooms for supplementary services are by contrast oriented towards the main square at the west end of the complex.

The lower ground floor contains, alongside various ancillary spaces, an underground car park with space for 51 vehicles, 28 of them using a stacked double parker system. Colour coded entrances identify the different staircases from the car park, helping both residents and staff to find their way.

The upper storeys (first to seventh floor) contain a total of 75 two, three and four room apartments ranging from 70 to 145 m² in size. All apartments are arranged front-to-back and open onto the harbour on one side and the interior courtyard on the other. High ceilings, 2.65 m on most storeys, 3.25 m on the 7th floor, lend the apartments a spacious feeling. All apartments are barrier-free and have at least one balcony or a terrace. The living areas are generously glazed affording a good view even when seated.

The design of a residential building for older people necessitates a sensitivity to proportion, scale

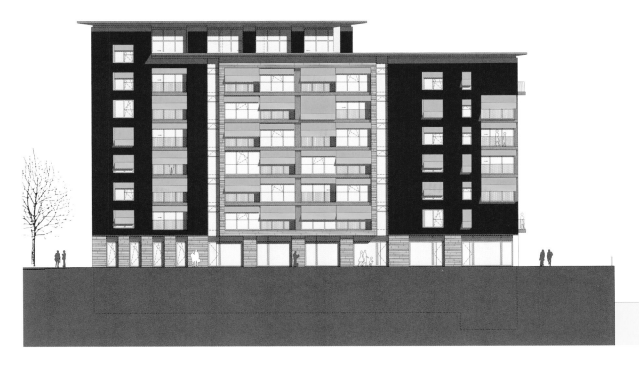

Elevation study showing shading blinds

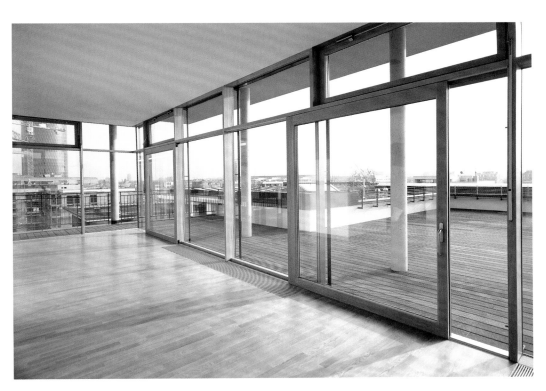

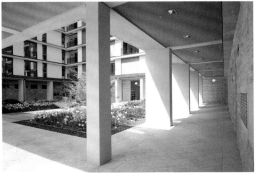

House library with comfortable reading corners | Light and barrier-free bathroom | Seventh floor penthouse with roof terrace and spacious outdoor area | The inner courtyard and arcade is designed as an inviting and semi-public space

and materials as these factors can strongly influence the living environment of older people and their sense of well-being. This principle informs the choice of materials and colours inside and outside as well as the proportions of the façades. The distinctive appearance of the Cronstetten House makes it readily recognisable and engenders a sense of identification among the residents. The cantilevered eaves also contribute to the building's distinctive appearance, strongly delineating the edges of the different sections of the building and how they relate to the main body of the building. Special attention was given to the design of the details: eschewing fashionable variety, the choice and demarcation of materials are used to denote certain purposes and underline a sense of quality.

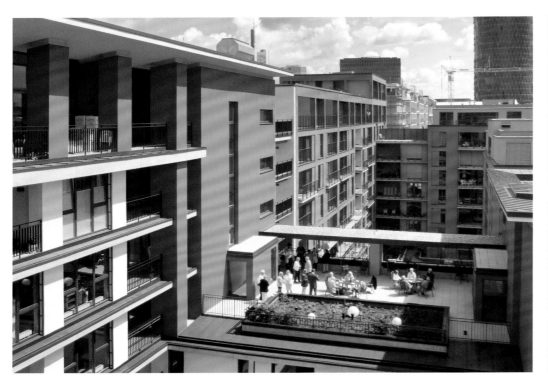

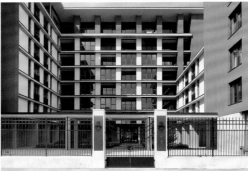

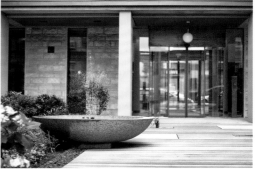

The terrace on the fifth floor connects the different parts of the building and serves as a meeting place for residents

Sheltered entrance from the north | High-quality materials denote the entrance area

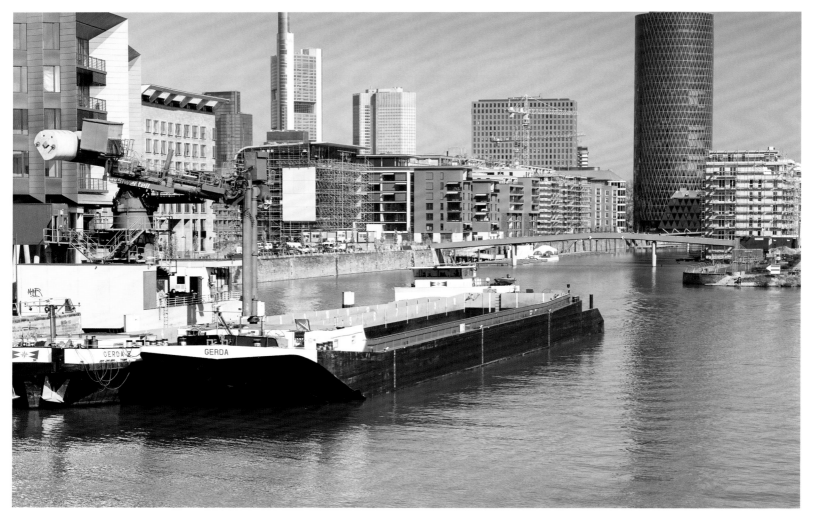

Urban location in the harbour in close proximity to the centre of Frankfurt

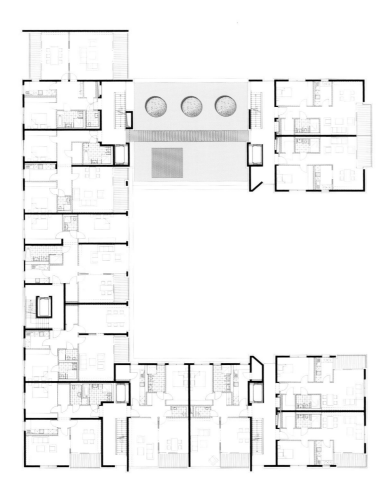

Fifth floor plan

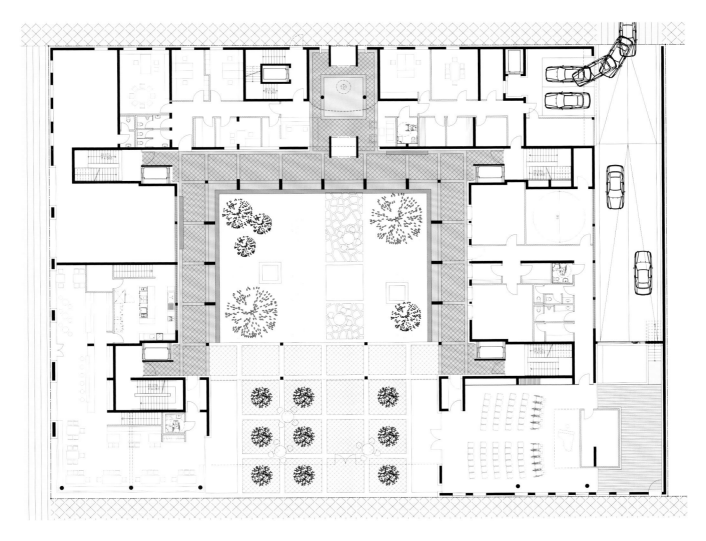

Ground floor plan

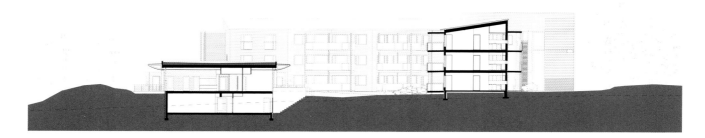

Section through the Activity Centre and housing

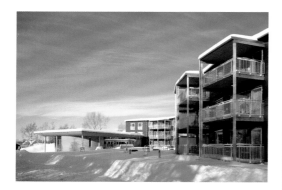

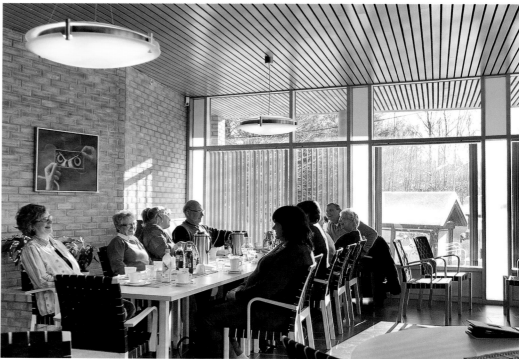

View from the road of the apartments with the Activity Centre in the background | Residents' common room | Sheltered walkway as access to the apartments | Entrance to the Activity Centre | Façades with south-facing balconies

Tårnåsen Housing and Activity Centre

Oppegård near Oslo, Norway

Architect	KVERNAAS ARKITEKTER AS
Client	Oppegård Community
Operator	OPAK AS
Completion date	2008
Useable floor area	3,500 m²
Units / Capacity	26 apartments 2 one-room apartments for short-term care

The brief for this project was to create a home for people with different needs. Old people as well as people who are connected to the community's Psychiatric Health Services and Relief Efforts for Disabled People live in the 26 sheltered accommodation units. In addition there are two units which contain staff rooms and common rooms for the residents.

The apartments have a net living area of about 56 m². They are equipped to enable the residents to look after themselves. All apartments are accessible for disabled persons. In addition eight of the apartments are further equipped for disabled use

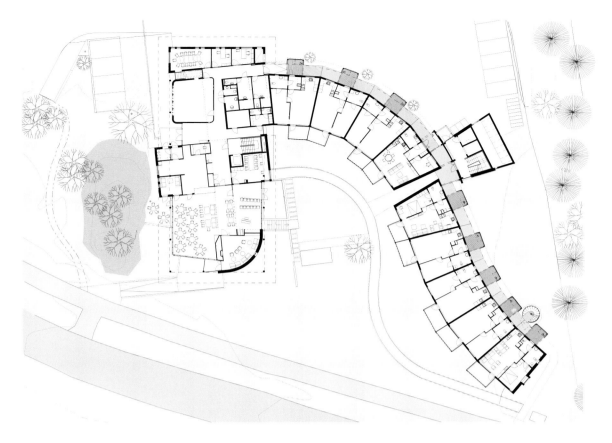

Ground floor plan

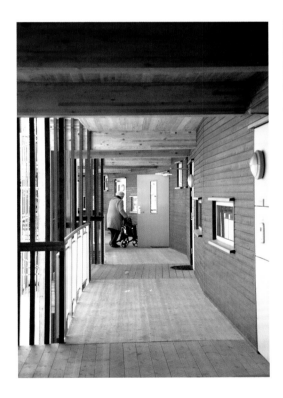
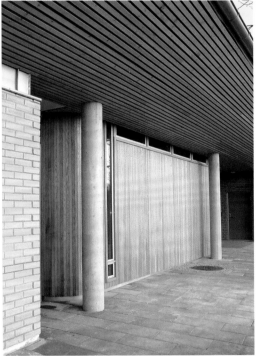
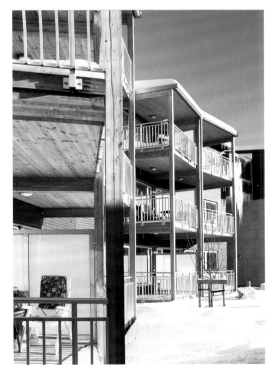

and therefore contain kitchens with worktops and cupboards with lift mechanisms. All apartments have balconies.

The accommodation also houses areas designed to encourage social interaction among the residents, visitors or people living in the neighbourhood. These areas include a café, a large communal kitchen, meeting rooms, a reading room, exercise rooms with variable facilities and a workshop.

The two functions of the scheme, the public and the private, are planned to intertwine but also to stand out as individual forms. Design and choice

of materials have been used to highlight this dualism, creating two separate buildings in one establishment: the long, curved, three-storey block of dwellings, whose external walls are clad with stained timber, contrasts with the flat, rectangular green planted roof of the Activity Centre, whose walls are clad in light-coloured brick. The curved apartment building intersects the Activity Centre, stamping its own imprint on the centre.

The apartments are situated along external galleries with a solid wood construction. Additional space at each private entrance provides a possi-

bility for charging electric wheel chairs. The main entrance is situated on the northern side via a free standing common staircase and lift. The curved apartment block divides the site in two, enclosing a common garden to the south and separating it from the parking area near the entrance.

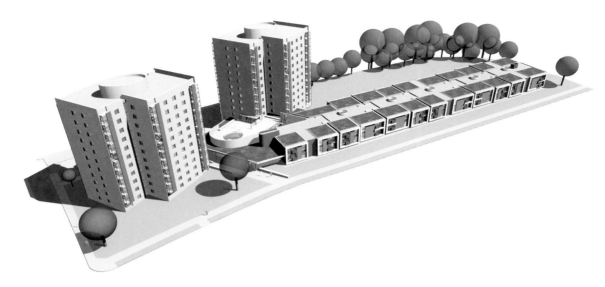

Two high-rise housing blocks, a two-storey new extension and central curved entrance building, 3D computer visualisation

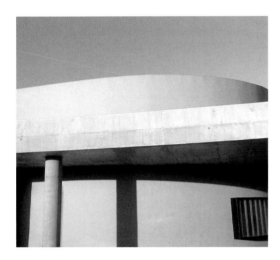

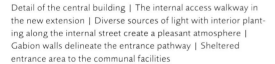

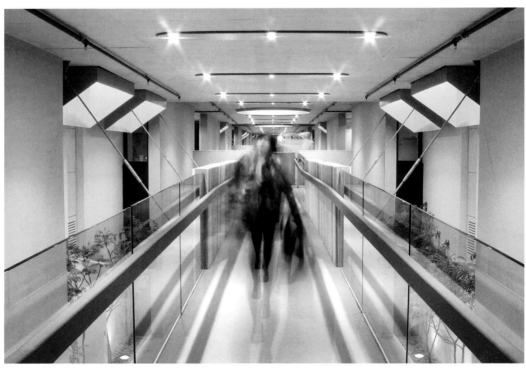

Detail of the central building | The internal access walkway in the new extension | Diverse sources of light with interior planting along the internal street create a pleasant atmosphere | Gabion walls delineate the entrance pathway | Sheltered entrance area to the communal facilities

Brookside House

Knotty Ash, Liverpool, UK

Architect	shedkm
Client	Liverpool Housing Action Trust, Housing 21
Completion	2004
Useable floor area	5,210 m²
Units/Capacity	42 units

The project consists of the replacement of the former housing with care apartments, the refurbishment of two existing 1960s tower blocks, and the construction of communal facilities for the elderly. The project is split into three separate phases, with the housing with care apartments having been completed in January 2004. The location is the suburb of Knotty Ash which is predominantly residential and remarkably "green".

The practice's winning scheme created a strategy that unites the whole site, utilising the analogy of a village with streets and a central green. The proposal involved the linking of the apartments within

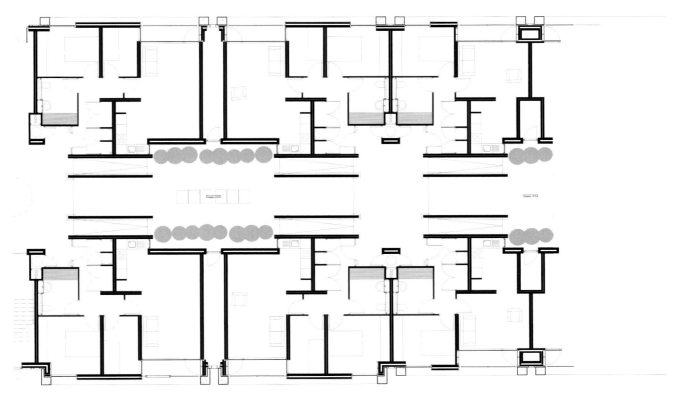

Ground floor plan

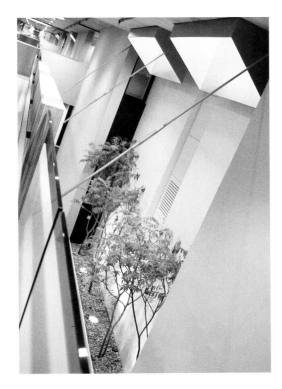
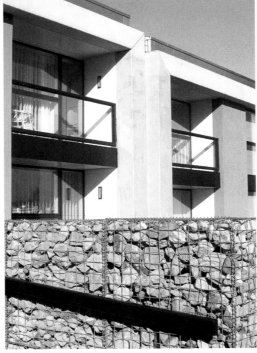
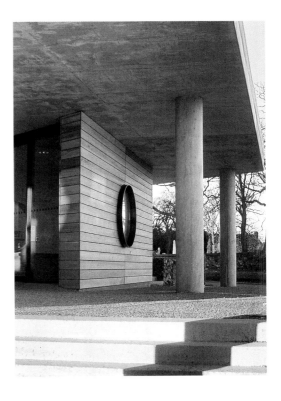

the existing tower blocks with the new sheltered housing apartments constructed either side of an internal street. Both elements converge at the central communal hub.

All apartments are positioned to benefit from an east or west orientation, with roadside or communal garden frontage. The two-storey housing with care facility consists of two banks of one/two bedroom apartments accessed from the safe environment of a central internal street. The internal street is designed as a common meeting place from which to enter individual dwellings. The heated linear route is lit and ventilated by a series of large rooflights

that illuminate double-height spaces with planting and seating areas. First floor access is via a series of walkways. The competition concept to integrate the landscape with the development has been retained throughout the tenant consultation and detailed design period. The green roofs are a reaction to both environmental issues and increased thermal provision for the inhabitants and also create a significant visual roofscape seen by the majority of residents who occupy the eleven-storey blocks.

The central hub creates a single safe point of access to the development. The curved, colour-rendered wall can be identified from all areas of the site and

provides orientation for residents with varying physical and mental ability.

The proposal for an integrated site, perceived and designed through commitment to the competition concept and responsive tenant participation, has been maintained. Indeed the ideas have been strengthened by existing residents who enjoy living in alternative forms of dwelling to the traditional house type, and wish to continue to live in modern examples of housing: "Just because we are elderly, does not mean we want to live in something that looks like an old people's home."

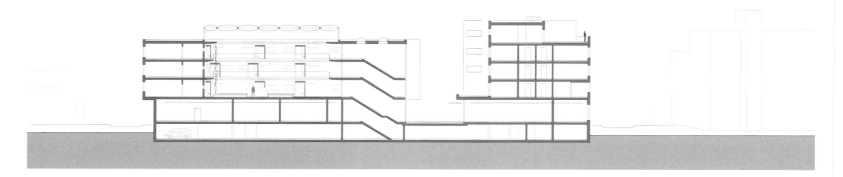

Section

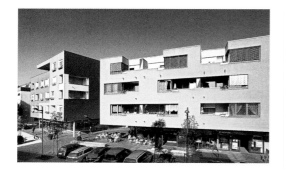

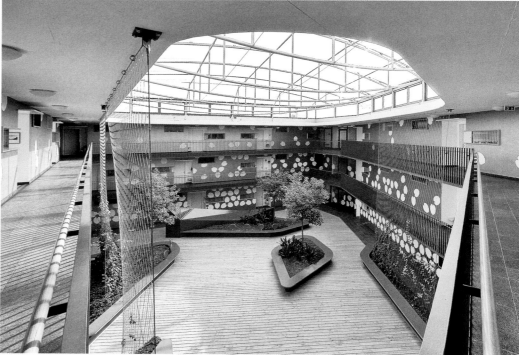

View of part of the complex looking north | View of the communal interior courtyard

"Stadtcarré"

Bad Rappenau, Germany

Architect	ASIRarchitekten
Client	Kruck + Partner, Wohnbau- und Projektentwicklung GmbH und Co. KG
Operator	Evangelische Sozialstation Bad Rappenau-Bad Wimpfen e.V.
Completion	2007
Useable floor area	residential: 3,562 m² offices: 375 m² shops: 1,936 m²
Units/Capacity	36 assisted living apartments (phase 1) 15 apartments suitable for old people (phase 2)

The new building complex in the centre of Bad Rappenau, designed by ASIRarchitekten, contains a mixture of public and private spaces and reconnects pathways within the city. In addition to numerous shops and apartments, the complex also includes 36 assisted living apartments for the elderly.

A key element of the design is a new public passage. Oriented towards the church spire, it re-establishes an important connection between the railway station and the town centre. In addition to public transport stops and short-stay parking the complex provides a large underground garage for the residents, located in the base of the building be-

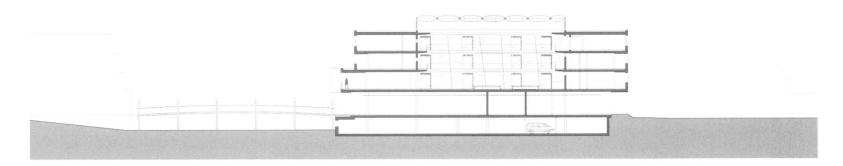

Section

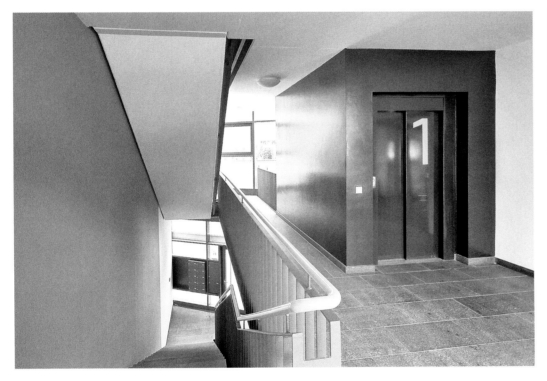

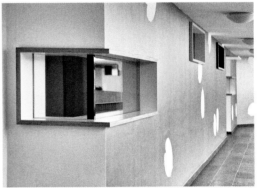

Main staircase | Entrance niche with kitchen corner window

neath the shops. A new bridge allows pedestrians uninterrupted passage from the railway station to the market square and provides a direct connection to green areas lower down.

The passageway through the centre splits the Stadtcarré into two parts. In the larger section on the east side, three floors house sheltered accommodation. The apartments vary in size, with a total of 29 two-room apartments of between 45 and 60 m² and seven three-room apartments of up to 90 m² in size. The apartments fulfil German barrier-free norms (DIN 18025 parts I and II) with 101 cm-wide doorways with no thresholds, and bathrooms suit-

able for disabled use with flush-mounted shower basins. In some cases, minor deviations from the norms have been accepted, for example, storage rooms are not always fully dimensioned for disabled-accessibility as this would have meant creating larger and therefore more expensive flats, or else cramped the indoor spaces.

Each apartment has its own loggia which, as an additional "room", forms a centrepiece of the flat and increases the sense of space. The bedroom adjoins the loggia and is connected to the living area via a large sliding door. The loggia can also be accessed from the living and dining room, which has large

windows that wrap around the corner and a low sill affording a view out onto the street.

Particular attention was paid to the design of the entrance niches which form a semi-private area in front of each apartment. A corner window in the kitchen overlooks this entrance area, giving the residents a greater sense of security. A door buzzer with video camera allows residents to see who is entering the building.

Care assistance is provided by the social care centre in Bad Rappenau which has offices and a kitchen, therapy pool and other care facilities on the

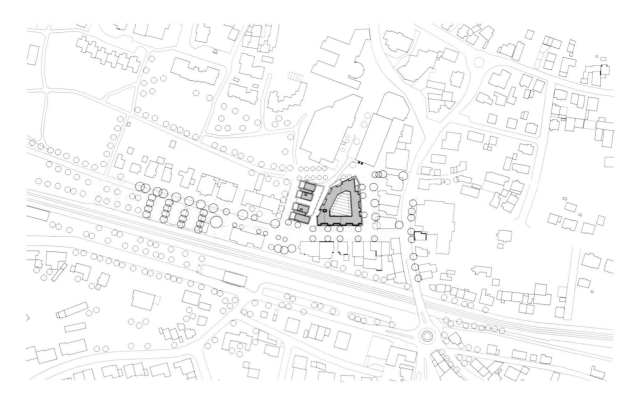

Site plan

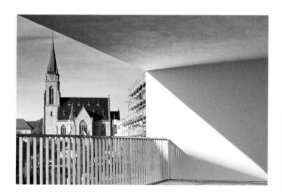

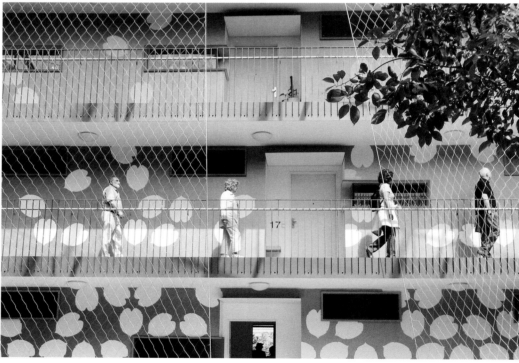

View from a communal terrace of the main landmark in the vicinity | Gallery walkways with personalisable entrances to the apartments

entrance floor of the building. Also on the ground floor is a communal space from which one can see the church, providing a visual connection with the city. It also serves as a conference space and, like the internal courtyard, can be hired out to organisations for events. In addition to its public uses, the interior courtyard also provides access via galleries to the apartments and serves as a communal area for the residents. Covered by a translucent membrane roof, the courtyard is an indoor space and can be used year-round by the elderly residents as a place to meet and chat. The atrium is supplied with fresh air that has been either pre-cooled or prewarmed by being drawn through earth ducts before

being distributed to the individual apartments to provide regular ventilation. Vents at the edge of the membrane roof can be opened or closed depending on the season and provide additional air circulation. A further special aspect of the building is the temperature regulation of the concrete core of the upper walkways, which serves to level out extreme temperatures in summer and winter. In summer the trees also provide additional shade in the atrium. The air climate within the atrium is further enhanced by the Bougainvillea which grow up vertical stainless steel netting and give off moisture through evaporation. Beside its climatic function, the communal, greened courtyard provides residents with

the equivalent of a garden of their own. The second part of the complex to the west of the central passage contains 15 apartments with between two and five rooms that overlook the town's park. The standard and kind of fittings is similar to that of the apartments for assisted living and they are therefore also suitable for use by old people.

Through its successful integration of housing for the elderly on an inner-city site, as well as the high degree of satisfaction among its residents, the Stadtcarré in Bad Rappenau can serve as a pioneering example for other cities.

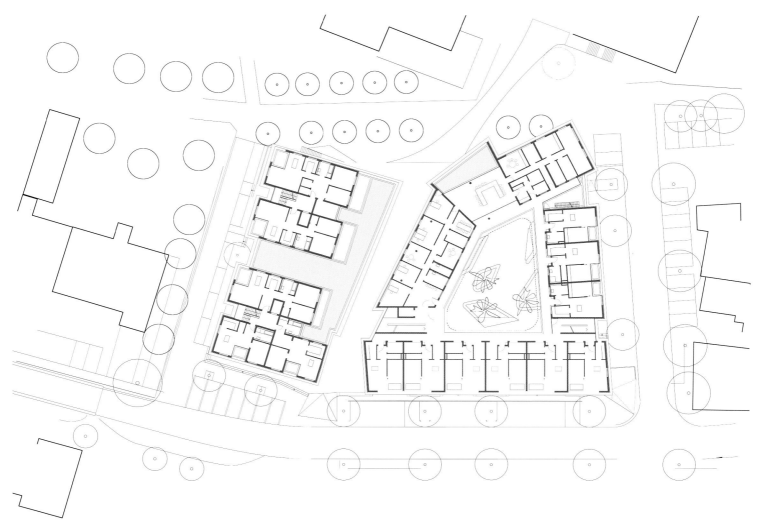

First floor plan (atrium level)

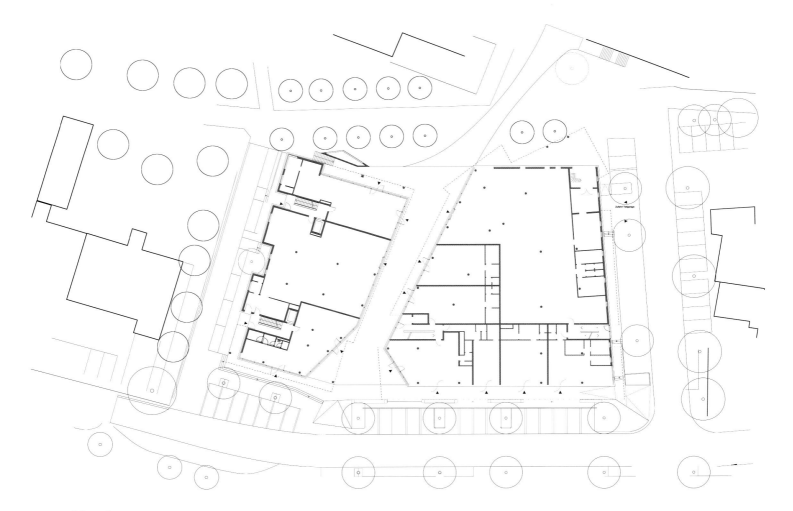

Ground floor plan

Left page
View from the interior courtyard to the communal facilities |
Detail of the foil-covered roof | View from the park looking south-east

Right page
Public passageway heading south | Interior courtyard with vents at
eaves level| Façade details | Interior courtyard at dusk

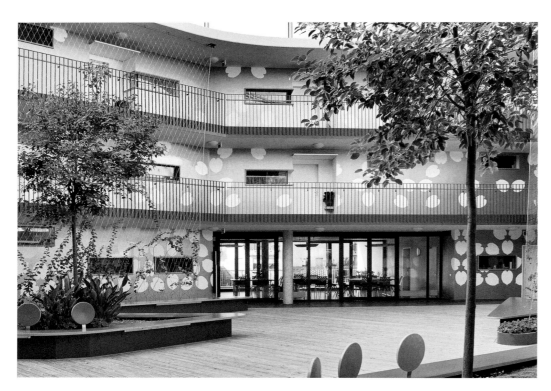
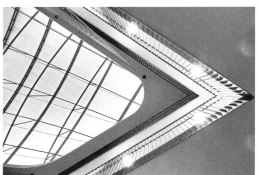
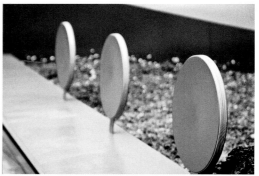
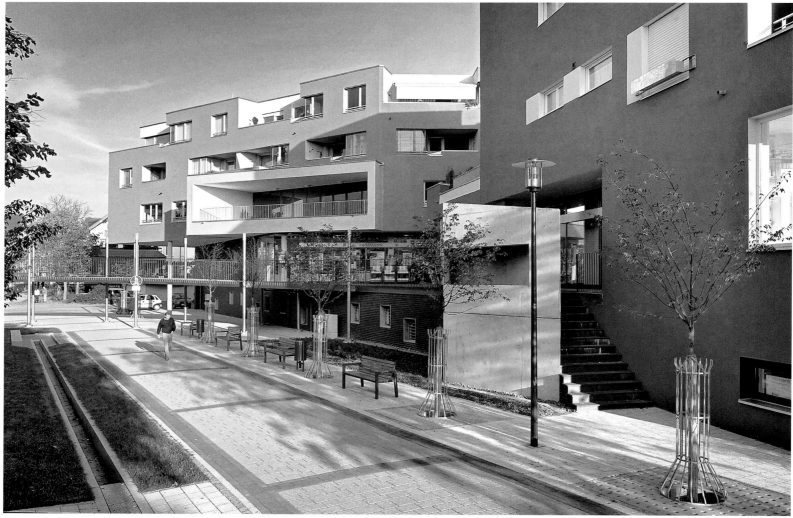

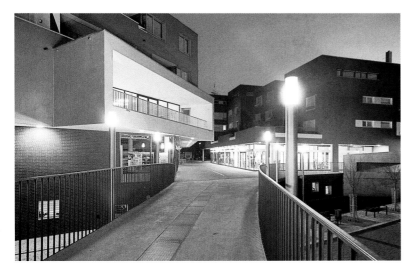

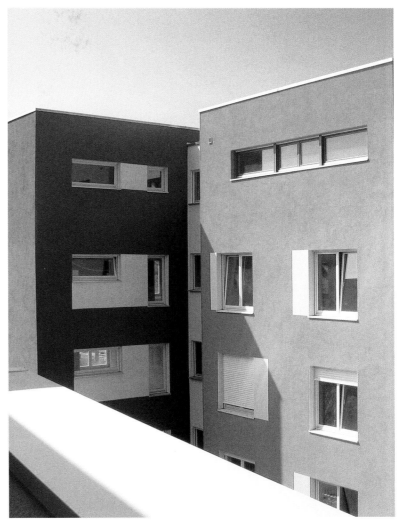

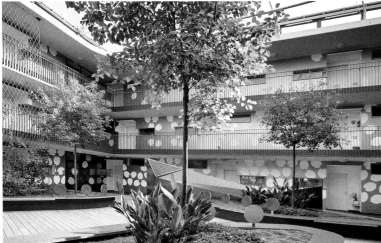

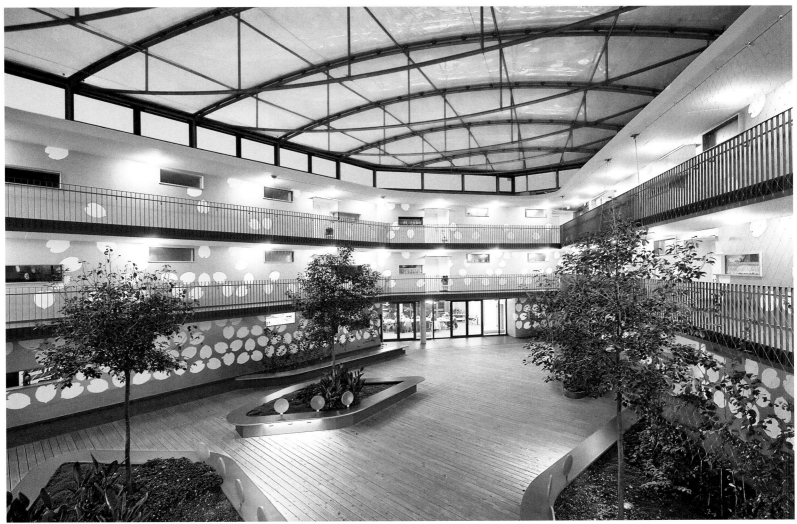

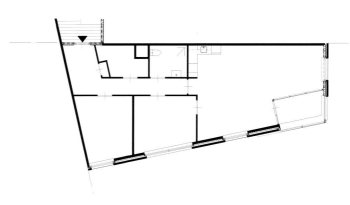

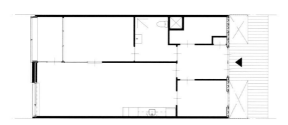

Floor plans of different apartment types

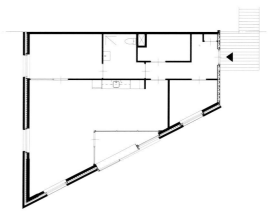

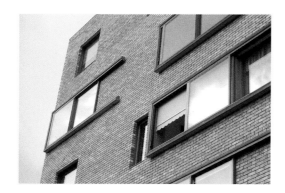

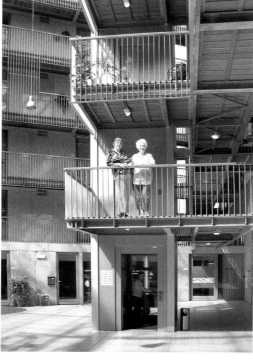

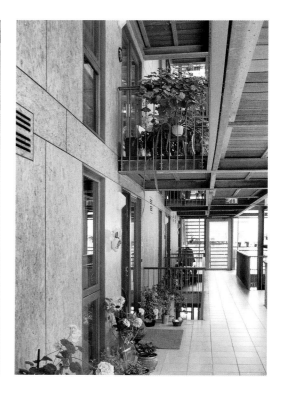

Exterior façade detail | Vertical access | The gallery walkways as semi-private areas | Central atrium covered by a glass roof | Urban context | Interior façades

Sheltered Housing Complex

Emerald, The Netherlands

Architect	KCAP Architects & Planners
Client / Operator	Ceres Projects
Completion date	2000
Useable floor area	7,675 m²
Units / Capacity	105 apartments

Emerald is a "Vinex" location, a large suburban area declared by the Dutch Ministry of Housing for large-scale new housing developments. Here, the apartment complex and the adjacent shopping centre, though clearly distinguished in terms of programme and function, both stand out from the rest of the urban fabric. In the shopping centre, shops are situated on the ground floor and flats on the upper floors. Care services such as physical therapy, elderly care and medical facilities have leased commercial spaces. The apartments are arranged over six floors around a collective atrium, which serves as a common service area. From inside, however, the form is

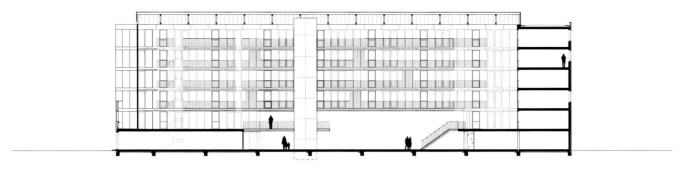

Section

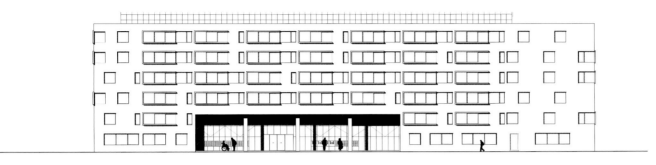

Elevation

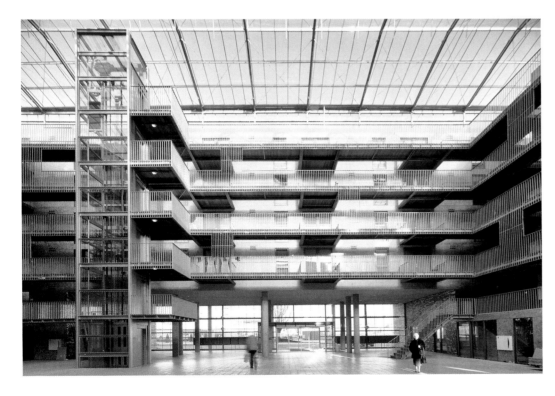

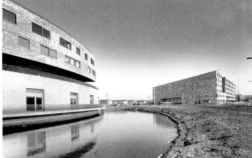

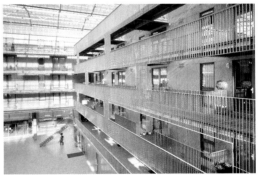

divided into four vertical blocks with open views to the outside. The wide two-storey entry lobby is designed as a continuation of the square outside.

The typical apartment floor plan has no hallway. Instead, there is a separate room, which opens via double doors onto the atrium and connects all rooms of the apartment including the living space. A balcony in front of this connecting space strengthens the relationship between the dwelling and the atrium. Apartments accessed via the gallery have their own winter garden, orientated to the south and west. Corner apartments have a

more indirect relationship to the atrium, but are larger. Due to the unusual shape of the building, the apartment layouts feature four different corner typologies, which exploit the specific corner situations.

The large living space windows of the typical apartments connect the living room either with the apartment's winter garden or with that of the neighbour. Two windows mounted in a robust timber frame can be slid to one side to fully open the winter garden. There are two variants of this sliding window: one pane of glass slides either in front of the other or in front of the brick façade

cladding. The resulting patchwork of variations creates a lively and dynamic façade.

Inside, the quality of the atrium as an interior space is enhanced by the use of timber for the interior façades. The balustrades of the galleries are woven into a continuous, transparent screen with wide window-like openings to the atrium.

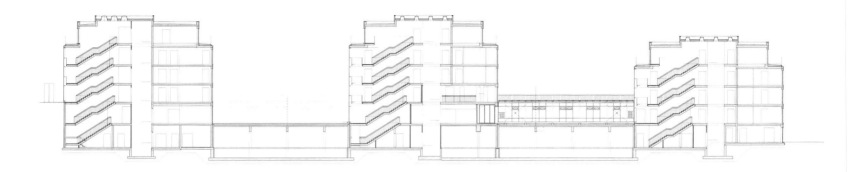

Cross section through the villas showing the connecting passageway

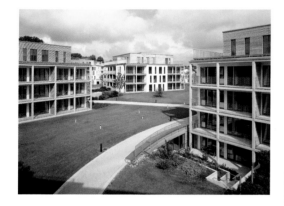

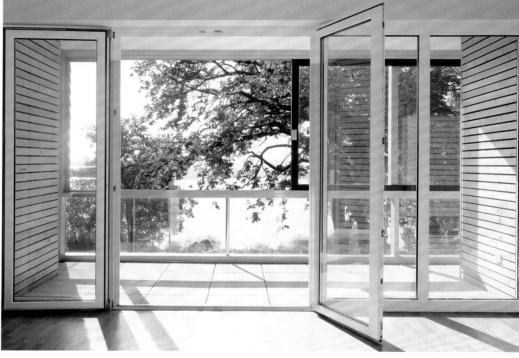

View of the urban villas at the rear of the complex | Full-height glazing and sheltered balconies create a relationship between inside and outside

Elbschloss Residences

Hamburg, Germany

Architect	Kleffel Köhnholdt Papay Warncke Architekten feddersenarchitekten architekten geising+böker
Client	Pensionskasse Hoechst
Operator	Elbschloss Residenz GmbH
Completion	2001
Useable floor area	21,347 m², wellness area 1,147 m²
Units / Capacity	167 units, 40 residents in care, 20 day-care

Waterside living has a long tradition in Hamburg. For Heinrich Heine, the Elbchaussee, which runs along one side of the river and connects Hamburg with the villas of the affluent suburb of Blankenese, was the most beautiful street in Europe. Situated about half-way along, slightly elevated, is the former Elbschloss brewery. The historic maltings with its long brick building and dominant tower characterises the extensive site on which the Elbschlösschen also stands, nestling under high trees.

In the middle of the 1990s, an urban design competition initially proposed up-market residences in conjunction with commercial uses for the site, all

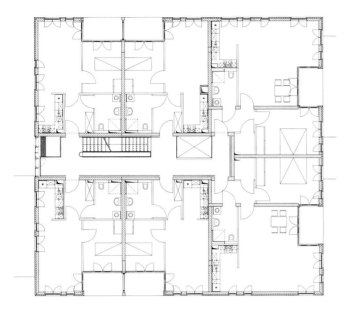

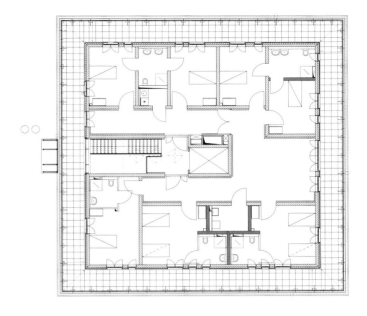

Typical floor plan, barrier-free apartments (first floor, house 2)

Roof-level plan, barrier-free apartments (house 1)

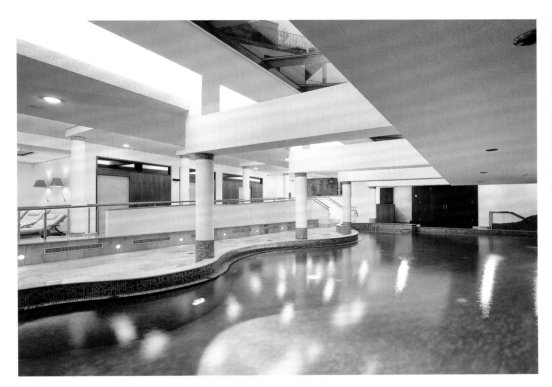

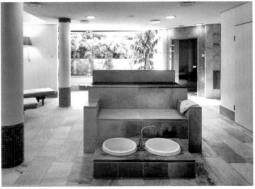

Wellness Centre for the elderly with a variety of technical assistive fittings

sensitively inserted into the protected historic context of the former restaurant building, the maltings and the Elbschlösschen. Although this concept won the competition for the architects, the site was later bought by a project developer and construction company who developed a proposal for luxurious residences for the elderly to be built for a pension fund. The shift in the nature of the planning task brought with it a stronger focus on economic considerations with the result that only the western portion of the site, still totalling some 18,000 m², was available for the project. The residences for the elderly are, with the exception of an additional nursing care facility, predominantly individual apart-

ments looked after by the elderly residents themselves. The residents can partake of further services as and when they wish.

The former Elbschloss Restaurant today also contains a restaurant and room for events that are open to the public, but otherwise consists of apartments. This is where old and new meet: the two rectangular new buildings, one faced with a glass cladding, the other with timber, wrap around, support and extend the remains of the historic building. The new glass building even "crowns" the old tower in more sense than one.

Taking their cue from the neo-classicist villa built by the Danish architect Christian Frederik Hansen, a total of seven freestanding rectangular urban villas were built behind the former maltings. These four-storey buildings, which contain a total of 167 apartments and nursing facilities for 40 persons, are distributed across the site, three parallel to one another along the edge of the site and four loosely arranged between the trees. Despite their historic reference, the new buildings, with apartments ranging from 50 to 81 m² in size, are nevertheless modern, light and transparent: the stepped back roof level is timber-clad with a large terrace around its perimeter, and on the floors below,

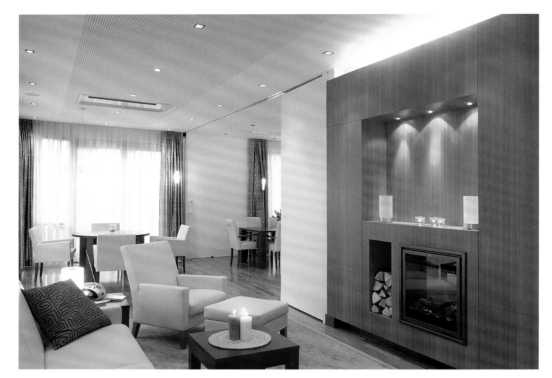

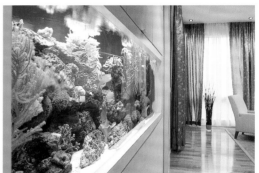

Day room for people with dementia: living area with fireplace |
Aquarium in the reading area | Adjacent area for relaxation |
Communal dining area

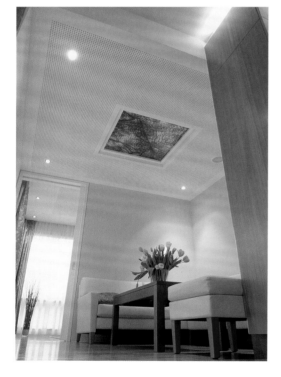

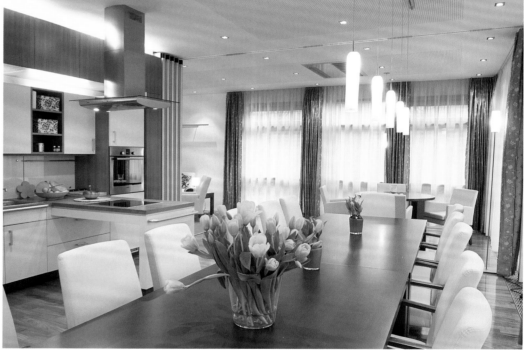

roofed-over balconies are inserted into the volume of the building. The vaulted cellars of the former maltings were demolished to make way for a meandering underground passageway that connects the different buildings with one another. Residents reach the restaurant on the Elbchaussee from their respective foyer, passing through the ground floor of the residences with the ground-level communal spaces. The passageway provides barrier-free access protected from wind and rain. Sections of the passageway are open to the outdoors, allowing sunlight in and giving the residents access to the gardens as well as providing natural ventilation.

The northern-most villa on the Elbschlossstraße contains the care facilities. Its plinth level and that of the middle residence for the elderly as well as both of the set-back connecting wings contain the foyer and access driveway to the Elbschlossstraße. This is where the reception is located, alongside the offices, lounge areas, a small shop and hairdresser, a therapy room as well as staff rooms. There is also a dining room; the adjacent kitchen services the restaurant on the Elbchaussee. The underground garage with entrance from the Elbschlossstraße is located beneath the plinth level.

The Elbschloss Residences is one of the first such facilities to have its own wellness centre, specially designed for the elderly by geising+böker. The heart of the 630 m² centre is a pool with a lift that allows the residents to bathe without needing assistance. The architects have integrated handrails and emergency call buttons into the interior design; they are intended to provide the elderly residents with a sufficient sense of security, even when overexerted, as they use the gym facilities with special sports equipment or the soft sauna with massage jets.

An approximately 100 m² day room by the Berlin practice feddersenarchitekten, designed for

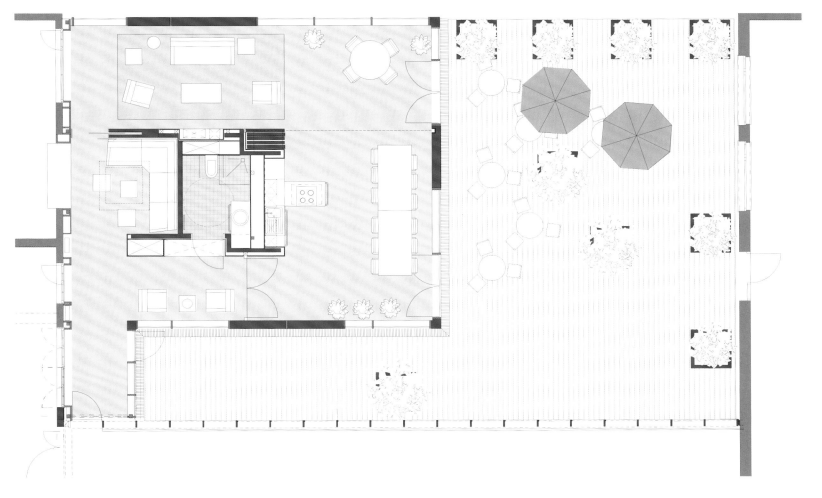

Ground floor plan of the day room for people with dementia

residents suffering from dementia, rounds off the facilities. Built as a timber and glass construction in the form of a conservatory, it sits on a part of the terrace. Inside it is arranged like a traditional apartment with a hallway providing access to the cooking, eating, living and sleeping areas distributed around a central core containing the bathroom, fireside and risers. The different zones provide the residents with spaces of differing degrees of intimacy. The various furnishings function as optical dividers between the spaces. Residents use mobile separating screens to "close the door behind them".

The entrance area is much like any entrance hall: two chairs for seating, a telephone, wardrobe for coats and key shelf create a homely feeling. The open kitchen with large windows and a glass door adjoins the terrace. The kitchen work surfaces also allow the residents to help with everyday activities such as washing vegetables, cooking and baking. The hotplate is built into a cantilevered worktop; the staff can watch over cooking pots from the "active" side with the kitchen sink, the residents from the "passive" side. The long table in the dining area with its light leather chairs serves as an invitation not just to eat together but also to socialise with one another.

In the living room, a fireplace let into a wood-panelled wall unit underlines a sense of homeliness. Recessed lighting at the junction with the ceiling creates a visual separation, lending the wall unit the appearance of a freestanding element. Similarly, sofas and chairs create a comfortable and intimate area, whose extents are marked by a large carpet. A small round table near the window can be used for playing cards or enjoying a coffee in a smaller group. Tucked around a corner, the bookshelves in the library communicate a sense of peace and contemplation.

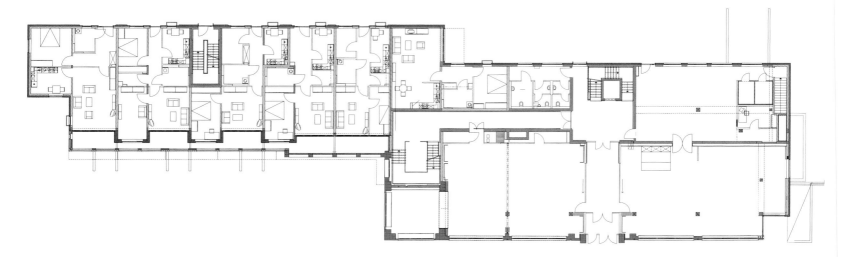

Ground floor plan of the former brewery building

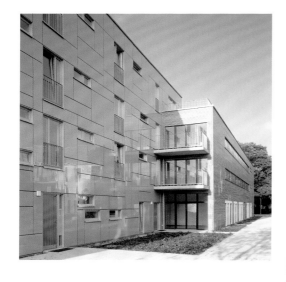

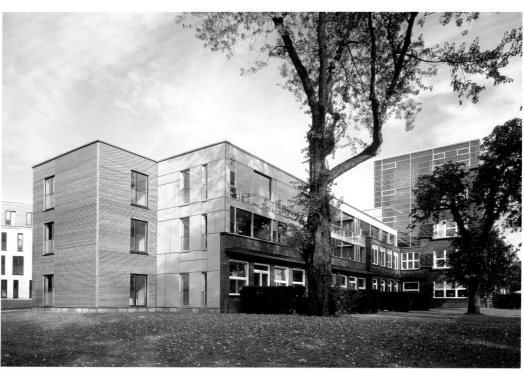

New residential buildings | Integration of the existing brick building in the new building with the landmark glass tower of the brewery in the background | Elevation of the new urban villa

In the neighbouring seating area, a wall painted a fresh green colour and an aquarium let into the wall create an atmosphere of calm and relaxation. A sofa in the corner is good for a snooze or a cuddle. Above them, an artificial skylight is let into the ceiling with a decorative three-dimensional tree motif that is intended to communicate the sensation of lying beneath a tree looking into the sky. Through an interplay of light, colour and sound this can be used to evoke different moods: yellow light and birdsong announce the onset of spring, the drumming of raindrops and flashes of light, an advancing thunderstorm.

Although the different parts of the space and their different characters contrast with one another, they all share a similar basic palette of colours and materials, in which wood, leather and earth tones predominate.

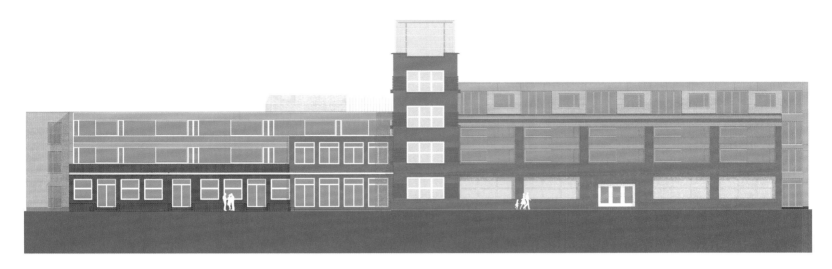

Drawing of the different parts and materiality of the building

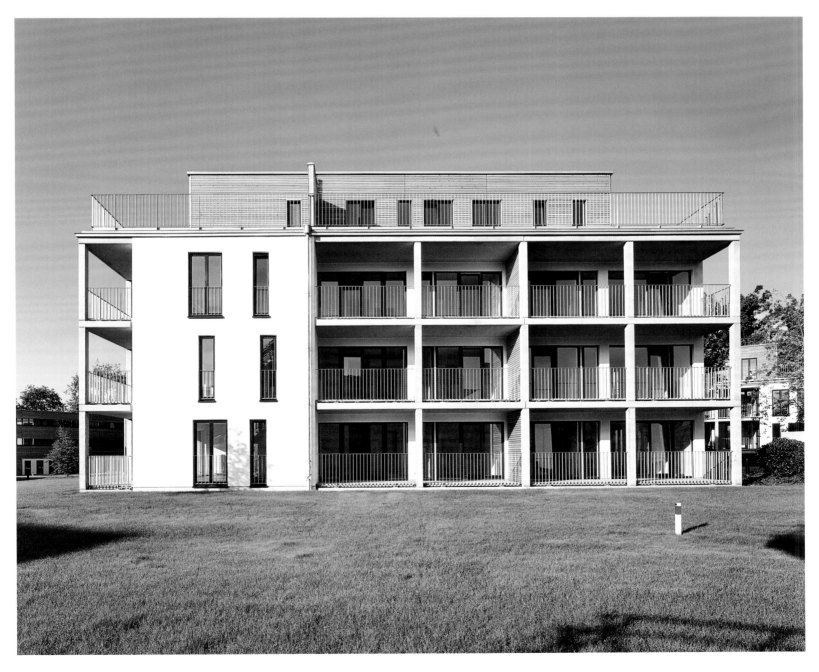

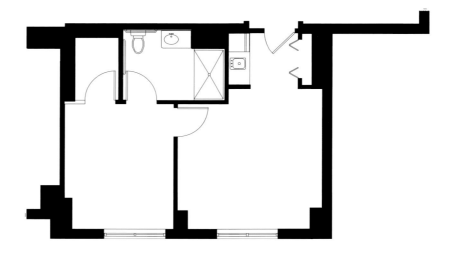

Plan of second and third floor dwelling unit

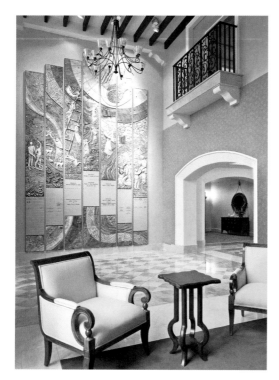

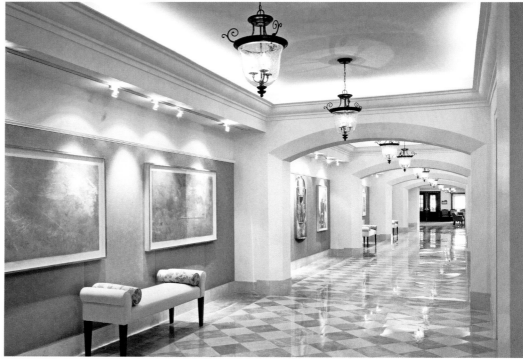

The Tradition of the Palm Beaches

West Palm Beach, Florida, USA

Architect	Perkins Eastman
Client / Operator	The Whiting-Turner Company
Completion	2004
Useable floor area	36,700 m²
Units / Capacity	144

The Tradition of the Palm Beaches developed a new approach for senior living facilities by expanding an existing long-term care campus into a full care continuum that offers a non-traditional flexible financial model with "pay as you go" options for services and housing.

The client's focus on the project was to incorporate specific themes like ageing-in-place, cognitive impairment, community-based programming and methods of service delivery into a care model that would meet the prospective residents' – the population of 85 plus – expectations without an overly institutional or clinical atmosphere. The geriatric

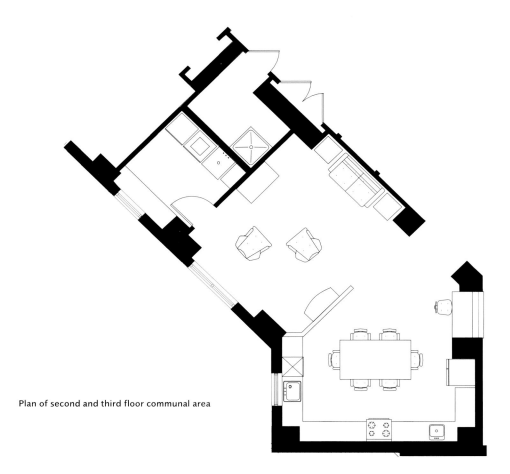

Plan of second and third floor communal area

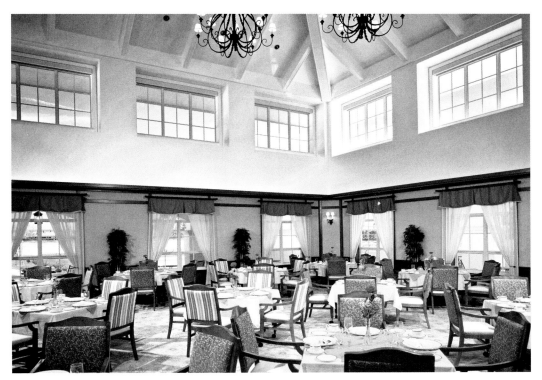

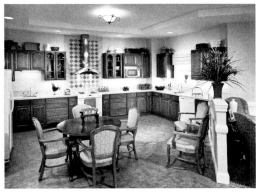

Large wall decorations in a lobby | Luxurious hallway |
Dining room on the ground floor | Homely design of a
communal kitchen

services centre offers training, assessment, home health and outpatient services for at-home seniors, with approx. 2,800 m² dedicated to a new network of services benefitting a broader community than just those residing on the campus.

The programmatic solution enhances a campus set on 11 ha, linking a 102-unit independent residential wing to a 42-unit assisted living wing that provides more comprehensive services and shelter for frail residents. While each wing has its own identity, all units incorporate universal design principles. Careful zoning of the site and building allows several communities to co-exist amid flexible services.

The overall design concept resulted in a contemporary version of gracious "grand hotel" living in the southern Floridian tradition: stucco arches, terra-cotta tiled verandas and intimate courtyards give way to interiors that express genteel hospitality and comfortable residential living reminiscent of The Cloister and The Breakers – palatial hotels constructed at the turn of the 20th century during Florida's own Gilded Age. A formal dining room overlooking one of the three man-made lakes is linked to a wellness and activity area, and other recreational amenities.

The Tradition of the Palm Beaches achieved 100 % occupancy in 90 days, triggering additional campus expansion. This can be seen as an indication for the success of a model that responds to consumers with flexibility, choice and a gracious style of traditional southern living. The project was mentioned as a Notable Project in the 2006 American Institute of Architects Design for Aging Award and in the same year won a Best of Seniors Housing Award from the National Association of Home Builders 50+ Housing Council as a Continuing Care Retirement Community – Overall Community of a small and midsize category.

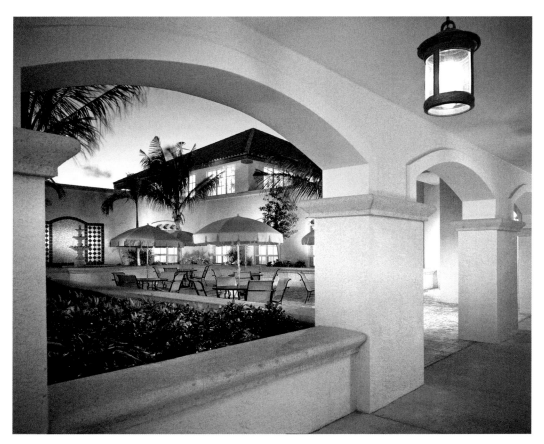
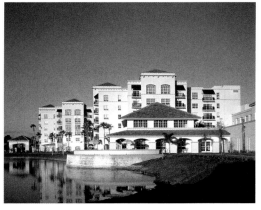
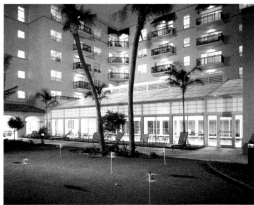
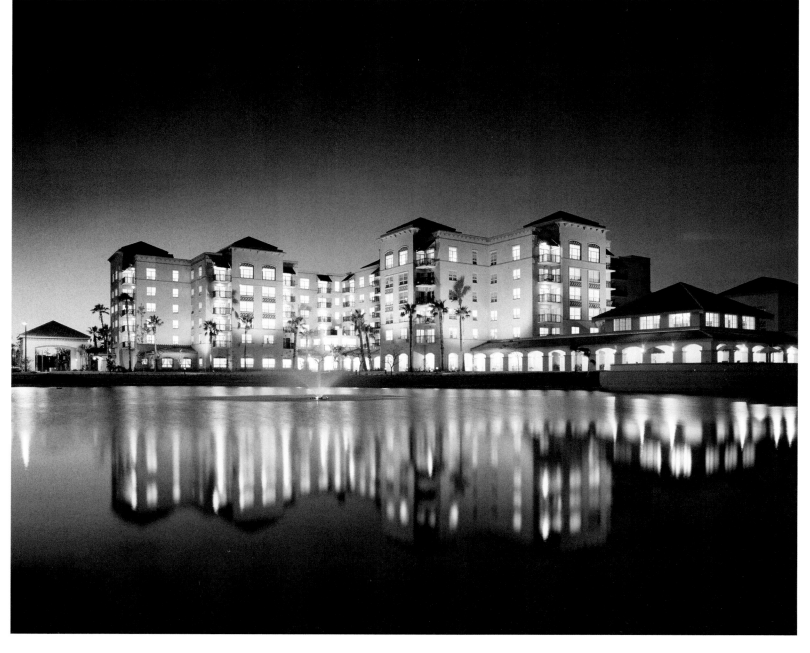

Left page
Patio with outdoor dining area | View of the entire complex
with viewing platform enclosed by a harbour wall | Rear eleva-
tion with swimming pool and small golf course | The complex
at night reflected in the artificial lake

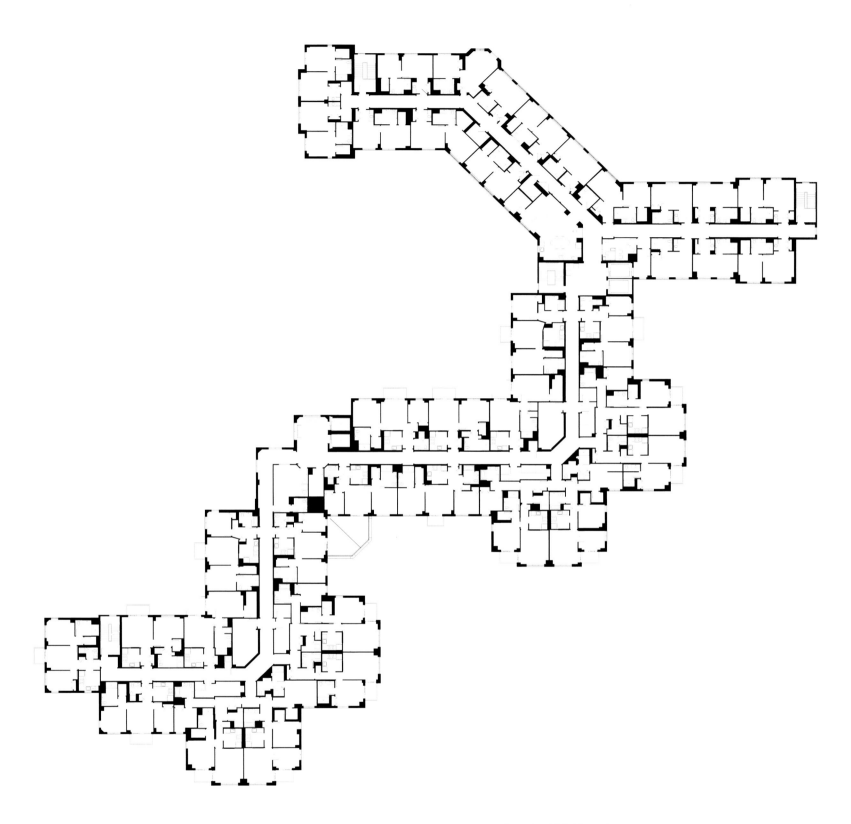

Second and third floor plans

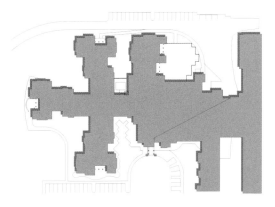

Overall layout plan

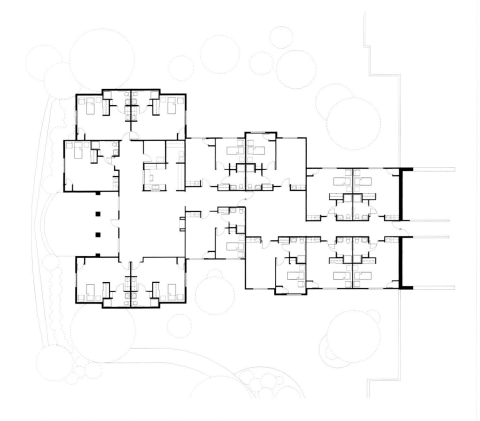

Floor plan of assisted living neighbourhood

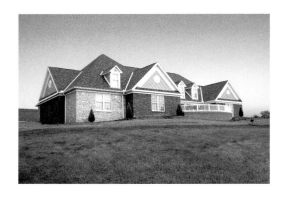

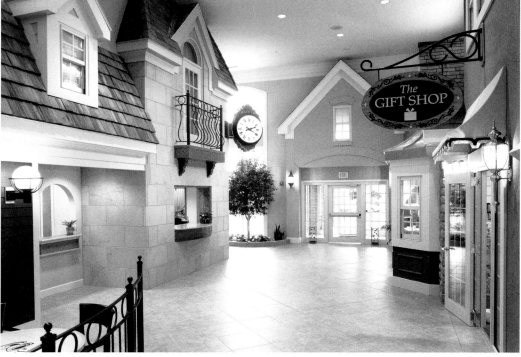

Exterior view showing the traditional domestic architecture used throughout the entire complex | An indoor "Main Street" connects the different areas of the complex | Entrance to the chapel in the "village" | Traditional, colourful and homely atmosphere of a communal space | The indoor "Main Street" leads onto an outdoor courtyard

West View Manor

Amish country, Ohio, USA

Architect	JMM Architects, Inc.
Building contractor	BCMC Inc.
Operator	West View Manor Inc.
Completion	2004
Useable floor area	new space: 4,642 m² renovated space: 150 m²
Units/Capacity	51 new units

West View Manor is an assisted living extension to a 1960s nursing facility. The traditional residential style of the extension complex updates the aesthetic of the entire facility.

The Town Square approach is the distinguishing feature of this project. An enclosed "Main Street" services both the assisted living complex as well as a new entry to the entire campus. The indoor streetscape resembles an early-1900s village. The completely enclosed space resembles a typical small town thoroughfare. The town centre establishes a connecting link between the assisted living residences and the nursing centre and incorporates

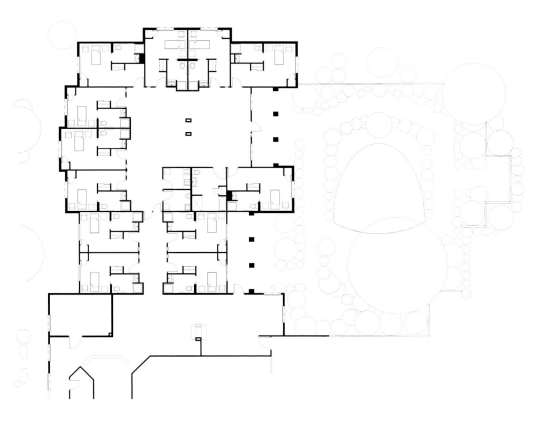

Floor plan of dementia neighbourhood

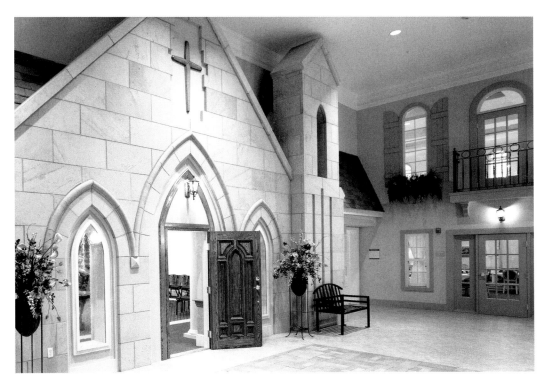

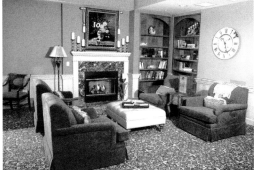

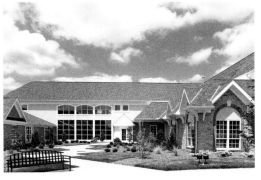

an array of service options. To foster inter-generational activities, "Grandma's House" provides children with a play area and encourages casual visits from friends and families.

The configuration of West View Manor in 15-unit clusters (the dementia cluster has 12 units) off the "Main Street Core" allows staff members visual access to all areas for easy monitoring. The complex is arranged into neighbourhoods. This helps foster a sense of familiarity and comfort among residents. The West View Manor Senior Living Community is comprised of The Villas as independent living apartments that offer single-story residences.

Town Square with its new assisted living units is a neighbourhood for the memory-impaired. West View Manor Nursing Center incorporates assisted living areas with skilled nursing sections.

The new assisted living community features spacious one and two-room suites. With the enclosed "Main Street" connecting the various wings of the complex, the inhabitants never have to brave rain or snow, while live trees, plants and perpetual blue skies are supposed to bring nature inside. Bridges, a special neighbourhood of twelve residences, provides memory support with careful attention to safety. Bridges uses "Snozelen", a therapy concept for the cognitively-impaired. Developed in Holland, "Snozelen" is a contraction of the Dutch words for "sniffing" and "dozing". A multi-sensory atmosphere incorporating sound, scent, colour and other sensory surprises is supposed to lift depression and calm agitation. Another form of technical assistance is Vigil®. This passive sensory system monitors the activities of the residents and alerts staff if they require immediate attention. The paging is silent and unobtrusive, maintaining the residents' privacy and dignity while keeping them safe.

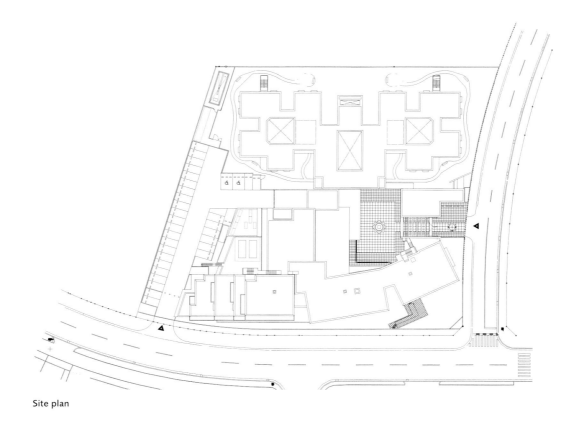
Site plan

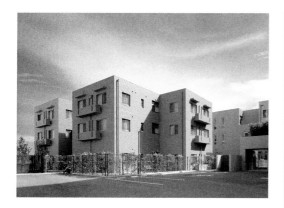

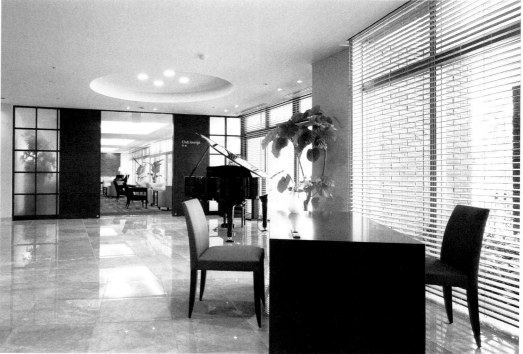

Exterior view from the north | Entrance lobby | A communal space for rest and relaxation | Resident's room in the assisted living wing with wheelchair-access washbasin | Japanese room for festivities with guests

Will Mark Kashiihama Residences for Seniors

Fukuoka City, Japan

Architect	KUME SEKKEI
Building contractor	Fukuoka Jisho Senior Life Co., Ltd.
Operator	City Care Services Co., Ltd.
Completion	2005
Useable floor area	14,352 m²
Units / Capacity	54 sheltered flats 105 standard rooms

The Will Mark Kashiihama Residences enjoy an exclusive location in Kashiigata Bay, 20 minutes by bus from the centre of Fukuoka, and are run according to an operating concept similar to that of a hotel, a format that is not uncommon in Japan and the USA. The project's concept can be attributed both to the architects KUME SEKKEI, who have long-standing experience in hotel design (the practice was founded in 1932), and the operator, who runs a number of hotels in the region as well as several facilities for the elderly.

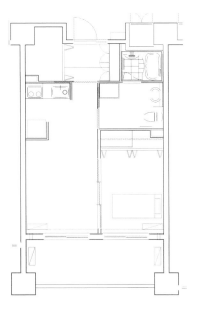
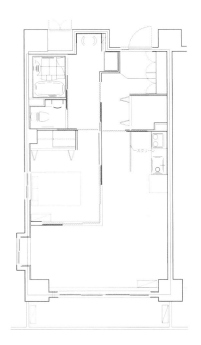
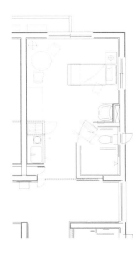

Floor plan of assisted
living room

Floor plans of standart apartments

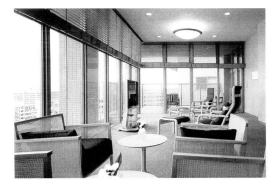
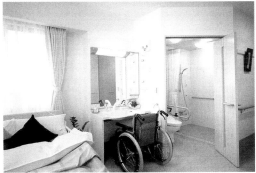
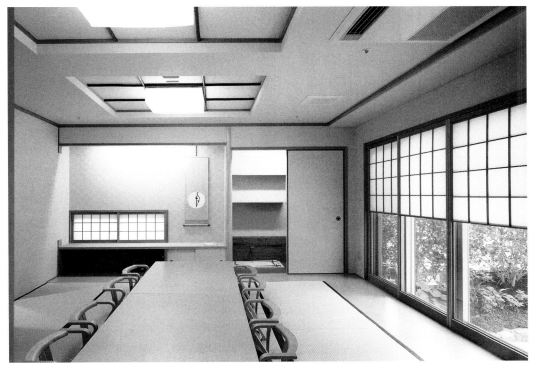

Although functional and rectilinear in its external appearance, the 11-storey brick-clad concrete building – with separate three-storey blocks on the north side with apartments for assisted living – resembles a high-class hotel inside. A wide variety of facilities are available to the tenants including a luxurious lounge with billiard room, a library, an event room, seminar rooms, hairdresser and beauty salon, fitness room and not least a bathing area with a panoramic view over the city. The interiors throughout have been given a distinct contemporary American-English style but are sufficiently structured to accommodate different needs and atmospheres. In addition, there is a "Japanese Room"

which is regularly used for family celebrations and larger gatherings.

The apartments in the high-rise block are for active and mobile senior citizens and have south-facing windows and balconies with sizes ranging from 48 to 80 m². All apartments have an open-plan arrangement and a fully-equipped kitchen which can be divided with sliding Japanese screens. Less able-bodied residents live in the low-level blocks adjoining the main building and have access to a 24-hour care service and a nearby clinic when necessary. These 24 m²-large single rooms each have two windows on different sides to ensure

sufficient illumination and to create an impression of space.

The rooms and bathrooms are designed for the elderly and equipped with a variety of technical installations; worktops and counters are designed so that wheelchairs can roll beneath them. Light wood surfaces and light green upholstery lend the entire assisted living facilities an open and friendly atmosphere.

Internal courtyards with different designs are interspersed throughout the complex and provide direct contact to the world outdoors. Along with

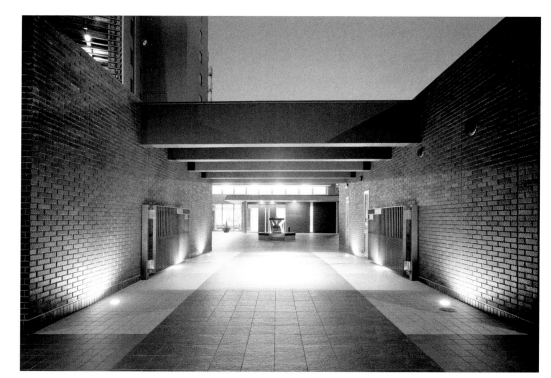

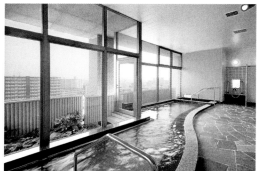

Brightly illuminated entrance area at night | Bathing area with panoramic view | Greened courtyard in the assisted living wing | Lounge with billiard table

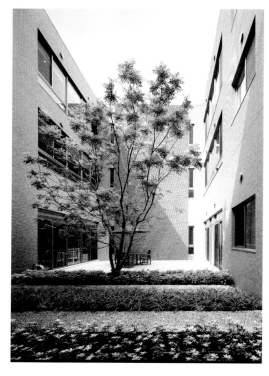

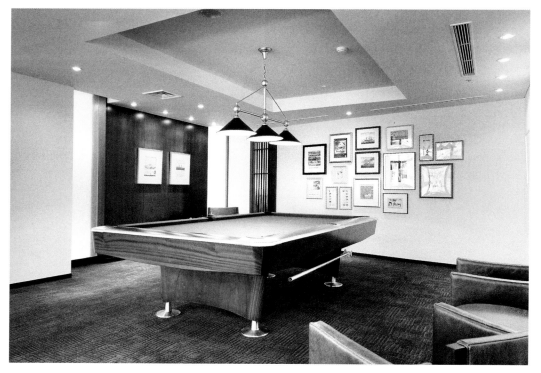

the common rooms in the main wing, they also serve to encourage contact between the residents of both buildings.

The entrance zones and parking spaces are fully lit to ensure the safety of tenants and guests even if they arrive home late at night, and the reception is staffed around the clock.

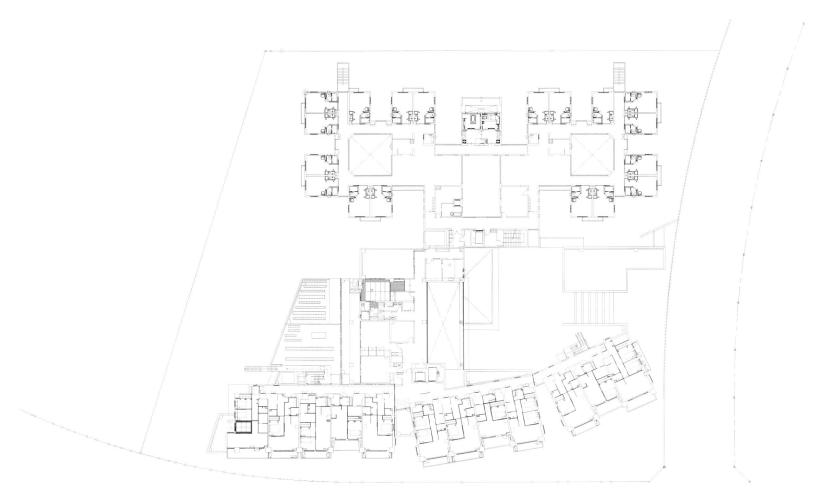

Second floor plan of the entire complex

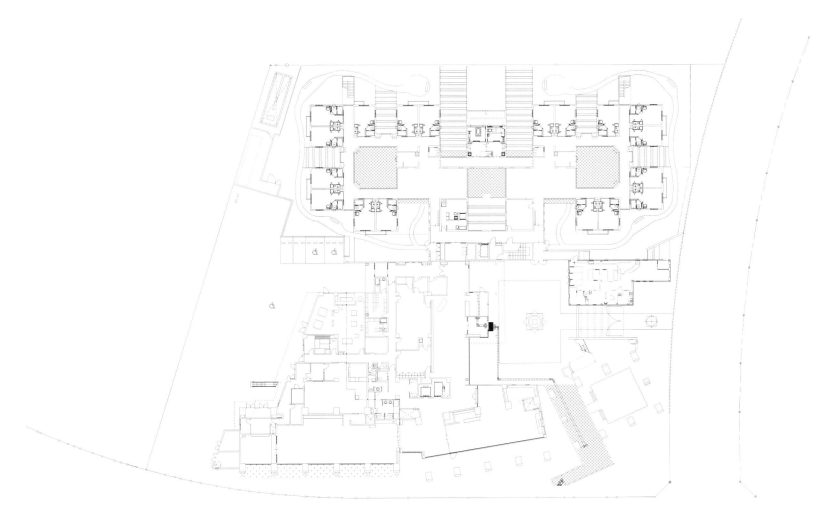

First floor plan of the entire complex

Living concepts
for specific user groups

Although a longer period of old age represents a chance to embark on new initiatives, it seems that where living in old age is concerned force of habit prevails and most prefer to pursue existing patterns of living. Despite the greater diversity of housing alternatives arising in response to increasing individualisation, one can observe a growing "birds of a feather flock together"-mentality as evidenced by emerging concepts for housing for specific social groups. These in turn are also easier for investors and providers to market.

In addition to long-standing inter-generational projects and women's housing, housing for gays and lesbians is gradually becoming more widespread, particularly in large metropolitan cities. As is already evident in the kind of lifestyle products targeted towards them, these social groups generally represent a comparatively affluent and aesthetically demanding section of society.

For many homosexuals, the thought of moving into a residential or nursing home has negative associations linked to worries of social exclusion. Accordingly, many have begun – often in the form of self-initiated projects – to club together as clients to find new ways of catering for their housing and living needs in old age and with increasing frailty.

The emergence of housing concepts for specific social groups can also be seen in other con-stellations: for example, home owners in the outskirts or suburbs whose children have left home may wish to move to a more compact and centrally-located urban apartment as they grower older. Similarly, concepts for people with similar biographical backgrounds, for example from similar professions, are beginning to appear on the market.

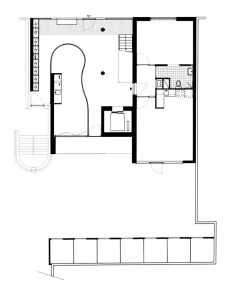
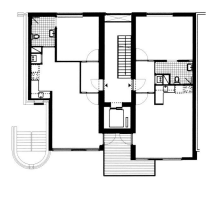
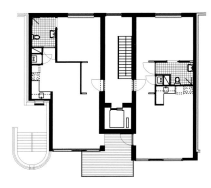

Floor plans of apartment types, Brouwersgracht

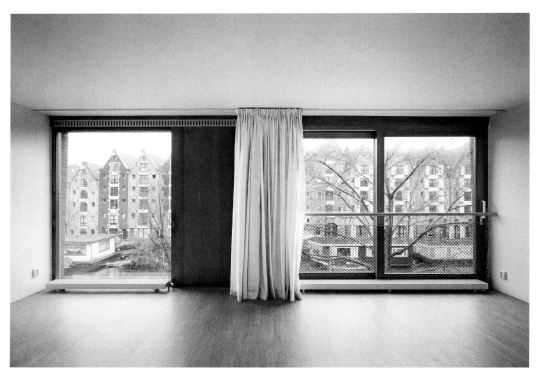
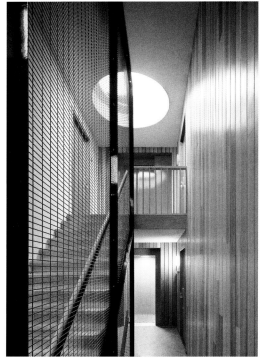

Brouwersgracht and L. A. Rieshuis

Amsterdam, Netherlands

Architect	mecanoo architecten
Building contractor	Aannemersbedrijf J. Scheurer & Zn.
Completion	1998
Useable floor area	Brouwersgracht 848 m² L. A. Rieshuis 555 m²
Units / Capacity	Brouwersgracht: 7 apartments, 1 studio L. A. Rieshuis: 7 apartments

The residences at Brouwersgracht and L. A. Rieshuis are located close to one another in the centre of Amsterdam. They belong to the same closed block of buildings.

The building on Brouwersgracht contains seven compact urban apartments and a studio. Each floor comprises two apartments – with different floor plans – reached via a staircase linked to the 4 m-high entrance hall. The kitchen and bathrooms are arranged so that the remainder of the space is as open as possible, much like a loft apartment. The top floor of the building contains a penthouse with a large roof garden. The ground floor contains ateliers.

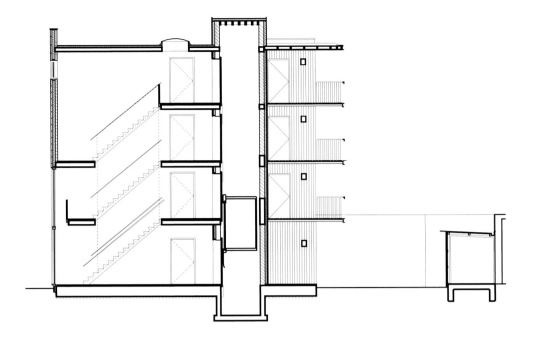

Section through the building on Vinkenstraat

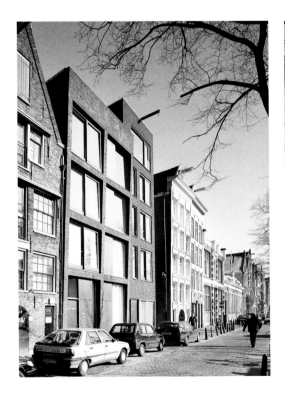

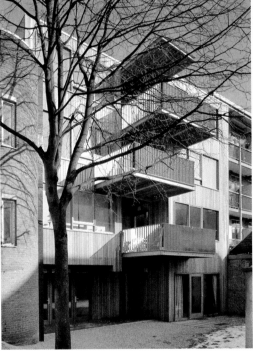

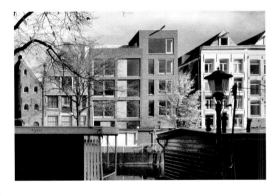

Interior of an apartment in the Brouwersgracht building | Narrow, 4 m-high entrance hall with stair | The new façade sits comfortably alongside its historic neighbours | Courtyard of the building on Vinkenstraat | View of the 11 m-wide façade on Brouwersgracht

The particular challenge of the design for Brouwersgracht was to sensitively insert the new façades into the existing historical structure of the inner-city canal houses where the existing plots are both narrow and high. The result is an 11 m-wide façade divided into two sections, one lower and wider, the other tall and narrow. The wider section, whose façade tilts slightly forwards, employs a combination of large sliding windows and timber screens to create outdoor spaces in the form of small French balconies. The right-hand section of the façade with its more regular arrangement of windows and characteristic brick cladding has a slender, elegant appearance.

In the Vinkenstraat, mecanoo architecten designed seven compact apartments with lift access. Together with a communal space on the ground floor, this forms the L.A. Rieshuis, a communal housing project for elderly homosexuals initiated by the L.A. Ries Foundation. The flats are designed for the needs of the elderly and look out over the courtyard garden and the adjacent nursing home. Each floor has a spacious, communal balcony. The even treatment of the façade emphasises the cohesiveness of the entire complex and is delineated only by a staggered arrangement of windows, which provide a different quality of light in each of the individual flats. The expressive brickwork of the street façade is contrasted with Western Red Cedar to the rear, where the slender steel balconies are located. Arranged alternately offset to one another, they maximise the available light and facilitate communication among the residents.

A communal space known as the "garden house", designed by the artist Marcel Kronenburg, dominates the ground floor of the building. Enclosed in corrugated plastic sheeting and floored with artificial turf, it allows the residents direct access to the nursing home next door. Via this entrance, the residents, who otherwise live independently, can make use of services provided by the nursing home as required.

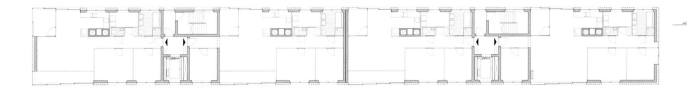

Typical floor plan

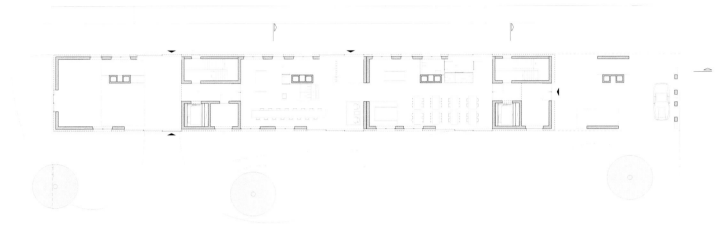

Ground floor plan

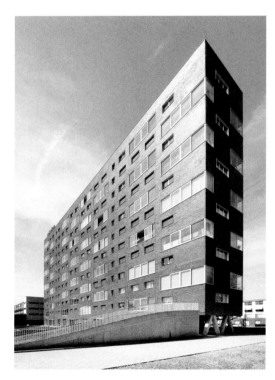

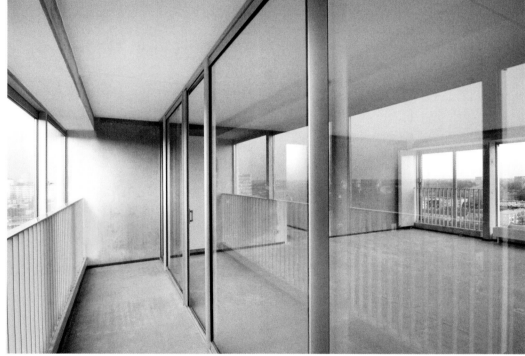

Palladiumflat

Groningen, Netherlands

Architect	Johannes Kappler Architekten
Client/Operator	Chr. Woningstichting Patrimonium
Completion	2006
Useable floor area	7,890 m²
Units/Capacity	44 residential units

The "Palladiumflat", designed by the German architects Johannes Kappler Architekten, is the first project realised as part of the "De Intense Stad" urban programme in Groningen. Differing slightly from traditional sheltered housing schemes, the building is conceived as residences for people above 50 who previously lived in a detached house, perhaps also in the suburbs, and are looking for a new environment more suited to their needs as they grow older. The design aims to combine the specific qualities of a detached house – privacy, generous outdoor spaces – with multi-storey living in an apartment block. Furthermore, all apartments were to be equally well lit.

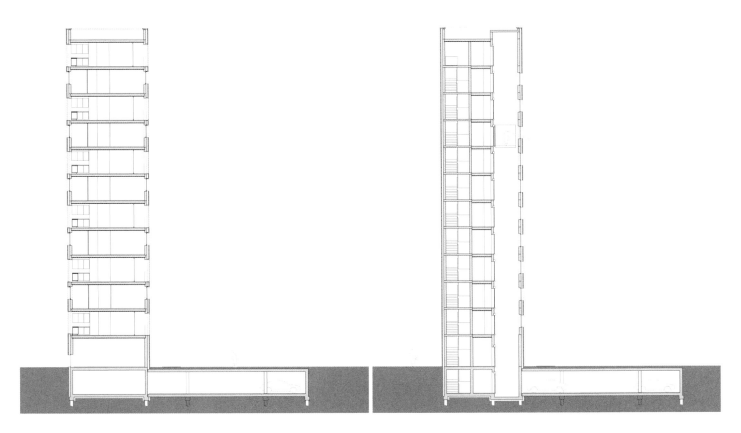

Cross sections

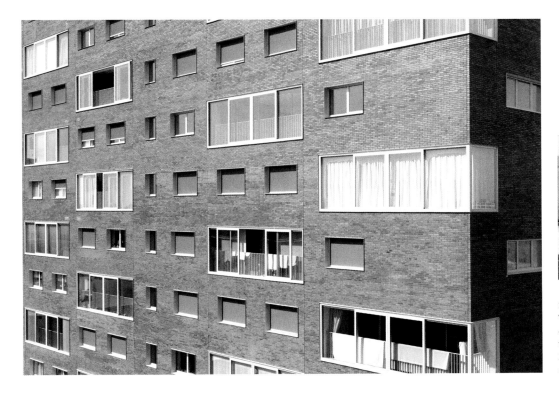

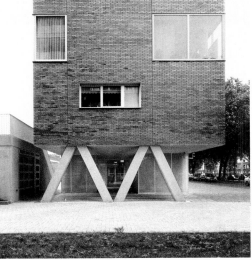

South elevation of the extremely narrow high-rise building | Winter garden on the south side that can be closed off as desired | Alternating pattern of fenestration resulting from the flipped arrangement of the dwellings in the floor plans | X-shaped columns support the end of the building and enclose an outdoor entrance area

The result is an elegant multi-storey building with two sets of lifts and stairs, each of which serves two flats per floor. With an extremely narrow depth of only 8.70 m, the building provides a variety of different atmospheric qualities – each flat looks over the street to the north and the peaceful communal gardens to the south. Instead of balconies, each flat has a south-facing conservatory that can be closed off and a large glass frontage to the north that can be opened as desired. All flats are designed for accessibility and are adaptable to the needs of residents with impaired mobility.

The arrangement of the floor plan is flipped from floor to floor, which can be seen in the alternating pattern of windows on every second storey on the façade. This makes it possible to incorporate eight different types of flats. None of the flats have internal columns, allowing the floor plan to be altered at a later date as required and maximising the use of space and daylight illumination. The building's stability is achieved via load-bearing external walls, which nevertheless feature large windows and even sections with corner glazing.

In addition to the two entrance lobbies, the ground floor also contains a community centre for the elderly serving the entire neighbourhood as well as the administrative offices of a seniors' organisation.

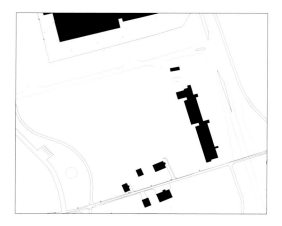

Site plan

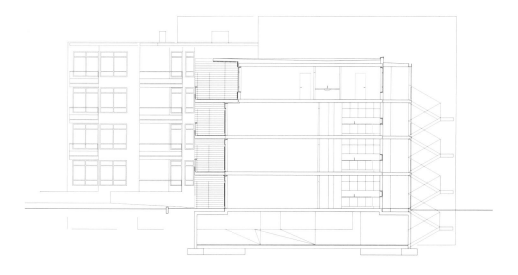

Section

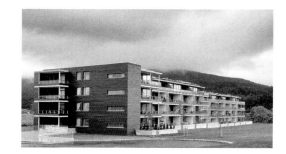

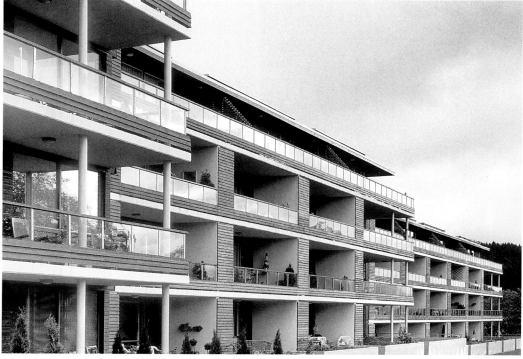

View from the south-west with open lawns in the foreground |
West elevation of the three building volumes | Access stair
with lift | Gallery walkways on the east side provide access to
the apartments

Nedregaard
Boligområde
Senior Residences

Ålesund, Norway

Architect	LONGVA ARKITEKTER AS
Client/Operator	Daaeskogen Eiendom AS
Completion	2006
Usable floor area	7,300 m²
Units/Capacity	45 units

Conceived especially for older people who wish
to move out of their private family house into an
easier-to-care-for, barrier-free apartment, this privately financed project is a response to the growing demand for living accommodation that caters
for the needs of the elderly. The project was
also supported by the State Norwegian Building
Society who provided low-cost public housing
loans to help individuals purchase an apartment.
For the architects this meant that the design and
detail planning of the building needed to adhere
to guidelines set down by the credit institute, in
particular with regard to accessibility and building cost.

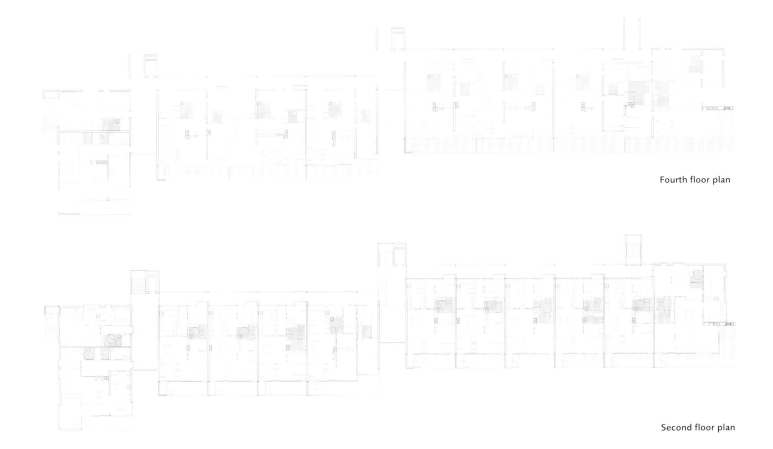

Fourth floor plan

Second floor plan

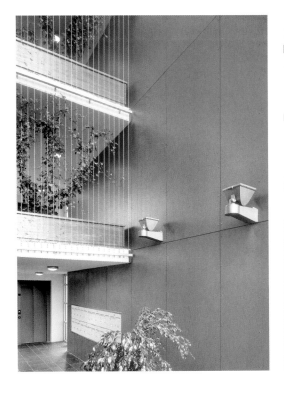
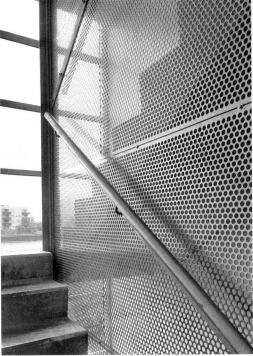
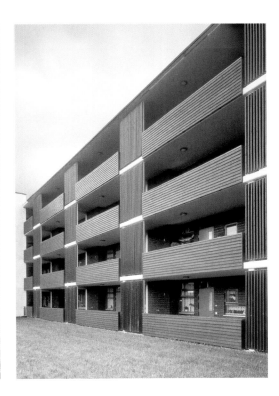

The plot lies on the edge of the town of Ålesund and looks out over open countryside to the west and south, providing an attractive view of the fjord and surrounding mountains from the sheltered terrace of the site. A band of vegetation to the east and north shields the apartments from a busy road and a shopping centre.

The apartments are arranged in three four-storey buildings, with communal facilities and access areas, including stairs and lifts, located between them. The two, three and four-room apartments ranging from 65 to 150 m² are accessed via broad 1.80 m-wide galleries that also serve as a screen against road noise. A storage cupboard outside each apartment creates a semi-private area in front of the entrance and kitchen. Each apartment, regardless of its size, has a spacious covered balcony which can be accessed step-free from two different rooms. Higher than normal ceiling heights compensate for the increased shading of the interior.

To meet cost constraints, a rational and straightforward construction system was employed with load-bearing concrete walls between each apartment. Arranged at intervals of 7.50 m, they provide optimal support without excessive wall thicknesses and match the arrangement of parking spaces in the underground garage. The timber construction of the external walls is clad with fir panels that have been stained black.

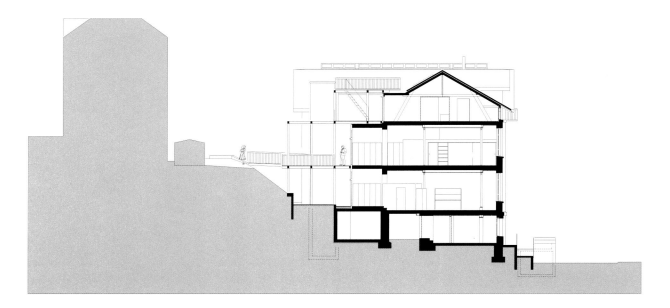

Cross section

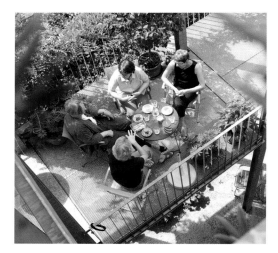

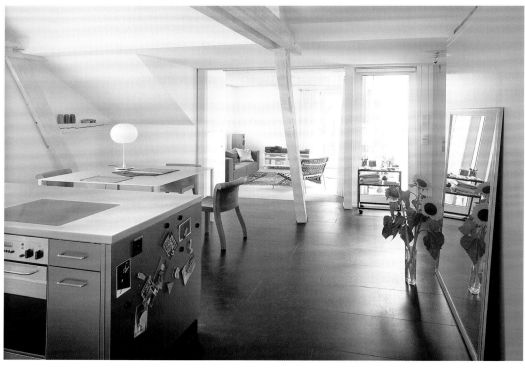

The courtyard provides an opportunity to communicate with neighbours | Roof apartment showing an example of the interior fittings and furnishing | Entrance and access area in the new addition | Communally used areas on the ground and basement floors | Former embroidery factory with extension, view from above

"Wohnfabrik Solinsieme"

St. Gallen, Switzerland

Architect	ARCHPLAN AG
Client / Operator	Solinsieme – Genossenschaft für neue Wohnform
Completion	2002
Useable floor area	1,440 m² (excl. circulation)
Units / Capacity	17 flats

The Solinsieme "Factory for Living" is a self-organised and communally financed project that was awarded the Age Award 2007 by the Swiss Age Foundation and represents an attractive example for anyone who, at the beginning of the second half of their lives, is thinking of combining their housing situation with a communal form of living. The name derives from the contraction of the Italian words "solo" (alone) and "insieme" (together) and signifies the conceptual as well as architectural concept. To realise such a project, the four initiators, all women, purchased a former embroidery factory near the centre of St. Gallen in 2000 after consulting with their architects Bruno Dörr and Armin Oswald.

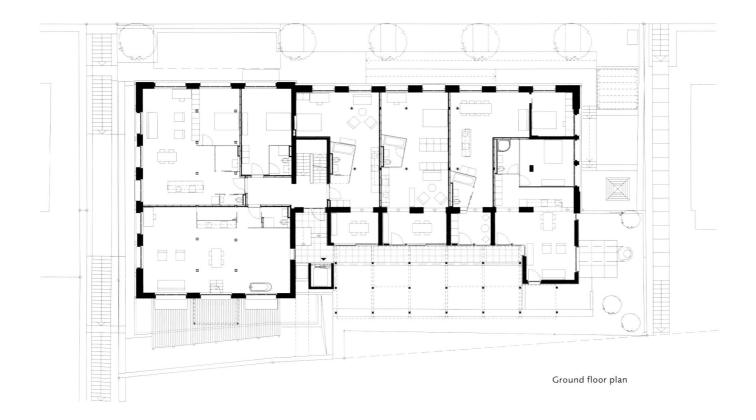

Ground floor plan

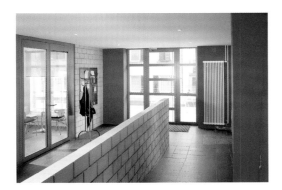

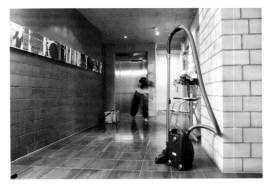

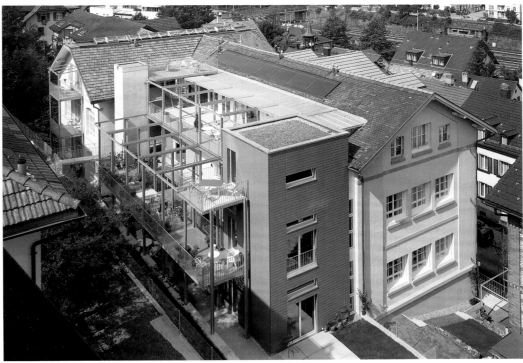

Over a period of 13 months of renovation and extension work, the existing fabric of the buildings from 1880 and the extension from 1887 were reutilised while the later extension on the south side dating from 1950 was replaced by a new building that serves as a communicative element containing the entrance and circulation, and terraces and outdoor areas. A total of 17 flats have been created, each a self-contained freehold unit following a Swiss ownership model, as well as numerous spaces for communal use which make up almost 20% of the overall floor area. These include the central communal room, called U1, with kitchen and bar, in which a variety of different events take place at regular intervals, as well as two ateliers, a guest room, a general-access roof terrace, a bicycle store and smaller utility rooms. The heart of the building is the access area facing the street with its inviting sun terrace.

The light-filled flats range in size between 56 and 93 m² and exhibit a wide variety of different floor plan arrangements and highly individual design solutions and materials, because the future residents were given a say in the design of their own living area. As there are no cramped bathrooms or corridors but rather freestanding sanitary cells, placed as boxes in the flat, and open kitchens, the flats feel very generous. Similarly the 3.80 m-high ceilings and tall mullioned windows in the historic building have been retained. To heighten the loft character, the upper section of the thin only 4 cm-thick partitioning walls are glazed.

Over 90% of the residents are very happy with their flats, but they are aware that the flats do have some deficits with regard to barrier-free access in old age, which was an initial motivation for starting the project. Evidently they are confident that together they will find an appropriate solution when the time comes and the need arises.

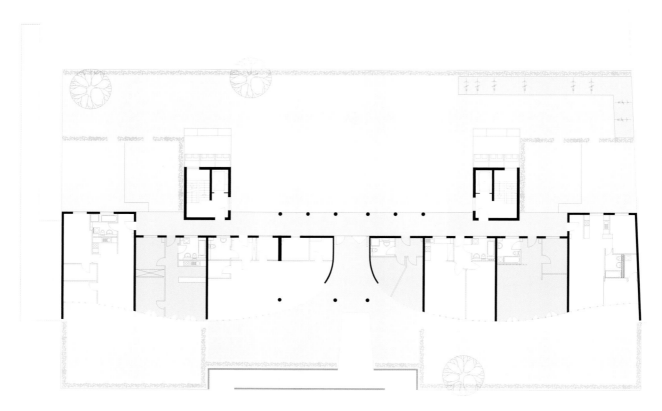

Ground floor plan

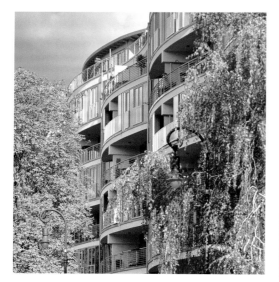

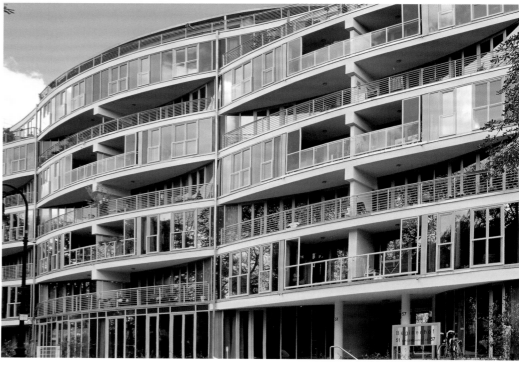

Street façade showing central entrance passageway | Full-height glazing in the interiors | Rooftop maisonette apartment | Gallery walkway facing the courtyard | Greened courtyard as private area for the residents | Plain courtyard elevation

Béguinage

Berlin, Germany

Architect	PPL Barbara Brakenhoff
Operator	Verein BeginenWerk e.V.
Completion	2007
Useable floor area	3,780 m²
Units/Capacity	53 apartments (incl. 4 maisonettes) 2 guest apartments

"Communality and individuality, freedom and security, closeness but not restrictive" is the motto of the house built in 2007 according to the tradition of the Beguines, who since the 12th century have lived together as independent women, not in cloisters but in relative freedom and independence in a community with other women.

Situated in a peaceful and attractive location near the Landwehrkanal in Kreuzberg, the building designed by the architect Barbara Brakenhoff is embedded in a vibrant, urban and functionally diverse district of Berlin. It fills a gap in the perimeter of an urban block alongside buildings from the turn of the

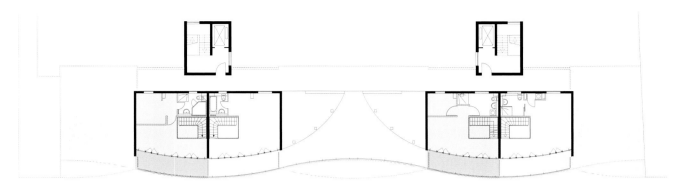

Seventh floor plan

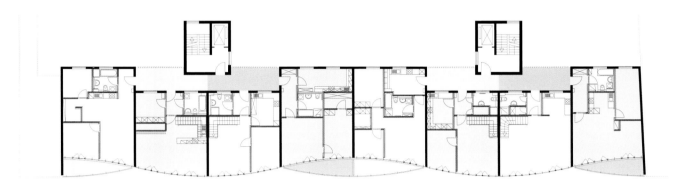

Sixth floor plan

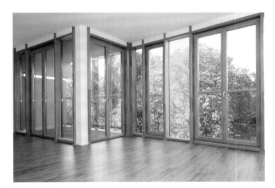
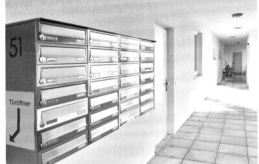
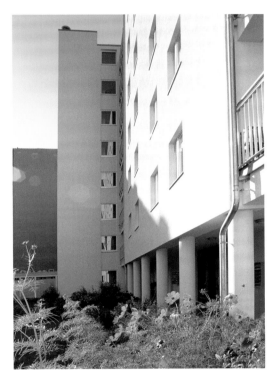
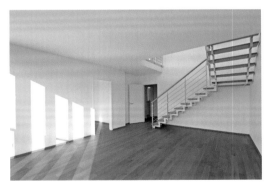
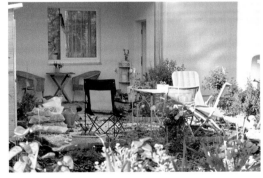

century and is conceived as a pair of seven-storey buildings with two sets of access lifts and stairs. The primary access to all the apartments is via an entrance passageway in the centre of the building which marks the boundary, via a gate, between the public street and the semi-public courtyard area for the residents at the rear. Four apartments on each storey are accessed via a balcony walkway along the rear of the building, reached from one of the two staircases and lifts. The ground floor contains the communal spaces as well as guest rooms and private apartments. The building provides a total of 53 wheelchair-accessible apartments. Three different groups of floor plan typologies were developed

with sizes ranging from 56 to 105 m². Of particular note are the ground-floor apartments, which have a small front garden facing the street as well as the courtyard, and the top-storey apartments, which are maisonettes with large terraces.

The spatial structure of the building is designed to facilitate and promote communication and social interaction: on each of the floors, four apartments are accessed via a joint balcony area which can be used and personalised by the group. The balconies that extend the width of the building and the loggias face each other so that they can be joined together as desired.

Commensurate with the specific needs of this communal living project, the building – which was developed in a process of intensive consultation with the residents about their different living requirements – creates a space for sociability and individuality, community and self-fulfilment specially for women.

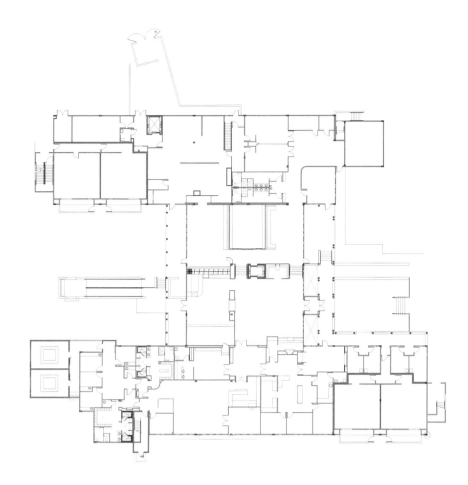

Ground floor plan

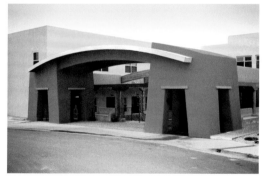

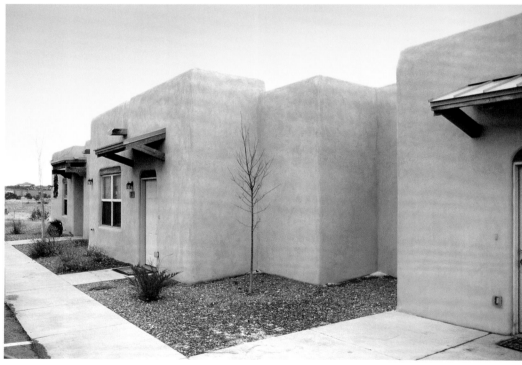

Entrance | Terraced buildings in the Mexican tradition of loam render | Inner façade | The complex in its surroundings

RainbowVision

Santa Fe, New Mexico, USA

Architect	LLOYD & ASSOCIATES ARCHITECTS
Client / Operator	RainbowVision Properties
Completion	2006
Useable floor area	Commons building (includes assisted living area) 4,188 m²; all other independent living units 11,731 m²
Units / Capacity	26 assisted living 120 independent living units

RainbowVision Santa Fe is the first retirement village by RainbowVision Properties aimed at gays and lesbians in the United States. Located in Santa Fe, New Mexico, it is in a well-known cultural oasis with a gay-friendly reputation. Communities tailored towards gay seniors have been a dream, gay advocates say, ever since the gay rights movement was born after the 1969 Stonewall riot in New York's Greenwich Village, when a fight between police and drag queens made national news after the police raided a gay bar. In today's world the GLBT community is welcomed into all-inclusive places like RainbowVision. There are several conventional subdivisions that market homes or lots specifically

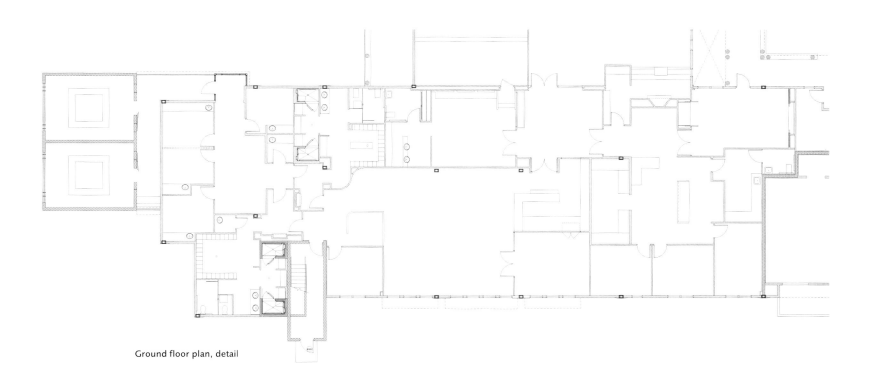

Ground floor plan, detail

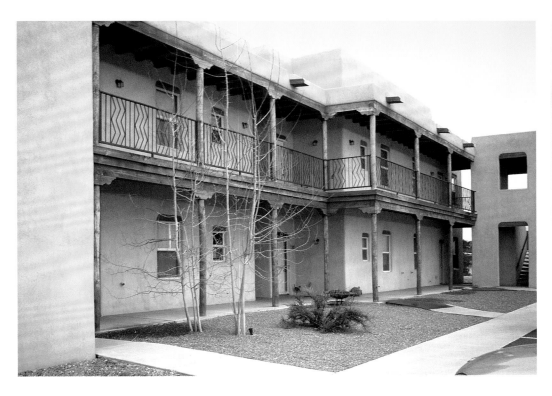

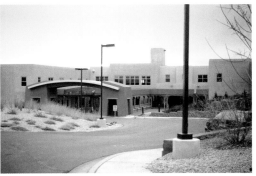

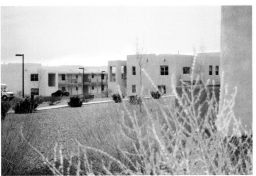

to gays, non-profit urban ventures that include af-fordable housing and combinations of all popping up throughout the country. "A few groups have acquired land and are moving forward", says the American Society on Aging, including subdivisions in Pecos, New Mexico, Zionville, North Carolina, urban condos and apartments in Boston and Los Angeles, and a lodge with cottages, town houses and nursing units in Santa Rosa, California.

RainbowVision counts 146 condos and rental units on approx. 2 hectares. Residents enjoy dining in the restaurant in El Centro, work out in a fitness centre complete with spa, massage services, yoga and

Pilates classes, physical therapy and acupuncture, or indulge in facials. There are art studios, meeting rooms, a lounge and cabaret. Assisted living apart-ments on the top floor are an option when residents grow frail but do not want to leave.

RainbowVision has attracted middle- and upper-middle-class gays from across the country. The gay-owned development company is building a second, larger project in Palm Springs, California. The gay senior market is large, but no-one knows exactly how large, given that census forms don't ask about sexual orientation. Gay senior communities do not exclude members of the straight community.

Like straights, most gays tell surveys they want to grow old at home, making RainbowVision and other gay projects extremely attractive to many gay retirees. This is significant especially considering that gays have different circumstances such as that almost 90% of gay retirees have no children, and nearly 80% are without partners.

According to SAGE (Services and Advocacy for Gay, Lesbian, Bisexual and Transgender Elders), a non-profit group that serves gay seniors in New York City, there are nearly 2.9 million gay men and lesbians over the age of 55.

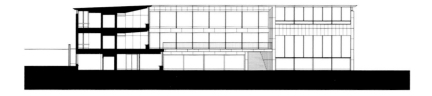

Cross section

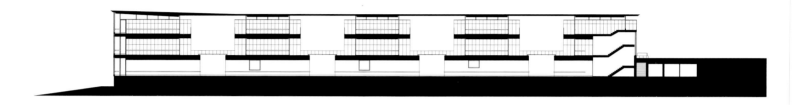

Longitudinal section

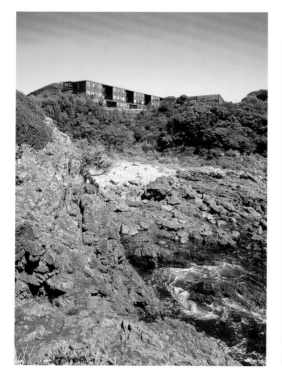

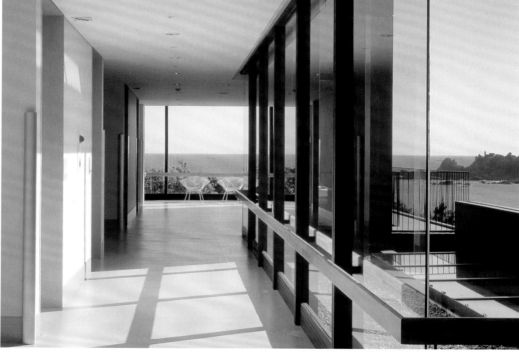

Kenyuen Home
for the Elderly

Wakayama, Japan

Architect	Motoyasu Muramatsu
Client	Tobishima corporation
Operator	KENYU-KAI Health care corporation
Completion	2001
Useable floor area	building 4,973 m², outdoors 15,490 m²
Units/Capacity	20 flats, 75 care places (62 single, 13 double rooms)

Kenyuen Nursing Home and Home for the Elderly is situated at the southernmost point of the Japanese mainland on a cliff overlooking the Pacific Ocean in Wakayama Regional Park and was designed specifically for residents whose lives revolved around the cycles of nature and rhythm of the seas, for example as farmers or fishermen.

Paying special regard to the particular needs of its residents, Motoyasu Muramatsu has designed a place to retire to "between the ocean and the sky" that responds to the unique topography of the site: a dark and rugged rocky landscape overgrown with blackcurrant bushes and dominated by the breath-

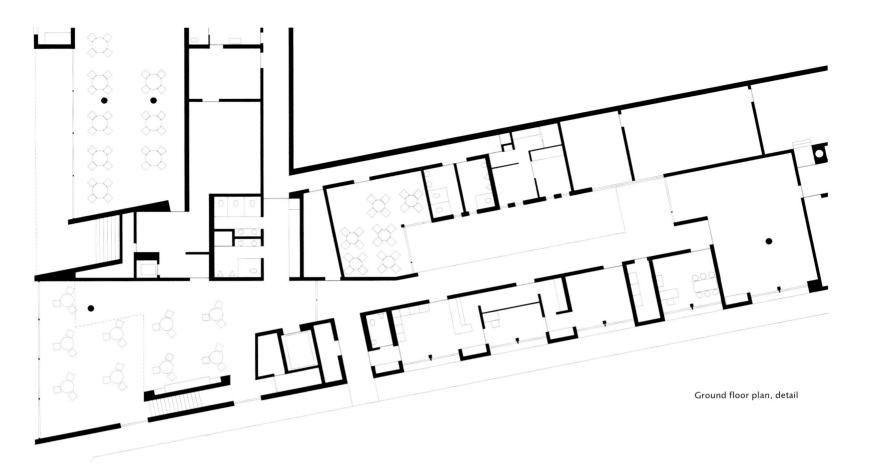

Ground floor plan, detail

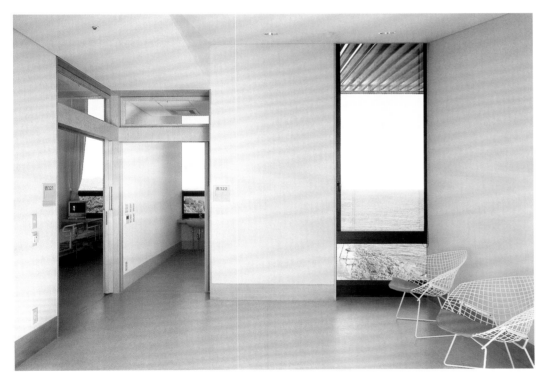

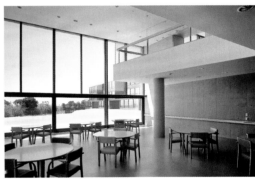

The building sits atop a rugged, rocky coastline | Full-height glazing affords an uninterrupted view over the ocean | Full-height windows with low cross-rails in the corridors and residents' rooms | Two-storey dining room with projecting gallery on the upper floor

taking presence of the ocean. The elegant reduced form of the building contrasts strongly with the wildness of the coastal landscape, lending it a discreet and sculptural quality.

The elongated Z-shaped building, faced with a dark pigmented concrete, is located next to a main road and arranged along a north-south axis between the mountains and the sea. The three storeys of the building are layered like bands of rock strata with a strong horizontality emphasising the extensive nature of the complex. Full-height glazing and the very narrow width of the building allow the world outside to permeate the world within and the nat-

ural surroundings, particularly sunlight, are allowed to flood the interior unhindered.

The residents are accordingly able to live out their affinity to the sea and wide expanse of nature throughout the complex and at any time. Combined with a variety of care provisions for improving physical condition – wellness offerings are, for example, standard in Japan – the home hopes to strengthen the residents' awareness of their own biography through their identification with the landscape. Indeed, staying at Kenyuen has some of the qualities of a rehabilitation, helping elderly people to find a way back into a "normal" way of life.

The attractive location and its good road connection also help to encourage relatives, most of whom live and work in the cities, to visit their family in Kenyuen regularly. A communal area in the central wing is conceived with this in mind and serves as a public area for visitors.

Despite its declared openness, the organisation of spaces within nevertheless caters for the needs of the elderly for peace and quiet, security and stability – and more importantly for the desire to grow old with dignity. The latter in particular cannot be taken for granted as old people, particularly those in need of care, are often subject to invasions of privacy and

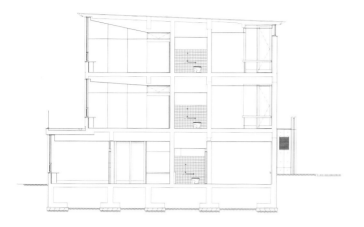
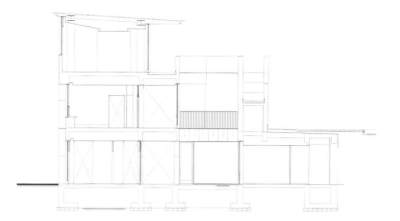

Sections

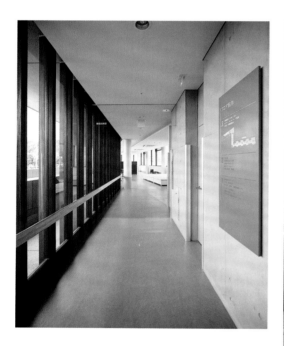
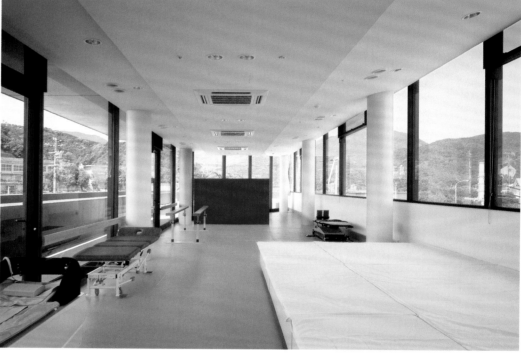

Light-flooded corridor | Therapy room

are wont to disguise their physical impairments. For the architect it was therefore important to create spaces with the fewest possible restrictions that allow residents to forget their predicament. All of the single rooms can be personalised by their occupant and the bed, a key element, is arranged so that residents are woken by the morning sun.

The extensive volume of the building resulting from its Z-shaped form made it possible to create a variety of spaces of different dimensions and degrees of intimacy and public openness. Numerous opportunities for private retreat exist alongside a hierarchical system of semi-public and public communal

areas much like in a village, allowing residents to retain their independence and seek out favourite corners. The central wing is the most public area of the building and contains an almost fully-glazed two-storey dining hall with gallery, as well as an extensive outdoor terrace and reception hall on the first floor. Therapy facilities such as a gymnastic room, swimming pool and the in Japan much-loved bathing room are located in areas adjoining the central wing.

In his design for Kenyuen, the architect has managed to turn an almost poetic idea into an architectural and care concept which can ultimately be

understood as a eulogy to the power and beauty of nature.

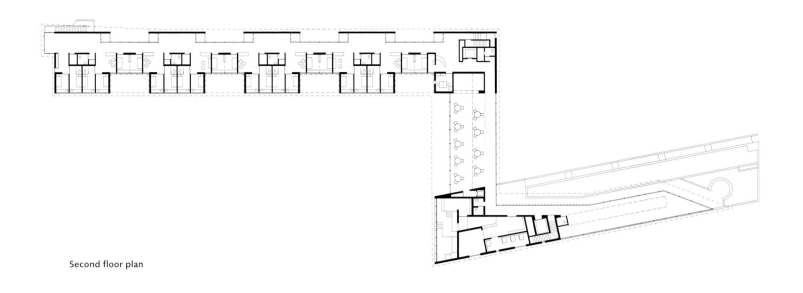

Second floor plan

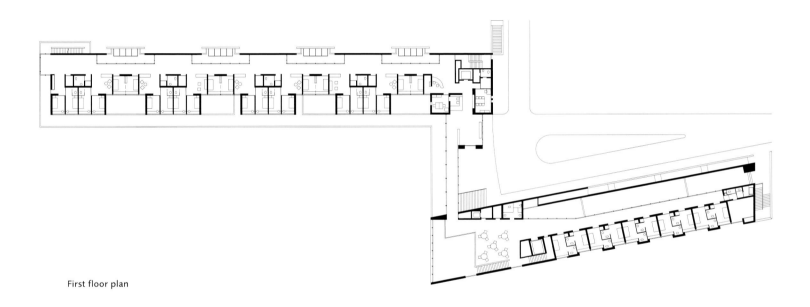

First floor plan

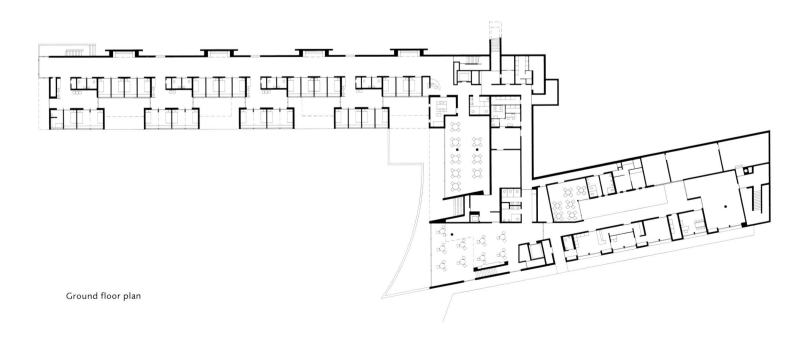

Ground floor plan

Left page
Site plan and topography | Façade detail | Therapeutic swimming pool on the second floor

Right page
Driveway from the north | The glass and dark-coloured exposed concrete façade creates an interesting contrast, even at night | The narrow zigzag of the complex underlines the horizontality of the building

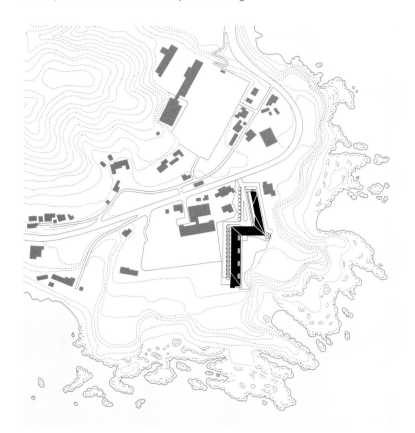

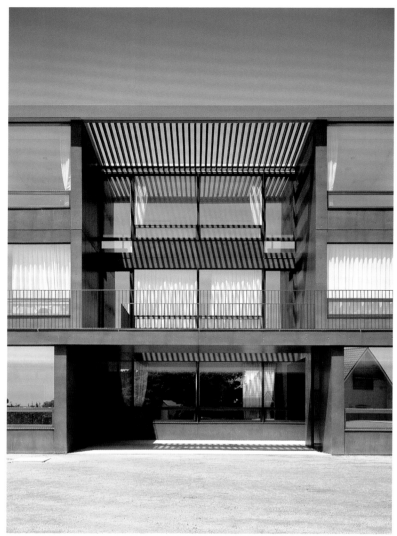

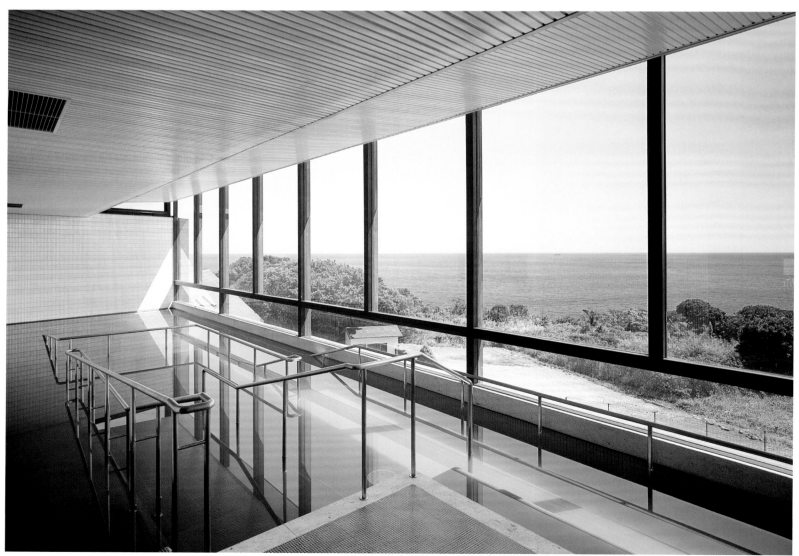

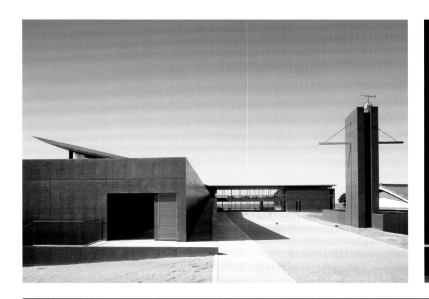
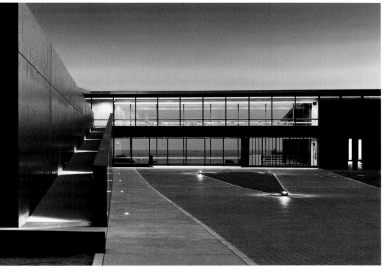
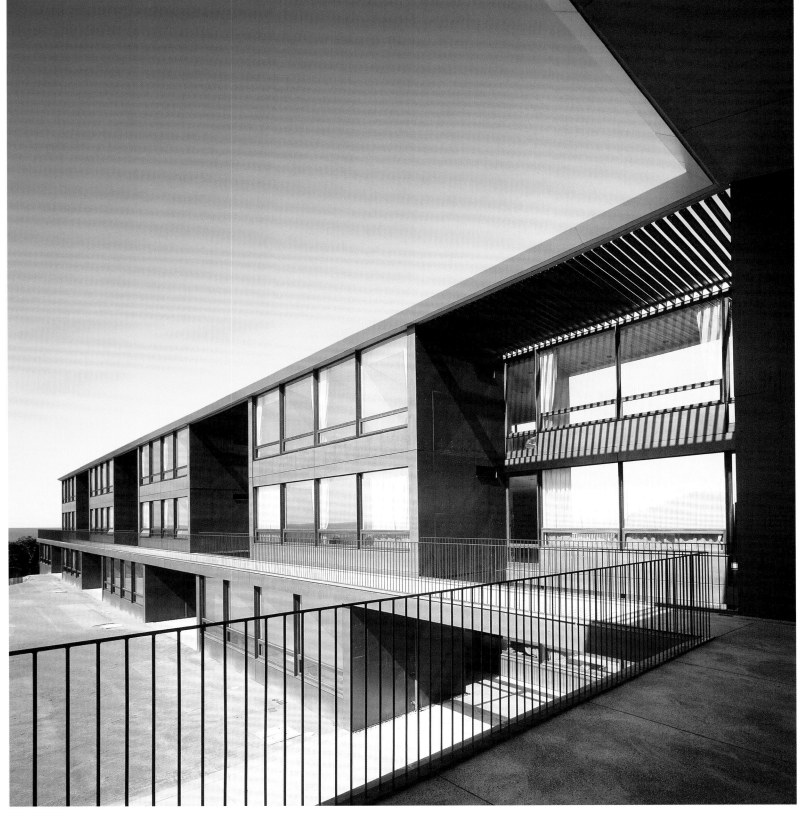

Living concepts for people with dementia

For nursing homes, the diagnosis of dementia among its residents – over 70% are affected – already presents a significant challenge. In view of the growing number of people with dementia and their particular need for a sense of security, inpatient facilities have more recently begun to adopt a system of so-called "communal care groups". These smaller, household-sized units, generally consist of spacious communal areas and individual private rooms for each resident.

This kind of "communal household" gives particular emphasis to places of contact and inter-action, such as hallways, the living room or an open kitchen-living area. Experience has shown that a daily routine in which communal activities dominate, is both stimulating as well as reassuring for residents within the group.

The day-to-day routine follows the familiar pattern of family life. The organisation of the floor plan and design of the interiors therefore resembles that of a traditional apartment. Although dementia sufferers have a less pronounced need for peace and solitude, their living environ-ment should nevertheless provide spaces for retreat and privacy – the resident's own room and secluded niches in communal areas for example – which likewise need appropriate archi-tectural treatment. The relationship between private and communal areas – between distance and closeness – needs to be carefully considered. Ideally, the residents' rooms are arranged around a central living and dining area with core care facilities and staff close by. This mini-mises the need for circulation space resulting in cost savings.

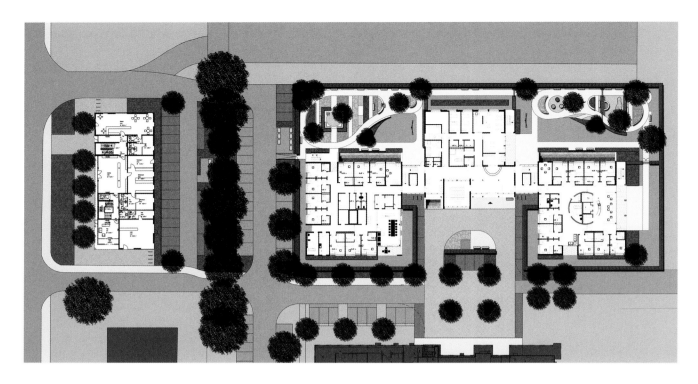

Floor plan with surroundings

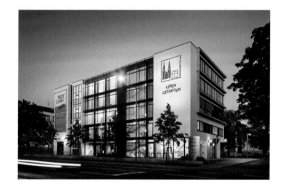

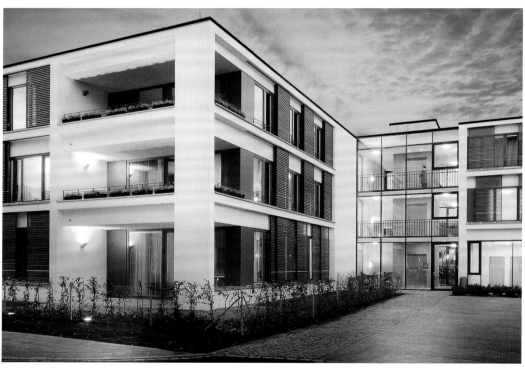

Glazed street façade of entrance building | Façade from the south

Competence Centre for People with Dementia

Nuremberg, Germany

Architect	feddersenarchitekten
Client / Operator	Evangelisch-Lutherisches Diakoniewerk Neuendettelsau
Completion	2006
Useable floor area	3,513 m²
Units / Capacity	96 residents in 8 households (incl. short-term care) 12 residents with day-care

The Competence Centre for People with Dementia in Nuremberg is the first initiative of its kind in Germany to establish a network of medical and nursing care professionals, relatives and the general public. Opened in 2006, the centre provides both information, advice and preventive assistance as well as care and therapy practice.

An architectural competition initiated by the care provider was won by the Berlin-based office feddersenarchitekten with a design which features a five-storey entrance building that, with its glazed street frontage, creates a strong symbol of the centre's open approach to dementia. The en-

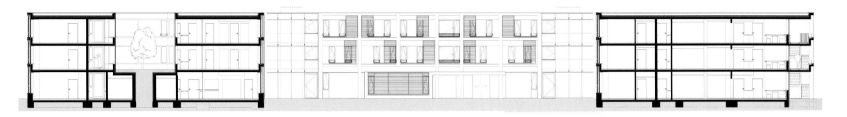

Section through houses A and C with elevation of house B

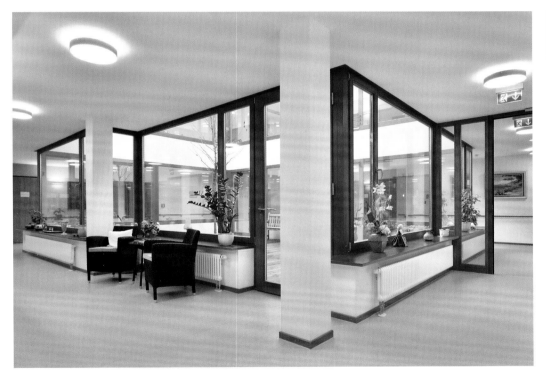

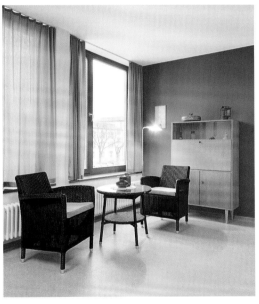

Patio on the first floor | An inviting corridor where one can while away the time

trance area contains a baker and a chemist, and above these rooms for consultation, events and care training, while the quieter, sheltered rear of the building provides a home for a total of 96 residents arranged in care groups on three storeys. The centre is a medium-sized facility of a size commonly found in German cities, often in the form of a headquarters with further smaller facilities in other locations.

Three pavilion-like buildings are clustered around a forecourt. A wide cantilevered canopy marks the central entrance to the lobby. With its white rendered façades and open frontage, the centre takes its cues from the neighbouring buildings and fits into the surroundings of the newly built residential neighbourhood "Tilly Park".

The outwardly restrained rectangular residential buildings are connected with one another, via fully-glazed staircases to form a complex and provide a differentiated series of internal spaces with quite different atmospheres: the "patio type" has a light and modern interior courtyard, the "janus type" has a dark, protective cave-like feel and the "rustic type" interprets a traditional rural living style. Each of the three floors feature variations on the three types by employing different colours and materials to create a variety of different atmospheres and living qualities.

Twelve residents live together in a so-called "residential group", much like in a large apartment. Eight single rooms and two twin rooms are grouped around a central living and dining area which adjoins a communal loggia. The entrances to the re-sidents' rooms are marked by indented niches, each creating a semi-public entrance area to a pair of rooms. The residents can sit here and chat or simply watch what is going on. Each of these niches has a different colour or wallpaper so that they are clearly identifiable. A wooden panel with

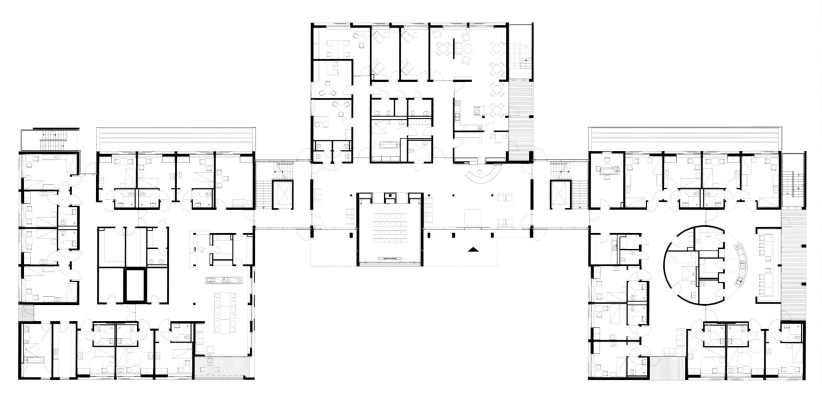

Ground floor plan

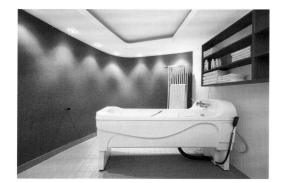
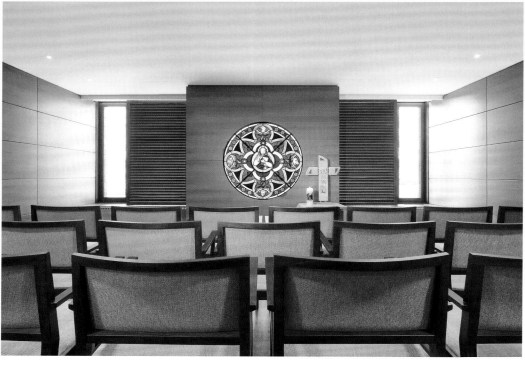

Wellness bath | Chapel

shelf next to each entrance can be personalised by the resident, for example with a photo or favourite object. A pigeonhole beneath the shelf serves as a post box where other residents and the carers can leave messages.

The floor plan arrangement minimises the use of corridors, keeping distances shorter and more economical and avoiding associations with nursing homes or hospitals. The use of "stable doors" where the upper section can be opened independently of the lower section, allows residents and staff to be aurally aware of activities outside their space, in the process making the occasional journey

unnecessary. The materials and textures used reinforce the residents' relationship to their surroundings. The hand-troweled plaster in the "janus type" or the timber panelling in the "rustic type" recall familiar environments. In the "rustic type" the masonry of the wall is even left exposed and not covered with plaster; the bricks are simply sealed with linseed oil so that the residents can feel the rustic quality in more ways than one.

The design of the outdoor areas, by the Berlin landscape architect Harms Wulf, picks up and continues the qualities of the interior. The garden provides a variety of opportunities for activity as well as con-

templation. Intimate seating areas arranged at intervals along the paths provide an opportunity to sit down on one's own or in small groups. Raised beds allow old people direct contact with plants without having to bend down, stimulating the senses of touch, smell, sight and taste. Large windows create a strong connection between inside and outside. Residents can therefore experience the change of seasons from indoors, either seated on a low window-bench or from their bed.

Through the establishment of the first Competence Centre for People with Dementia in cooperation with the local hospital centre, a counselling associa-

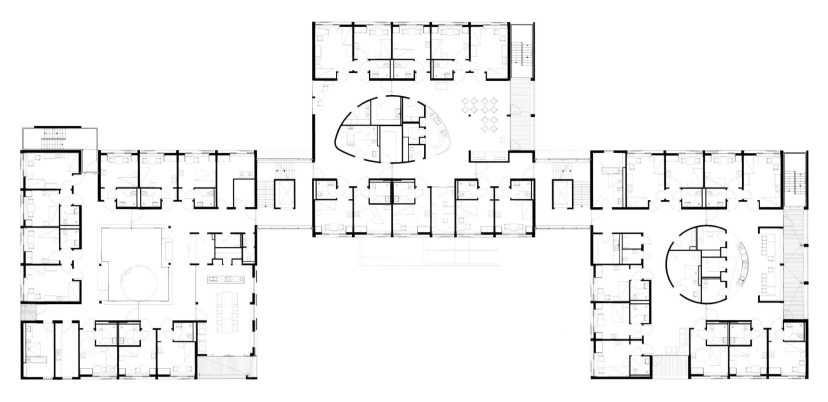

Upper floor plan

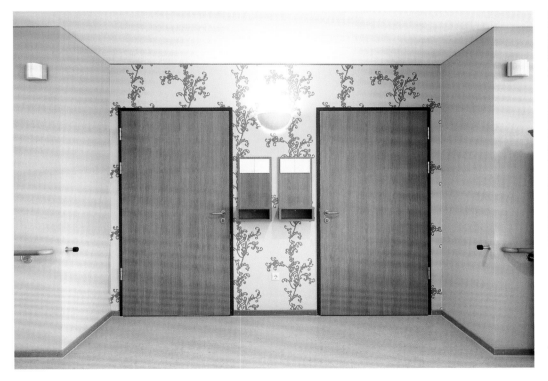

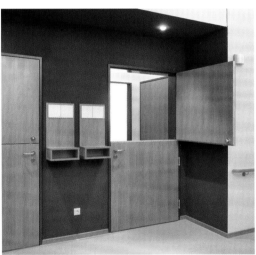

"One's home address" | Entrance to residents' rooms with open stable door

tion for relatives, the Psychogerontological Institute at the University of Erlangen-Nuremberg and the Bavarian Alzheimer Society, it has been possible to provide a broad spectrum of offerings for all those affected by the illness. Accompanying research projects and initial evaluations have confirmed the sustainability of the concept and further centres modelled on the same concept are now planned for Munich and Upper Franconia.

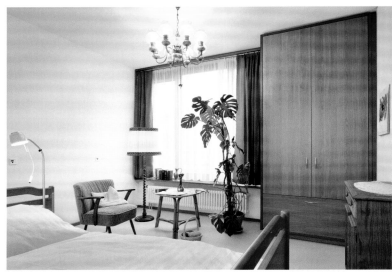

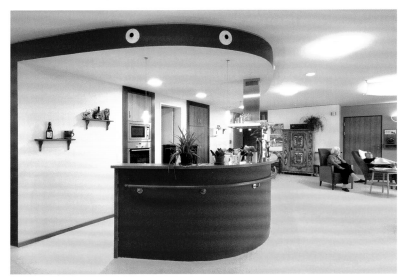

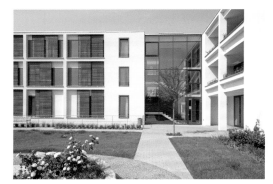

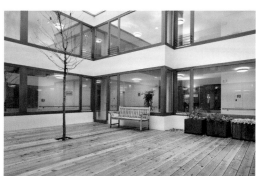

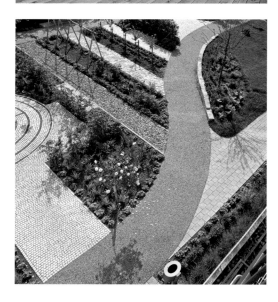

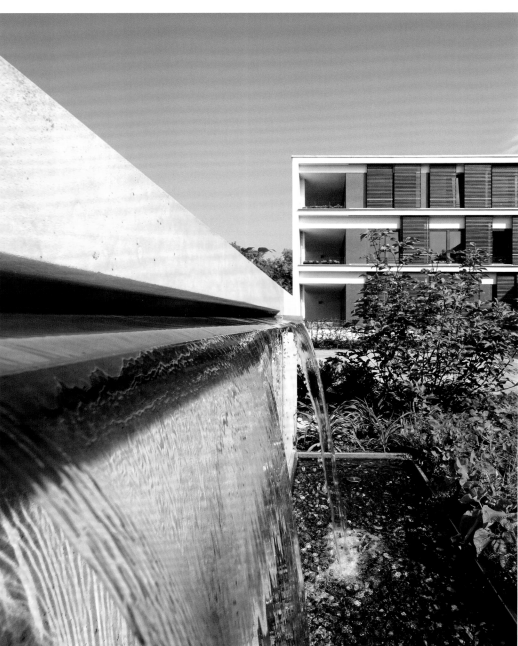

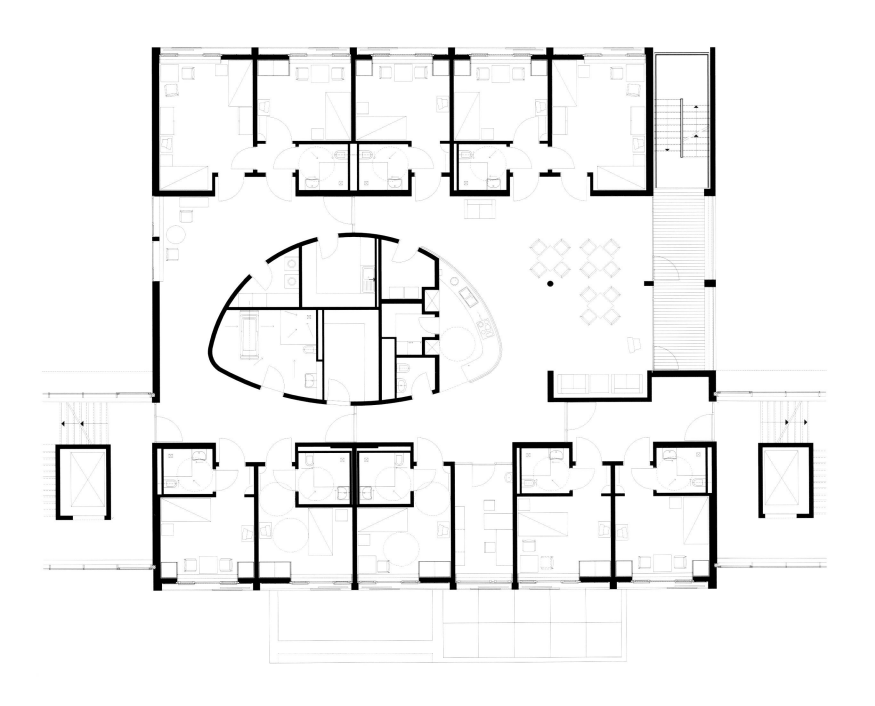

First floor plan house B

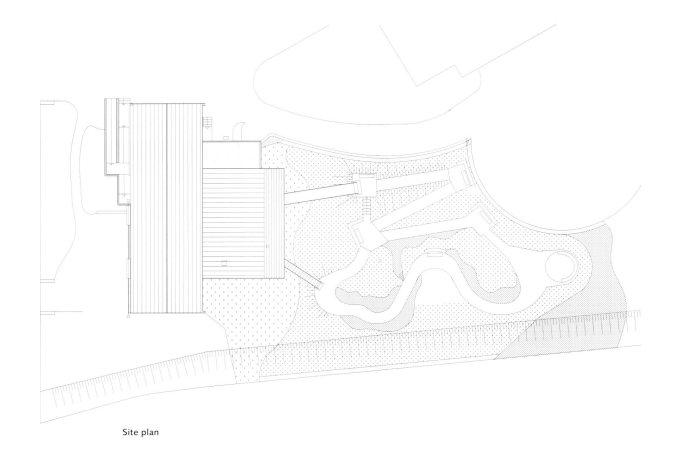

Site plan

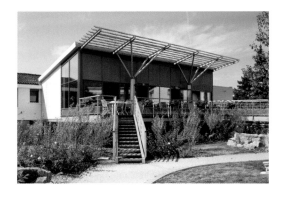

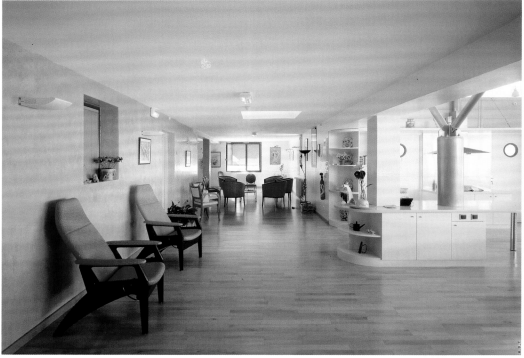

New extension on the north side supported on columns | Connecting corridor adjacent to the open kitchen (foreground right) is wide enough to sit in

Day-care Centre with Therapeutic Garden

Le Creusot, France

Architect	Dehan + Spinga Architects
Client/Operator	Éhpad du Creusot
Completion	2006
Useable floor area	350 m²
Units/Capacity	12 residents

Opened in 2006, the day-care centre is part of a complex of buildings of different periods and styles belonging to the regional nursing home for the elderly, and is exemplary both in terms of its care concept as well as its architectural solution and realisation. The plans for the conversion and extension of a freestanding building dating from the 1950s were developed by the architects Philippe Dehan and Benoît Spinga in close cooperation with the staff and future users, a dialogue that also brought forth the idea of creating a therapeutic garden. The "Projet de vie du Creusot" attempts to provide a semblance of "normal" everyday life in the day-to-day care of Alzheimer

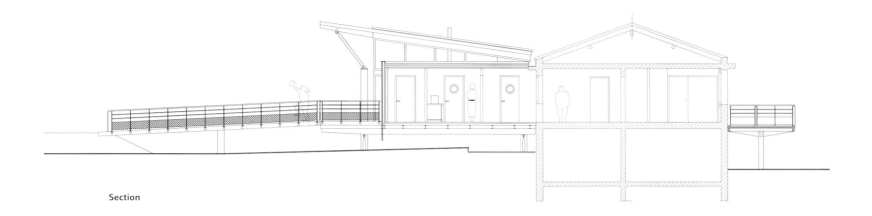

Section

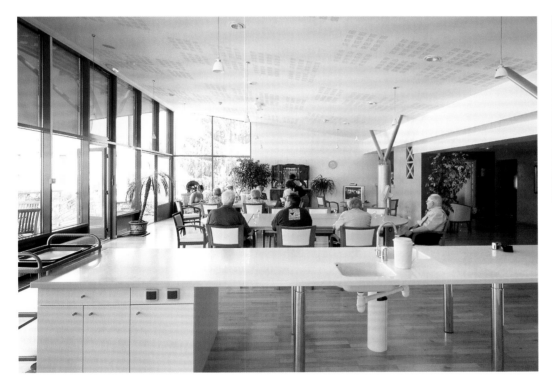

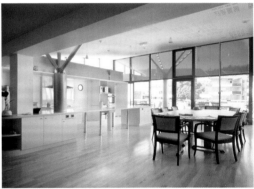

Dining room with therapeutic kitchen in the foreground |
Full-height glazing on the north façade of the dining room
that opens onto the terrace

patients. The project also aims to extend and complement the conventional care concept model in France, derived from the Cantou concept, by providing an environment specially adapted to the needs of dementia sufferers, with spaces and experiences that can serve as points of orientation in the lives of the residents. As such, the day-care centre offers residents from the neighbouring pavilions a regular succession of diverse activities, providing both variety as well as a weekly rhythm for those who visit once or several times a week. Alongside a therapeutic kitchen, the centre offers physical exercises, games and creative activities that help stimulate the senses and memory.

A beauty salon also caters for the residents' cosmetic needs.

The existing single-storey house on the edge of the complex was completely restored and extended on its north side with a new elevated extension and terrace. Although north-facing, the large window openings are equipped with blinds to reduce glare for residents suffering from cataracts. The main functional areas are arranged around a large open space and have different ceiling heights, wall colourings and levels of illumination. The light and spacious common room with its high ceilings contrasts with the more intimate living room which has

warmer colours and smaller windows. The offices, animation spaces and beauty salon are similarly illuminated via light wells to provide a calm and stress-free environment. The terrace is a popular place to sit outside and enjoy breakfast in good weather.

The garden – enclosed by a timber fence and hornbeam hedge – is designed in the form of an outdoor circuit that invites residents to enjoy the sensations of nature while remaining sensitive to the various physical impairments of the residents. Accessed directly from the terrace via a narrow stair with shallow steps and railing on one side and

Connection between the existing building and the extension, seen from the west | Therapeutic garden | Warm colours and gentle light levels in the living areas | Breakfast on the terrace

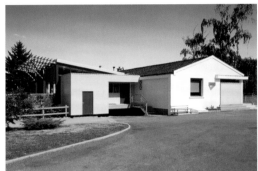

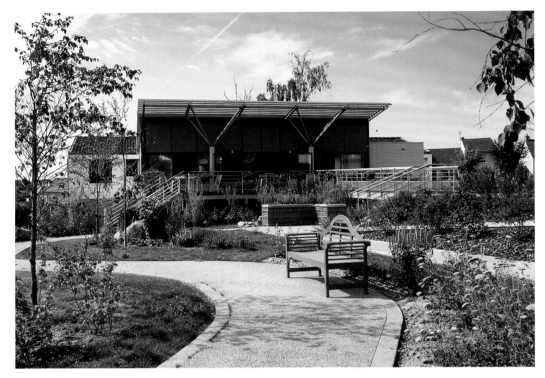

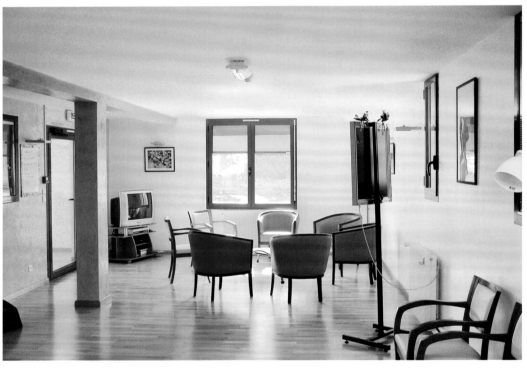

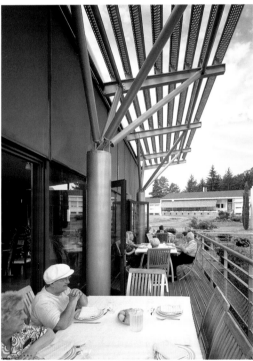

a gentle ramp on the other, the lush planting and benches at regular intervals invite the residents to immerse themselves in nature. Raised beds enclosed in woven chestnut fibres contain aromatic plants that stimulate the senses and allow the residents to do their own gardening without having to bend down. The garden culminates in a pergola draped with honeysuckle.

The way in which the project was realised was similarly inclusive. A considerable part of the internal finishing works as well as the planting of the garden was undertaken by the staff under their own initiative. In addition to keeping costs down this also increases the sense of worth for the residents and users. By all accounts the effort has paid off: since the opening of the day-care centre, instances of both aggressive as well as anxious tendencies among the residences have reduced considerably.

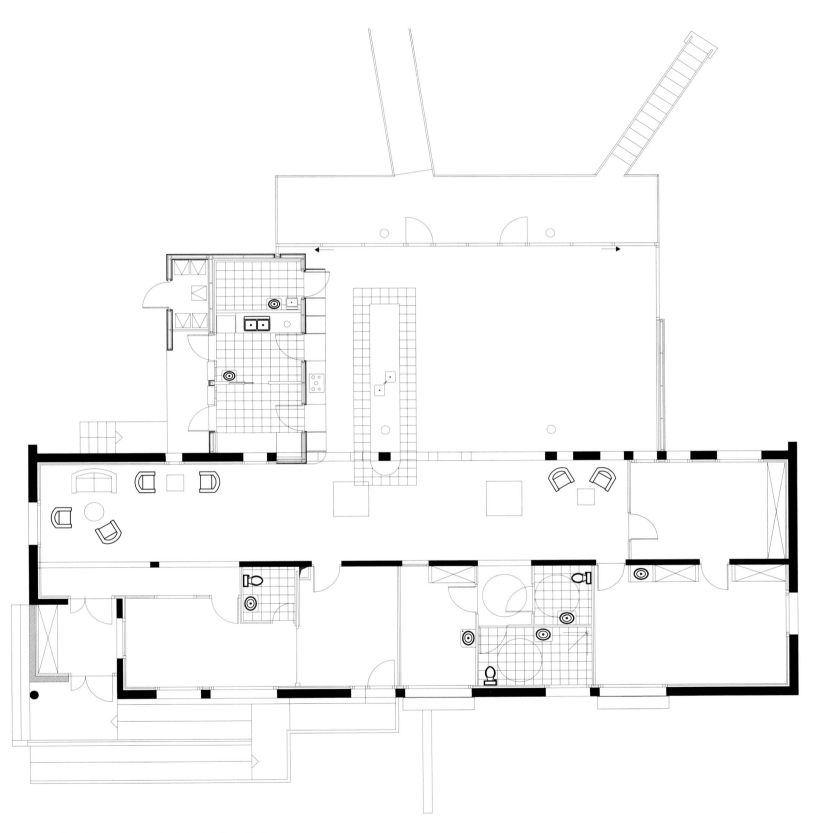

Floor plan of the extension and existing building with therapy rooms
to the south and the therapeutic kitchen and dining area to the north

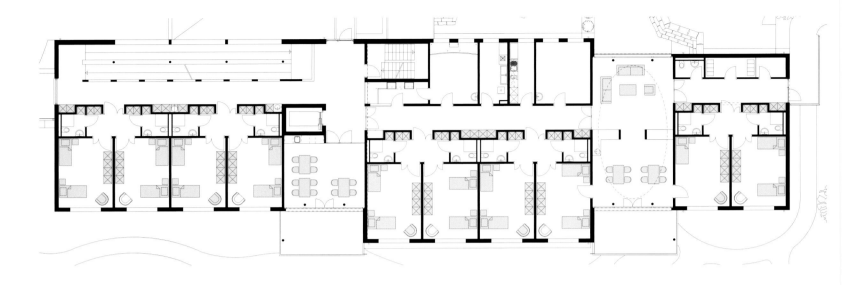

Third floor plan

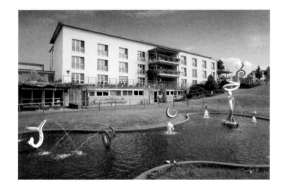

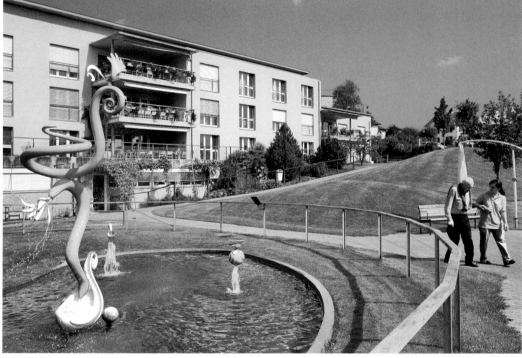

Main building with stimulating and diverse outdoor areas |
The "oasis" in the new building features a vaulted ceiling and
light furnishings made of maple | Light-filled corridors and
ramps | Older "care oasis" in the main building

Sonnweid Nursing Home Extension

Wetzikon, Switzerland

Architect	Bernasconi + Partner Architekten AG
Client / Operator	Sonnweid AG
Completion	2001
Useable floor area	5,010 m²
Units / Capacity	150 residents

Sonnweid Nursing Home, a privately-run institution in Wetzikon in the canton of Zurich, opened its second new extension in 2001. In both its care concept and its living arrangement, the home successfully pursues new directions for the care of people with dementia. The residents live according to their own "rules" and are no longer subjected to our conventional system of values, which for them have limited relevance. The guiding principle for the operation as well as the architectural concept of the home – where residents may stay until they die – is to recognise the residents' confused state as an immanent part of their being.

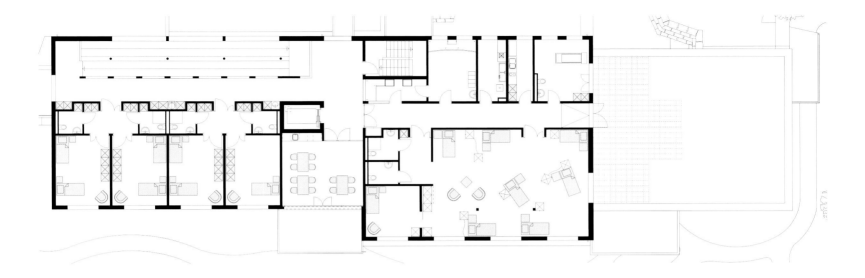

Fourth floor plan with "care oasis"

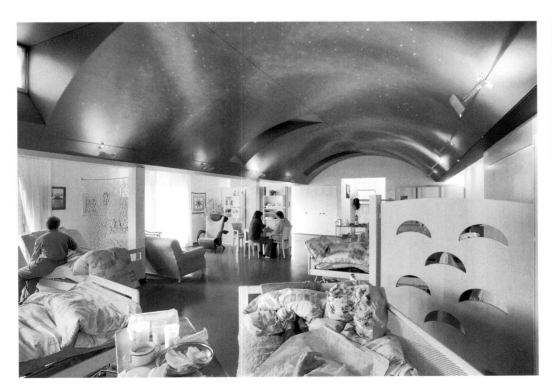

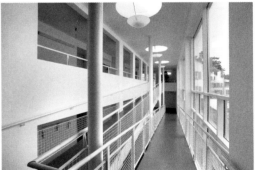

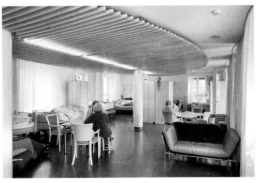

The new extension is a three-storey volume with a single-loaded arrangement of rooms and additional accommodation as well as a terrace at roof level. An important part of the building, which is connected to the main building that dates from 1933 via a glazed connector, is its circulation concept. Instead of using stairs, a system of ramps allows residents to move from floor to floor safely on foot. This reduces the risk of accidents while simultaneously allowing residents to move around freely and independently without being limited to the interior. Its continuation leads outside to a system of pathways that form a circuit through the garden. Due to the slope of the site the building provides several points of access to the gardens from each floor. Taken together, the paths indoors and outdoors form an "endless loop" with an overall length of more than a kilometre along which the residents can move around freely.

Clearly arranged floor plans with obvious circulation and light and friendly colours characterise the interiors. It is important for the residents that they can readily identify where paths lead and what goes on in the building. All the residents' rooms are south-facing. Ancillary spaces such as the kitchen on each floor, bathrooms and activity spaces are arranged on the north side. Large windows ensure that light illuminates the rooms entirely so that there are no dark rooms. Round skylights in the generously dimensioned corridors and above the ramps illuminate the circulation spaces which always lead towards daylight. Suspended ceilings made of perforated plasterboard and curtains absorb a lot of the noise. Tactile elements such as tree trunks, sculptures, water, colours and winding paths provide both variety and stimulate the senses with their different materiality. Even memories of holidays in earlier life are addressed in the design of the "Arven-stübli" which features an abstracted form of wood panelling – without the chalet kitsch – on the walls and ceilings, intended to stimulate associations and bring back memories.

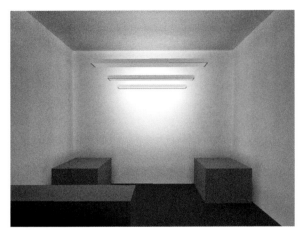
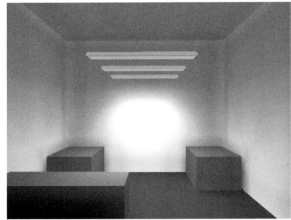

Morning
- Low proportion of direct light
- Indirect light with warm, orange component
Gentle wakening and comfortable begining to the day

Noon
- High proportion of direct light
- No ceiling illumination, additional indirect light according to ambient weather conditions
On sunny days, alert and full of motivation

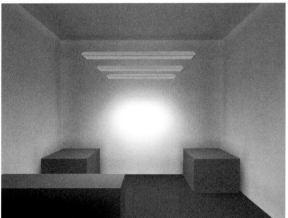
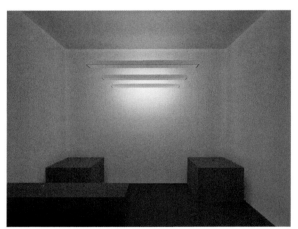

Afternoon
- Dimmed direct light
- Indirect light with cool, blue component
Gently stimulating while marking the progression of the day

Late evening
- Low proportion of direct light
- Indirect light with blue component
Peaceful and calming for sweet dreams

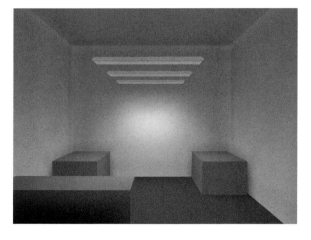

Night-time
- Low proportion of direct light
- No ceiling illumination, no indirect light
Support without being overly intrusive

Lighting that adapts to the rhythm of day and night

In Sonnweid, every resident is cared for according to their specific needs. To help reduce conflicts, behavioural problems and overburdening of the residents, the home is divided into three living areas, with care provision and therapies aimed at activating the residents' still active faculties appropriate to each phase.

Residents in the early stages of the illness may no longer be able to live alone at home but can still relate, at least partly, to "our" reality and can undertake all manner of everyday activities. In Sonnweid, these residents live in small residential groups.

In more advanced stages of the illness, often typified by an urge to move around, the residents live in a care group. These residential units are accessed via a common entrance and consist of a pair of two-bed rooms with a common entrance lobby and two bathrooms. The level of illumination in the rooms can be regulated according to the residents' state of well-being.

The "oasis" on the upper storey is for residents who are most seriously affected by dementia and require the highest level of nursing care. The oasis is arranged as a single room with several beds, with adjoining single-bed rooms. The ceiling is arched and

punctuated with 1300 points of lights reminiscent of the night sky. The furniture, made of maplewood, is mobile and can be moved around to create niches and intimate corners as required.

To the north and to the road, the building is mostly glazed so that residents are aware of everyday life in their immediate surroundings. The rhythmically arranged windows on the yellow-rendered south façade look out over the landscape. Several terraces with planting provide transitional spaces between indoors and outdoors.

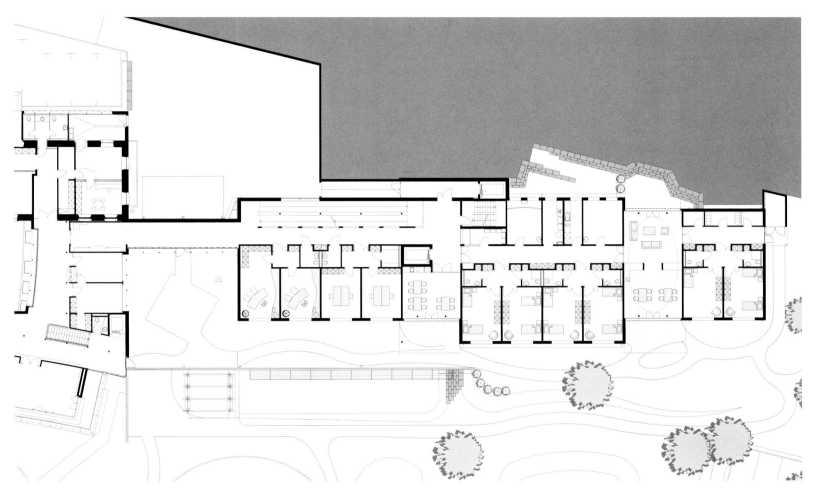

Second floor plan

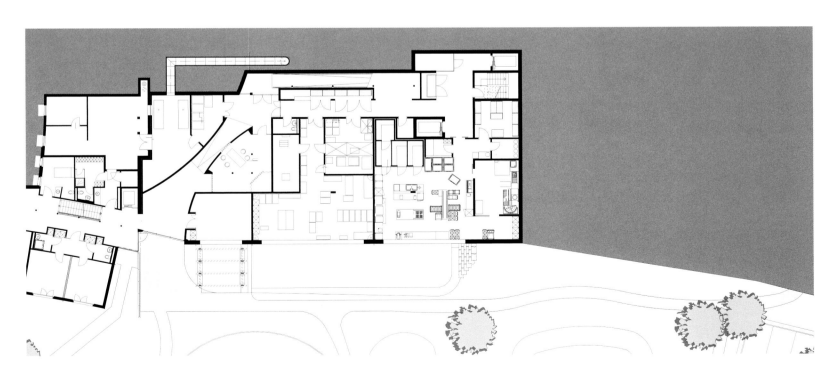

First floor plan

Residential and nursing homes

The size and organisational structure of residential and nursing homes often bear typological similarity to those of institutions like hospitals, with the primary difference that they serve a residential function (see also Living concepts for people with dementia).

Most conventional design approaches for institutionalised care facilities exhibit floor plans that are merely rational and often bear similarity to rows of terraced housing. This is largely because 60–70 % of such facilities consist of rooms which in their repetition follow the pattern of a hotel or hospital. Very often, floor plans of this type exhibit an L, H or U-shaped arrangement to keep corridors as short as possible. Winding amorphous arrangements are often regarded as bad for orientation and too long for staff. Although closer inspection shows that this is not necessarily so, competition juries often seem to rule out such arrangements for this reason. Furthermore, the economic constraints on institutionalised nursing homes are so great that their functional character leaves little room for any semblance of beauty. Occasionally, the choice of materials reflects regional influences in a last remaining attempt at aesthetic enhancement.

As the serial repetition of rooms very quickly becomes monotonous and care institutions have limited financial resources, particularly those at the lower end of the social scale, many designs, which we will not consider here, are of a poor quality. Unlike low-cost hotels, which exhibit similar problems, little attempt is made in such cases to find an individual aesthetic expression, and dull and even bleak interiors are the result. More adventurous artistic expression is the exception for institutionalised care facilities.

However, an unmistakable desire for change is afoot, which can be summed up as a need for greater homeliness and comfort: new care facilities are moving away from cold and sterile environments towards a more homely atmosphere in which the specific character of the individual as well as a sense of belonging to a group or a particular biography are accorded equal expression. This includes the design approach whereby a facility should not differ from the houses around it and as such effectively be invisible. While not particularly adventurous, this is nevertheless a better solution than an excessively large and intrusive building. The more successful examples, many of which can be seen in Austria and Germany, exhibit an increasingly free experimentation with window openings and façade proportions more reminiscent of residences in Mediterranean regions. Similarly, a tendency towards better quality materials such as brick façades and wood or natural stone can be observed. In the 1970s, many nursing homes were built with balconies, a feature that disappeared from the 1980s onwards and only made a welcome return more recently.

Special attention should also be given to the continuity of the design outside and inside. Today's initiatives strive to achieve more than just prettifying the outside, employing deliberate and coordinated design strategies that are met with greater acceptance by society.

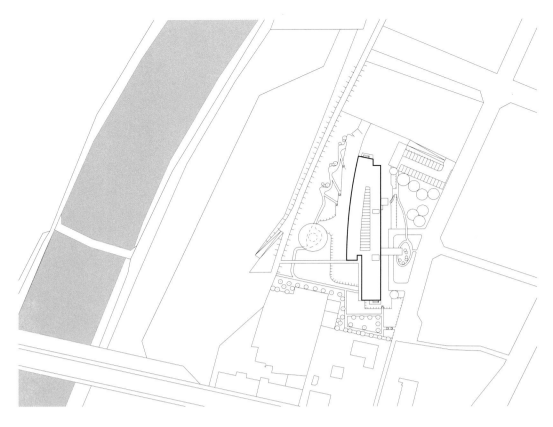

Site plan

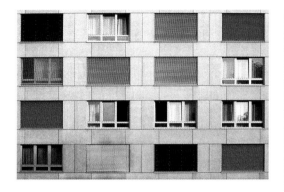

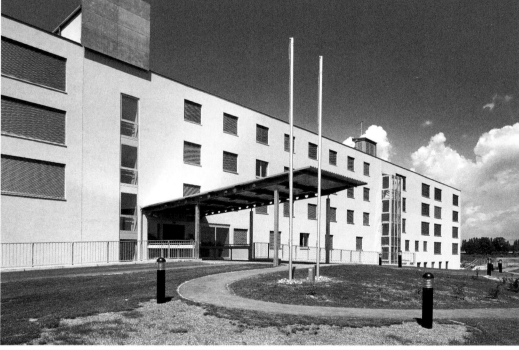

Coloured blinds on the west façade | Yellow-rendered east façade | A kitchenette and dining area is located at each end of the corridors | Each resident's room features an entrance door made of light-coloured maple wood with an adjacent vertical window strip with shutter

Home for Pensioners and Nursing Home

St. Pölten, Austria

Architect	Georg W. Reinberg
Client	Pinus/Hypoleasing of Lower Austria; Regional Administration Depts. of Lower Austria: Abt. 2HB2, Abt. 4.HB4, GS7 Nutzer
Operator	Landespensionistenheim des Landes Niederösterreich
Completion	2000
Useable floor area	5,220 m²
Units/Capacity	121 residents, day-care for 15 persons

The brief for the design of a new building for an existing nursing home in St. Pölten, the capital city of the State of Lower Austria, required that the building be user-friendly, barrier-free, have a functional arrangement and exploit modern technology. For the architects, this was a unique opportunity to bring together all the conceptual components and integrate not only the operator but also the future residents and their relatives in the planning process. Based on a design by the Viennese architect Georg W. Reinberg – selected in an expert review selection procedure commissioned by the State of Lower Austria in 1996 – a "sun-filled house for the elderly" was developed.

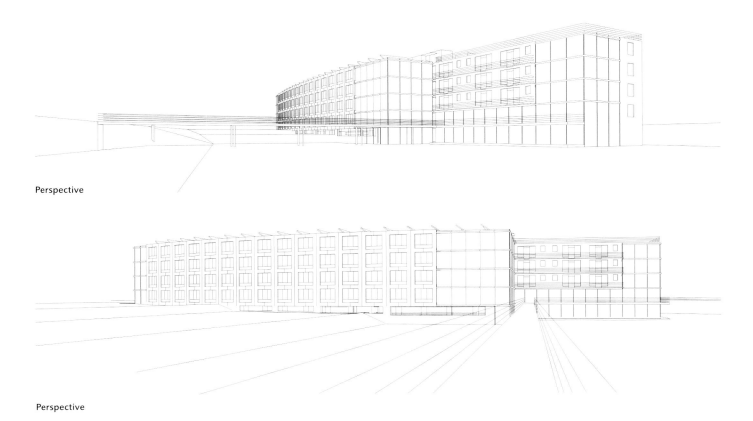

Perspective

Perspective

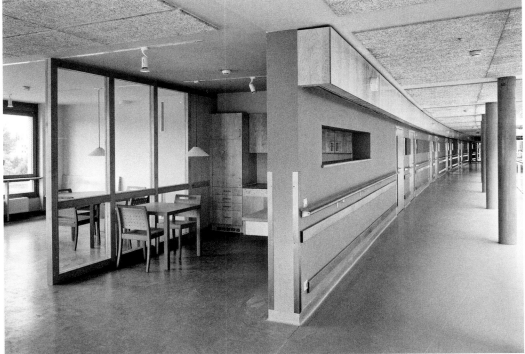

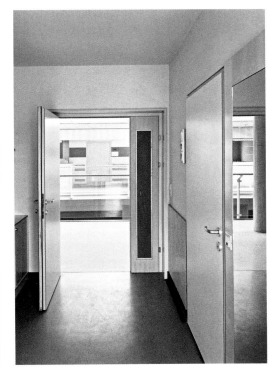

Taking the restricted mobility of the residents and the typical image of an old person seated at a window as its starting point, the design is oriented around the principle of seeing and being seen. The compact volume of the building serves as a mediator between the world outside, i.e. the manifold views of the public spaces in the neighbourhood, and the public areas in the interior world of the home. The latter is particularly apparent through its full-height, sun-filled and richly greened atrium, which is open to the sky and serves as an entrance area and central access and circulation space within the building.

The five-storey nursing home and home for pensioners is situated on the banks of the River Traisen only a short walking distance from the old town and near to the government district. It adjoins pasture land that is used as a popular local recreational area. With a straight, yellow wall on the east and a curved grey façade on the west, the building is realised as a concrete frame construction with brick infill and curtain walling. Coloured blinds, with individually adjustable shading elements, enliven the grey rendered façade. The building rests on a base that contains all the services, plant rooms, kitchens and storage rooms as well as communal facilities such as the chapel and hairdresser.

The entrance level is on the first floor, with day-care centre, administration, café, therapy rooms and small nursing ward, over which three further wards are stacked. The majority of the 51 single-bed rooms and 25 twin-bed rooms face onto the River Traisen and the town to the west; additional rooms are oriented eastwards. The central section of the east wing houses the various service facilities such as the nurses' rooms, bath, washing facilities and further ancillary functions.

The nursing home and home for pensioners offers numerous means of predominantly barrier-free access via bridges and lifts. The main entrances

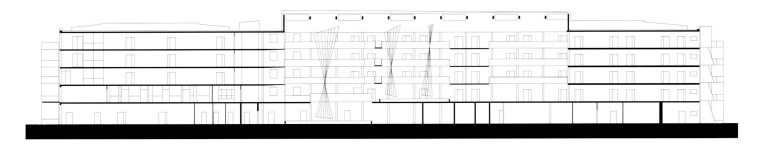

Section

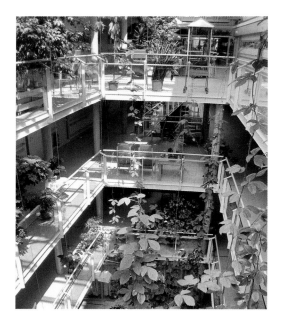

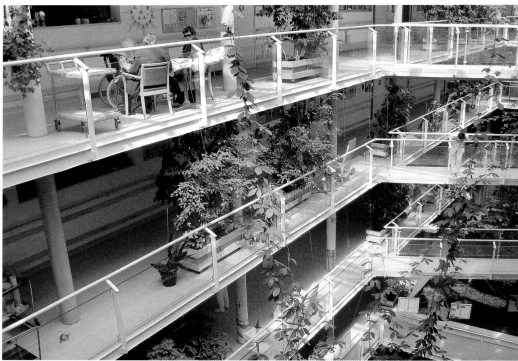

The entrance hall and greened atrium extends the height of the building and is crossed via diagonal walkways | Public café on the first floor

on the east and west open onto a "platform" on the first floor from which all parts of the clearly-arranged interior of the two-wing building can be seen, making it easy for residents to ascertain where they are. The popular sun terrace and fully-glazed winter garden and dining room with kitch-enette lie on the outer south and west ends re-spectively to encourage residents' to make their way there and be more mobile. The diagonally arranged narrow bridges through the atrium, by contrast, provide quick and direct access from the nurses' room to the individual resident's rooms.

The design of the rooms, also by Reinberg Archi-tects, is pleasant and light with wall panelling and furniture made of maple plywood and a green lino-leum floor. Next to each entrance doorway there is a tall narrow window which can be closed with a "shutter" from the inside. Like the glazed balus-trade of the interior walkways, it provides a view into the "world of the elderly residents" within. The upholstery of the chairs in the public interior space has been given slightly different shades of colour to create a sense of variety in the interior, especially as the day progresses and the interior is aglow with light.

In addition to the use of environmentally-friendly building materials and high-quality thermal insula-tion, Reinberg Architects also paid special atten-tion to energy efficiency: a mechanical ventilation system employing a system of controlled ventila-tion and heat recovery from the outgoing warm air, leads not only to a reduced energy demand and cost savings of around 35% but also helps improve the indoor air quality and with it the comfort and health of the residents. The air supply is routed vertically in prefabricated installation risers and ducts and horizontally within the suspended ceil-ings. Pre-filtered fresh air enters the room via a valve outlet and is also pre-cooled in summer.

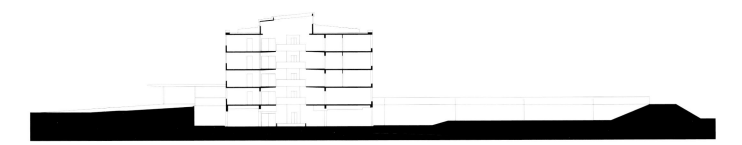

Section

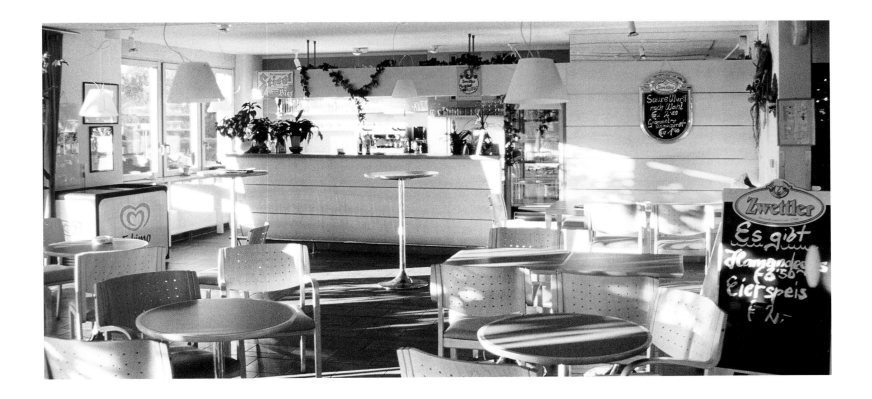

The latter is achieved using water-filled pipes laid 2 m beneath the ground, which utilise the natural coolness of the soil to cool the water using underground earth collectors.

The complex also has its own well which is used for watering the gardens and for process water. The water heating uses an energy-saving system using a twin-tank arrangement with a standby water tank and hot water storage tank, together with a stratified charging system. Airquality tests undertaken after completion of the building in the year 2000 showed that the building was free of hazardous substances.

All these qualities have rapidly become well-known and the nursing home in St. Pölten is now one of the most popular care homes in Austria. Plans are being made for a further extension and the addition of a hospice.

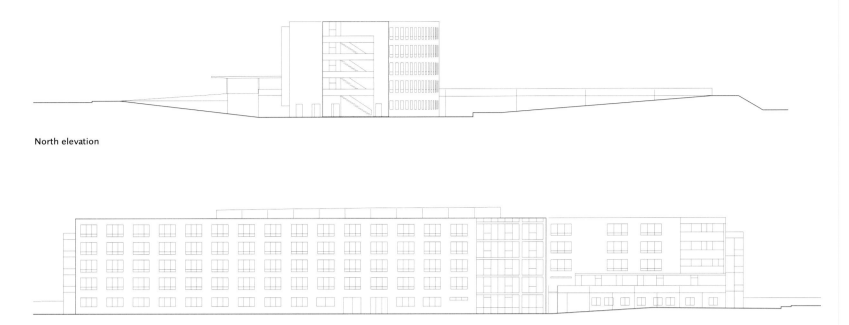

North elevation

West elevation

Direct barrier-free access from the Traisendamm along the river to the first floor

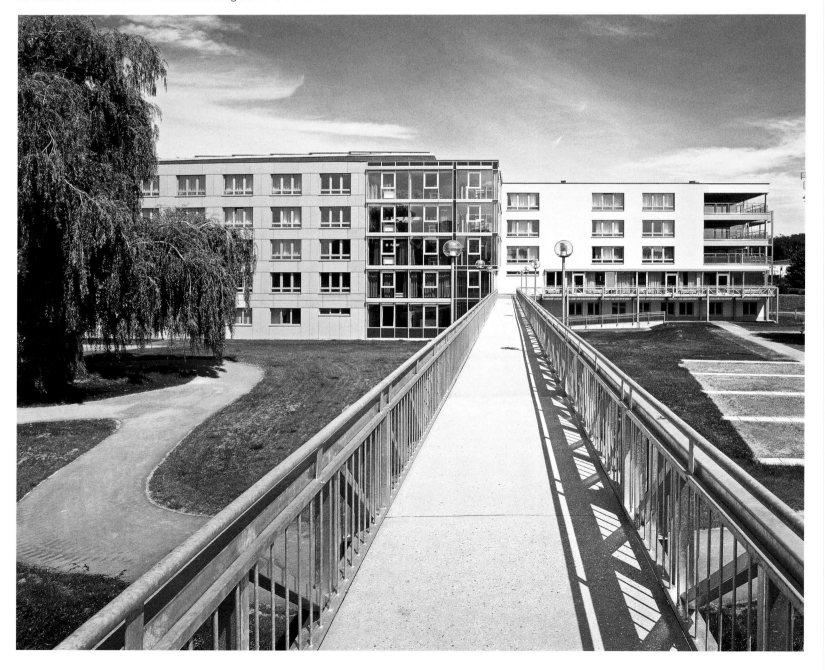

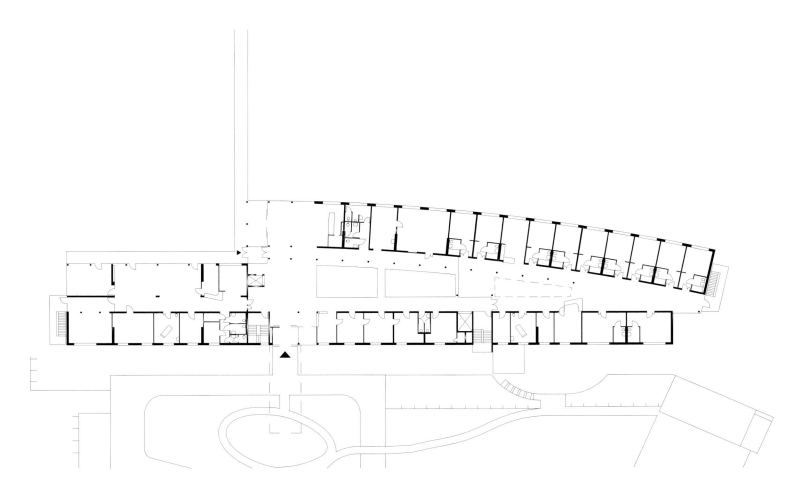

First floor plan

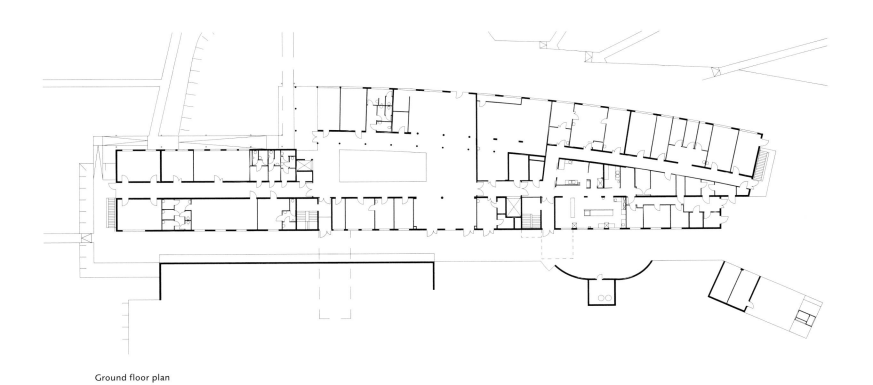

Ground floor plan

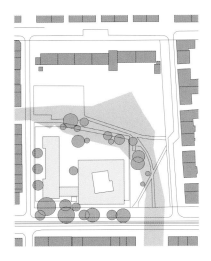

Site plan

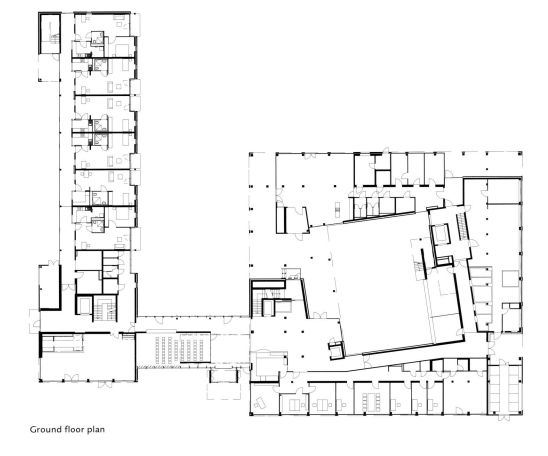

Ground floor plan

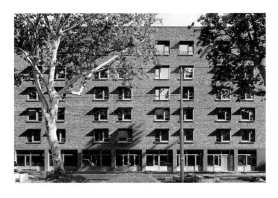

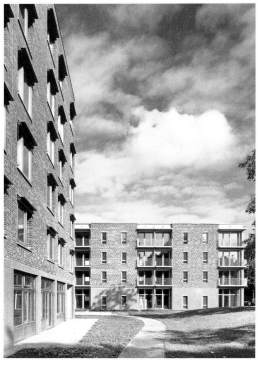

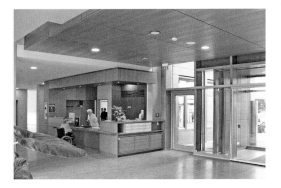

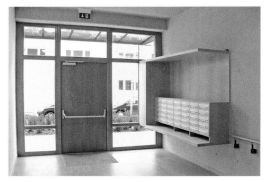

Street façade | Garden façade with rearward courtyard | Entrance area and reception | Entrance to the building with letterboxes

St. Anna Nursing Home

Karlsruhe, Germany

Architect	PIA-Architekten, Prof. A. Löffler, R. Schneider, M. Schmeling, G. Leicht
Client/Operator	Orden der barmherzigen Schwestern vom heiligen Vincenz von Paul
Completion	2005
Useable floor area	approx. 7,200 m²
Units/Capacity	120 persons in care 47 assisted living units

This complex of buildings, situated on a green site in the centre of Karlsruhe, is a model approach that aims to provide a home for elderly residents with a variety of different needs. In order to integrate the building into the greenery of the surroundings, all of the large trees were carefully retained, creating the impression that the building has stood on this spot for decades. Similarly, the subtle polychromatic colouring of the brickwork gives the building's face a delicately aged appearance, lending the complex a timeless dignity.

Both the sight lines and entrance situation as well as the massing of the building take their cue from

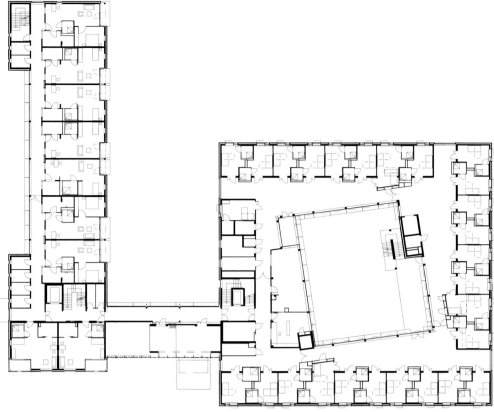

Upper floor plan

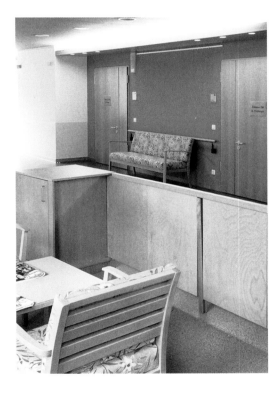

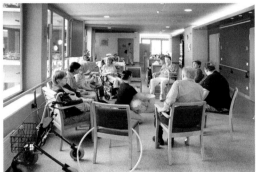

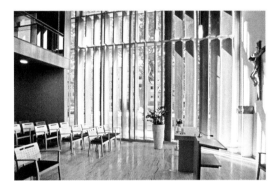

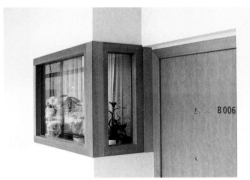

Example of the design of a residential corridor | Residential corridor with space to sit and chat | An entrance niche in the assisted living wing | Chapel

the local surroundings: the main building with a height of six storeys overlooks the street, while a second wing along a side street steps back and down to a height of four storeys to avoid blocking out the sun from the south for the neighbours. The square building is home to the nursing area, which is grouped around a central courtyard and can cater for 120 residents. On the fifth floor it contains a further 12 sheltered apartments. Day-care facilities are on the ground floor. A separate long building to one side houses a further 33 residences. Between the two parts, a connecting section contains all the public and communally used areas such as the foyer, chapel and consultation rooms.

The connecting building ensures that living areas and care facilities are closely linked so that residents who are in need of increased care do not have to leave their own four walls. The care area, with its single-loaded, glazed corridors arranged in a ring around the central courtyard, is designed to provide plenty of daylight as well as sufficient opportunity for movement. The rectangular courtyard is rotated with respect to the square plan of the building so that the corners of the corridors widen, creating lounge-like spaces that can be used for a variety of purposes. The corridors are analogous to street frontages, with benches in front of the entrances which are set back slightly from the

"street". Corner windows mark each "house" in the row. Using the internal staircase in the courtyard or the lift, resident dementia sufferers can descend from their storey and reach the courtyard and garden on their own without having to leave the building. In this way they are spared the feeling of being locked inside.

The compactness of the building, its economical use of space, the conservation of the trees and the solidity of the materials form the basis for a sustainable concept. Heat demand simulations were conducted during the design phase in order to optimise the building's performance.

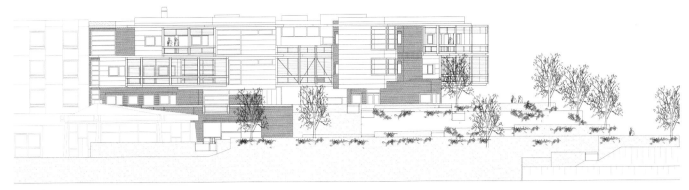

West elevation

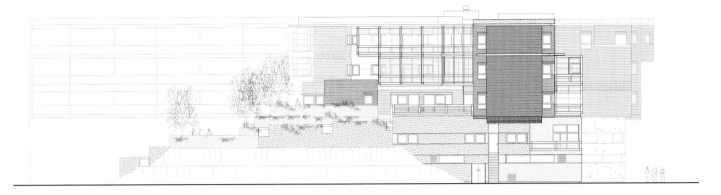

South elevation

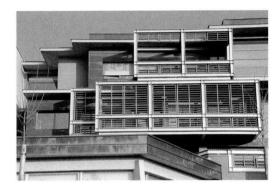

The two upper storeys, rotated by 30°, determine the building's appearance | Full-height glazing creates a relationship between indoors and outdoors | Unusual copper cladding grille on the volumes of the south-west façade

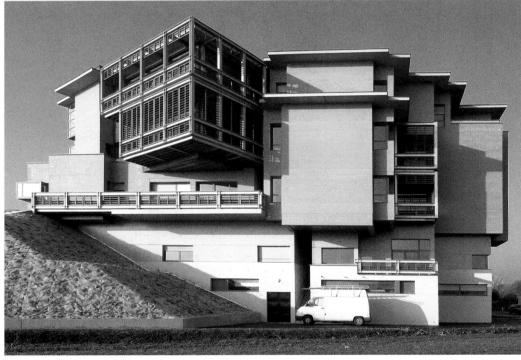

"Plaine de Scarpe" Nursing Home and Home for the Elderly

Lallaing, France

Architect	Yann Brunel
Client/Operator	Société de Secours Minière du Nord
Completion	2006
Useable floor area	new extension 3,978 m² existing building 7,065 m²
Units/Capacity	140 geriatric residents, 17 Alzheimer residents

The elongated L-shaped complex is capped by a distinctive stepped, pyramidal extension at its south-west end and is a modernisation and refurbishment of the existing "Plaine de Scarpe" nursing home built in the 1970s that no longer fulfilled contemporary requirements. In addition to providing disabled access, the competition submission in 2000 divided the existing three-bed rooms into a series of single rooms of different character and proposed a new extension providing space for a further 53 residents, including a wing for Alzheimer sufferers, modern therapy rooms and communal spaces. Yann Brunel's design exceeded the requirements of the brief and

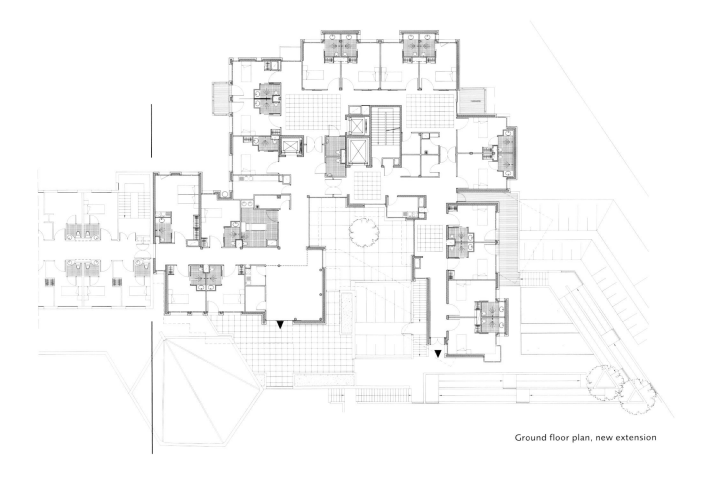

Ground floor plan, new extension

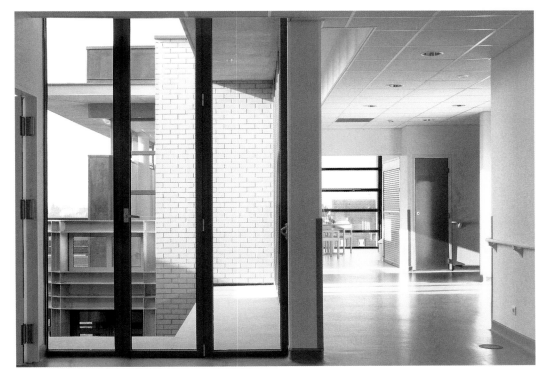

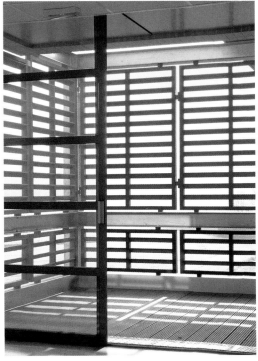

challenged the wisdom of generally-applicable uniform solutions for housing for the elderly. His design aims to provide a variety of quite different spaces that cater for residents with different characters and needs.

Four different types of accommodation were designed: a "conventional living area" with a spacious bathroom designed to accommodate the needs of geriatric residents; a "terrace type" featuring direct access to an outdoor space; a suite, also known as "therapeutic studio", that can be arranged flexibly, for example using sliding doors, and is conceived especially for couples;

and lastly a "communicative living area" for more gregarious residents with a greater desire to interact with one another. Double doors, which can be left open as required, entrance areas in front of the rooms, and corridors that widen to form communal areas with seating encourage contact between the residents and their neighbours.

The solidity of the brickwork and the high quality of the materials communicate a feeling of homeliness and comfort. The 30-degree rotation of the two upper storeys and the indented frames of the galvanised steel balconies lend the building a distinctive external appearance.

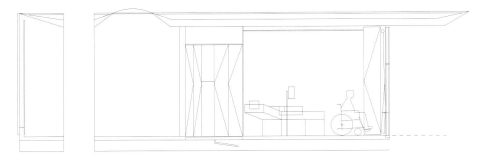

Concept of resident's room

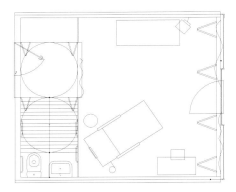

Plan of resident's room

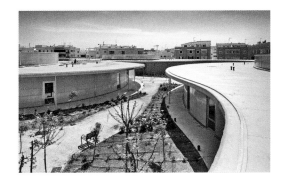

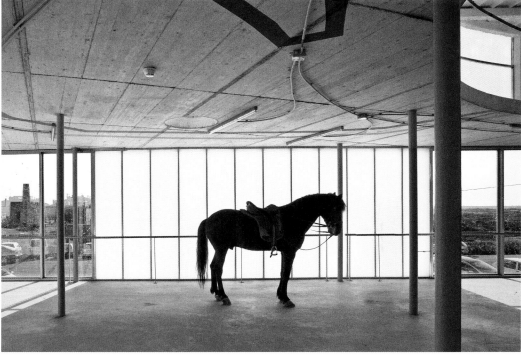

The ring of rooms encloses an internal courtyard garden |
Generously proportioned circulation space | View of the
complex, which is situated on a filled-in gravel pit

Santa Rita
Geriatric Centre

Ciutadella, Menorca, Spain

Architect	Manuel Ocaña del Valle
Client /Operator	CIME / Conseil Insular de Menorca
Completion	2007
Useable floor area	building 5,990 m², external works 6,200 m²
Units /Capacity	70 residents, 20 day-care users

In addition to creating a facility that provides residents with the necessary privacy, accessibility, security and independence in the last phase of their lives, a primary concern of the architects was to design a building that does not look like a hospital. Long monotonous corridors in particular were to be avoided. Manuel Ocaña's design is instead characterised by a sense of openness: access and circulation areas are generous and promenades non-prescriptive in their direction, opening up multiple perspectives that stimulate the residents, encouraging them to "discover" their environment. The distinctive form of the building, a loop inscribed in the topography of a filled-in quarry, was

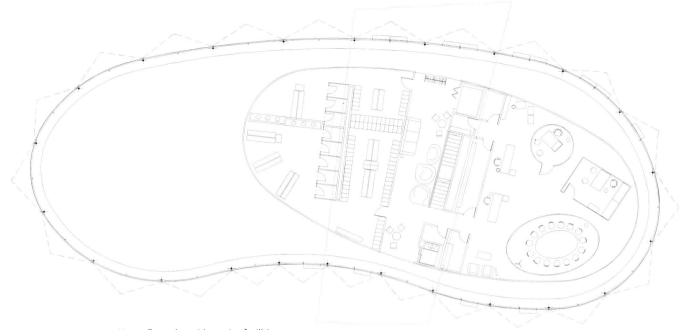

Upper floor plan with service facilities

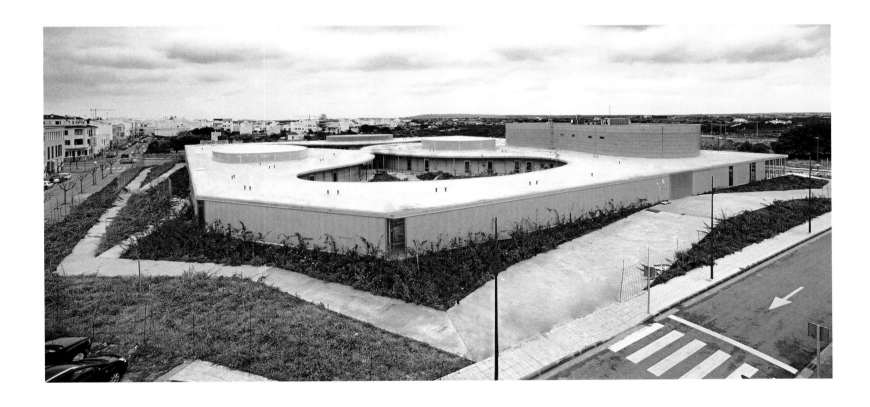

developed outwards from a basic core unit: the resident's room. Each room is generously proportioned with light and modern furnishings and two separate means of access. Arranged one behind the other, the rooms are strung like beads in a free-form loop that encloses a large interior garden accessible from each and every room.

The snaking band of rooms sits inside a rectangular plot with an exterior façade made of translucent double-wall polycarbonate sheeting, with additional shading elements depending on orientation. Coloured surfaces and plastic panelling emphasise the respective atmospheric effects of

the light: blue and green tones for the cool light to the north, yellow for the warmer light on the south and west façades. The ceiling consists of a bare slab of reinforced concrete painted with coloured lines that pick up the contours of the topography of the former quarry below.

Colour highlights are also used to provide additional orientation in each of the three "living loops" and their respective courtyards as well as in the different therapy areas in the geriatric centre: the walling of the freestanding disabled toilets, the lines on the ceilings and even the planting outdoors follow a consistent palette in each of the zones.

The space between the rooms and the outside walls of the building runs around the entire perimeter, varying in width and extending sometimes deep into the interior. It forms a flowing, open and connecting space in which all manner of activities can take place. Rather than having to follow prescribed routes, one can move around the building freely, going from A to B without always following the same path. The atmospheric qualities of this connecting space also change from zone to zone, making moving around an experience that stimulates the senses. The different zones, their changing degree of enclosure and lightness, allow the residents to decide spontaneously which way they

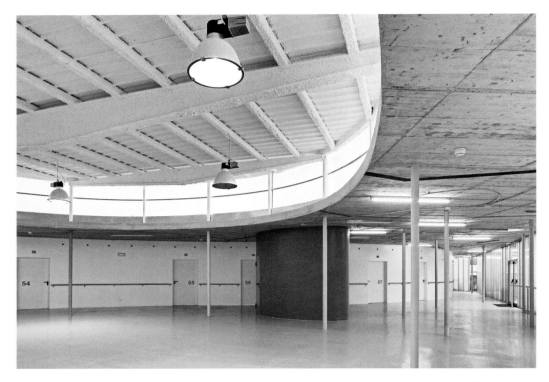

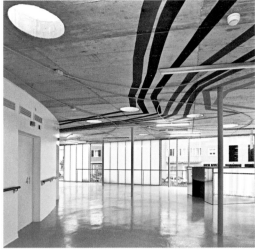

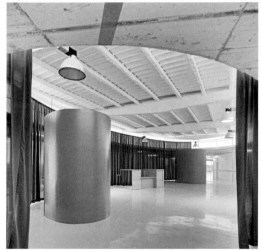

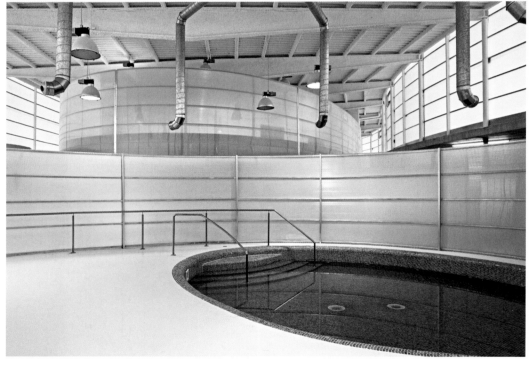

Three views of omnidirectional circulation spaces in the green, orange and red zones | Swimming pool in the blue zone of the two-storey service facilities

would like to go and where they want to rest, according to their mood and physical constitution.

The project was realised on a very tight budget – 6000 m² were realised for the price of 4000 m² – and priority was given to providing key geriatric facilities and the most essential fittings. Most of the furnishings and finishes, in particular the technical installations, have been left exposed, almost bare. The architects have tried to be as economical as possible with the construction in order to free up remaining funds for supposedly "pointless" things, citing the Dadaist credo that it is the pointless things which one can least do without in life.

The centre opened in 2008, and it remains to be seen whether this comparatively cool and futuristic facility will be embraced by its users in the warm climes of the island of Menorca.

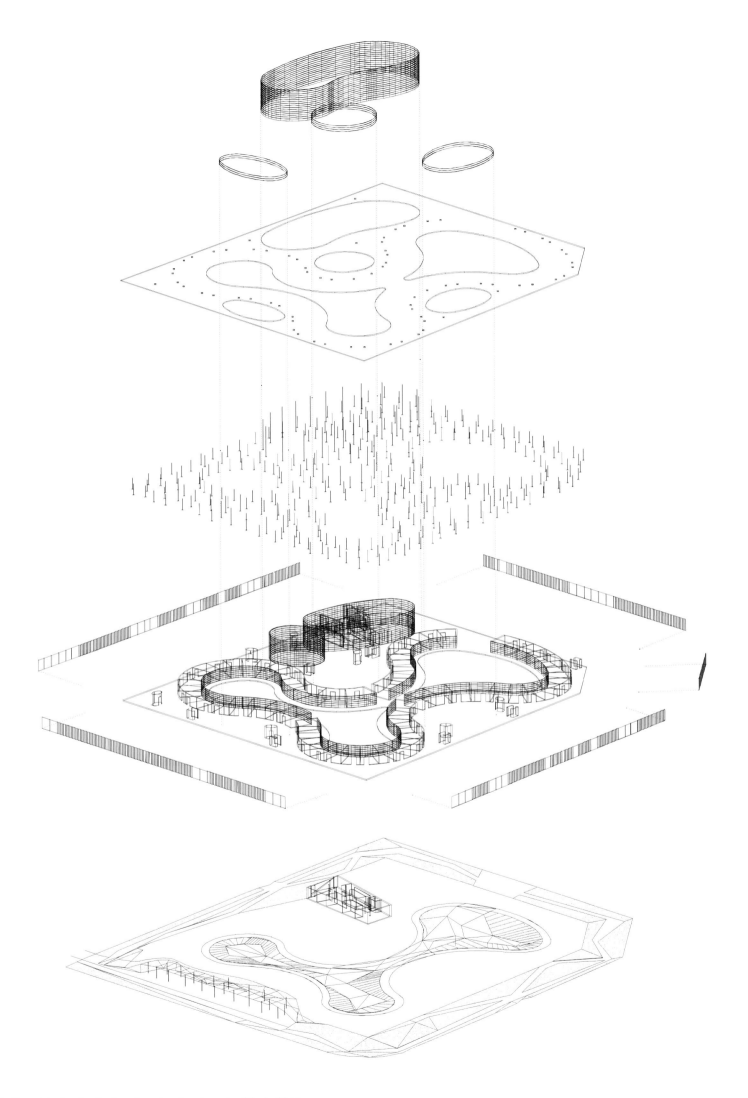

Exploded isometric showing the formal construction elements of the building

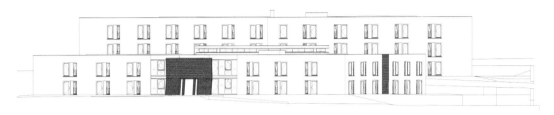

West elevation

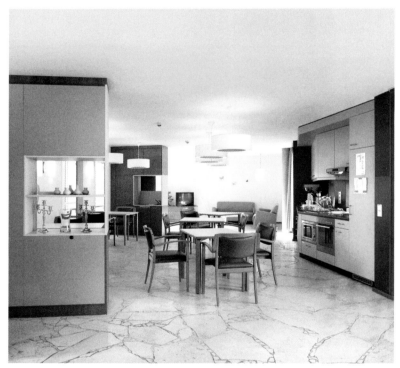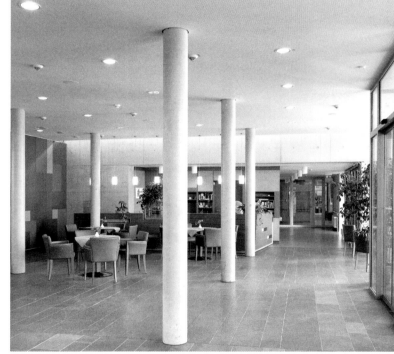

St. Michael Centre for the Elderly

Berlin, Germany

Architect	GAP Gesellschaft für Architektur und Projektmanagement mbH
Client	St. Hedwig Krankenhaus
Completion	2004
Useable floor area	6,117 m² (net useable floor area)
Units / Capacity	120 residents in care 6 two-room and 7 single-room assisted living apartments

Situated on the south-east outskirts of Berlin on a sloping site, the design by GAP Architekten responds to the contours of the site through a stepped arrangement of the buildings. The site borders a public landscape park to the north and a housing estate to the south and west. An existing hospital on the eastern part of the site adjoins the St. Michael Centre for the Elderly, constituting a functional unit with it.

The topography of the site and the terraced arrangement of the buildings provide expansive views out over the landscape. The central element is a glazed entrance hall which serves as

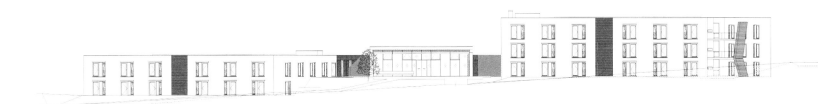

South elevation

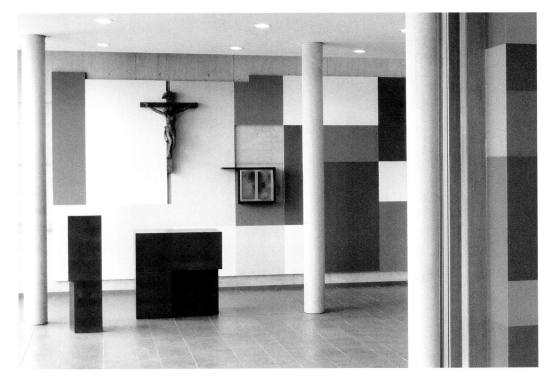

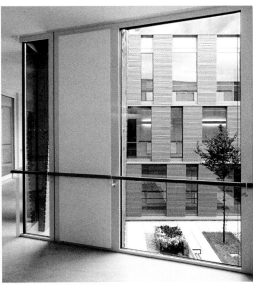

Open communal kitchen | Café in the entrance hall | Chapel on the ground floor with orthogonal pattern of yellow, orange and red panels on the wall | The light-filled access corridor overlooks the interior courtyard

a meeting and communication area with a café, a multi-purpose hall and a chapel. The nursing and care areas lie on each side of the spacious foyer along with 20 apartments for assisted living, which can also be accessed via an entrance of their own.

In contrast to the rendered external façades that face the neighbouring buildings, all private areas and interior courtyards have been clad with façade panels made of timber and glass. The larch timber has been stained grey to counteract the uneven ageing of the wood, and the premounted, storey-high timber façade elements are also slightly in-

clined to reduce the degree of weathering. The timber sections alternate with storey-high glass windows and are divided horizontally by metal weather strips on each floor. The terraces on the external façades have also been given a slatted larch cladding, setting them apart from the rendered façades.

In the design of the care areas, the architects have followed a therapy concept that motivates the residents, each according to their own ability, to remain mobile. This fundamental principle begins in the rooms themselves with the design of the windows, which were developed especially

for this building. The low sill affords a good view out over the landscape from the resident's bed, allowing the eye to wander, while a shelf integrated in the window invites residents to decorate and personalise their window with items of their own. As an interface between inside and outside, the window is an especially important element for people whose ability to shape their own environment has become increasingly limited. The window element is therefore the centrepiece of every room: it functions as a "display window", as a "flower window" and as a "platform for items of personal value". This effect is visible from inside as well as from outside, giving passers-by

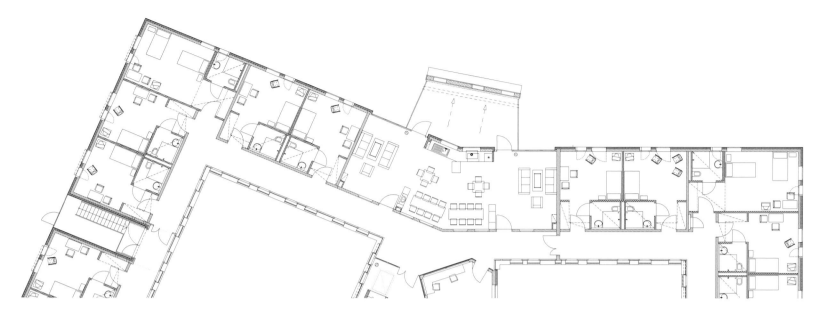

Ground floor plan, detail

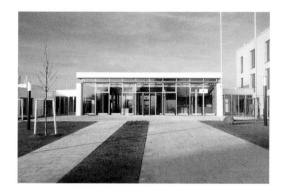
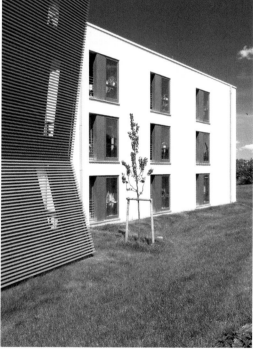
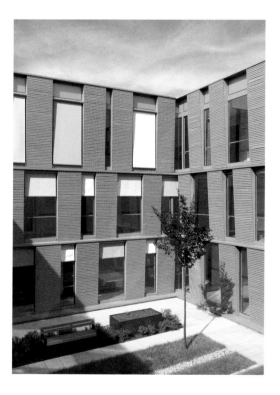

Glazed entrance area on the south side of the complex |
Timber elements in front of the balconies screen them from
view | Alternating pattern of closed and open surfaces and
adjustable blinds

and visitors an impression of each individual, and at the same time helping residents to identify with their surroundings.

The corridors are light-filled, glazed walkways, arranged in a ring around the courtyard gardens, which have been planted by the residents themselves. Various seating areas provide an opportunity for residents to spend time outside. The gallery leads past a common room with its own small kitchen and a sheltered balcony with a view out over the landscape. The slatted timber front of the balcony provides a sense of privacy for the residents. The staff rooms are situated so that

the staff can always see the residents moving around, providing additional reassurance for the residents. The residents are, of course, free to leave their floor, meet up with others in the common areas in the entrance hall or spend time outside in the garden. To aid orientation, the wall that leads from the entrance hall to the care areas has a special glass-fibre wall-covering that is painted and has a random structure.

A further visual highlight is the chapel, which, with its orthogonal arrangement of yellow, red and orange colours on the walls, is clearly differentiated from the other spaces in the build-

ing. It is used primarily as a space for prayer and meditation, but sometimes also together with an adjoining hall for larger events.

The construction of the entire complex varies with the load-bearing capacity of the soil and its position with regard to a water conservation area. The buildings containing the care facilities are predominantly masonry constructions and have no underground cellars, only an installations channel made of water-impervious concrete along the line of the bathrooms which can be accessed for maintenance purposes. This avoided the need for expensive double-wall sheathing for all the

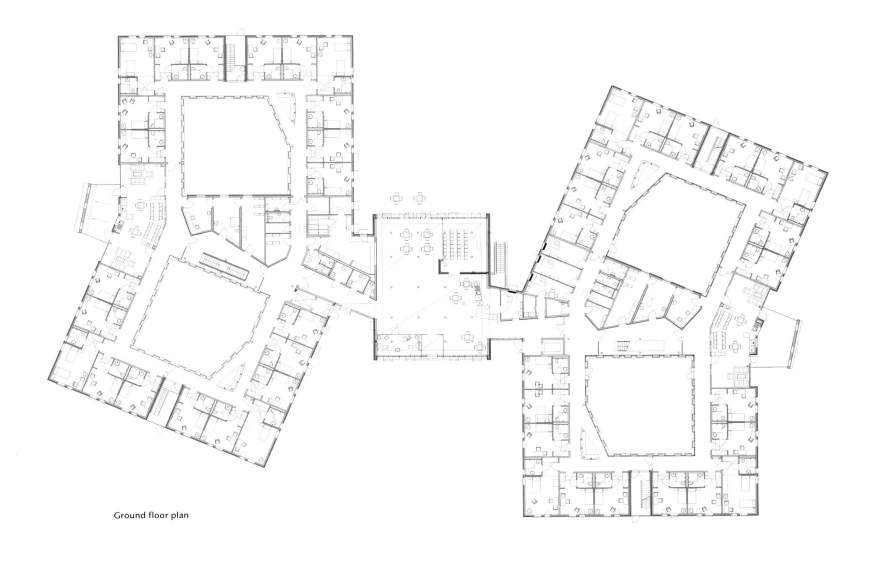

Ground floor plan

subterranean drainage pipes. Only the reinforced
concrete frame construction of the entrance hall
has a cellar for storage purposes, staff changing
rooms and plant rooms.

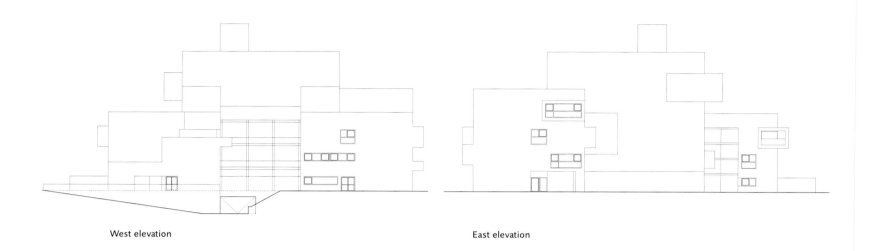

West elevation

East elevation

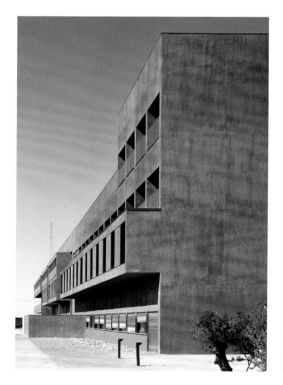

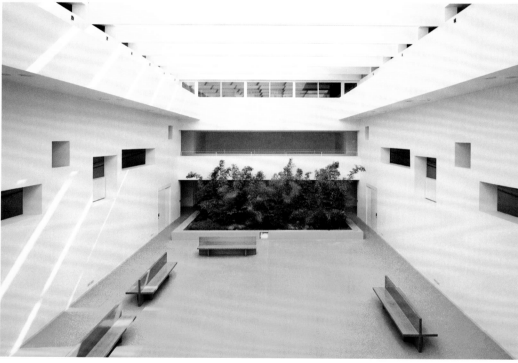

Residencia Alcázar Juan Hermanitas Ancianos

Alcázar de San Juan, Spain

Architect	Ignacio Vicens y Hualde José Antonio Ramos Abengozar
Client/Operator	Congregación de las Hermanitas de los Ancianos Desamparados
Completion	1997
Useable floor area	15,000 m²
Units/Capacity	150 residents

Two key factors determine the appearance of this large architectural structure in the Spanish province of Ciudad Real, which serves as a home for the elderly: firstly, the specific requirements of the extensive programme of spaces for the interior of the building, which follows the rules of the order of the Congregación de las Hermanitas de los Ancianos Desamparados (Congretation of the Sisters of the Elderly and Homeless), who own and run the old people's home; secondly, its specific location between the city and the open landscape in an area otherwise occupied by light industry and the municipal sewage treatment works. The provincial town of Alcázar de San Juan is situated in the middle of

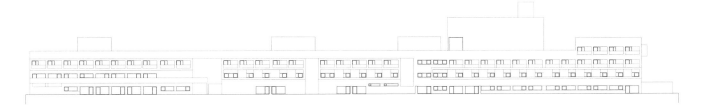

North elevation

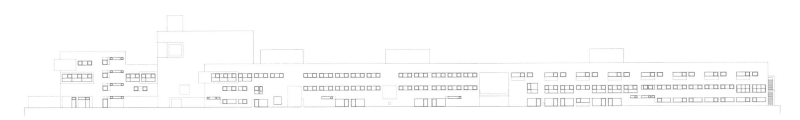

South elevation

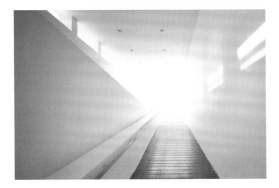

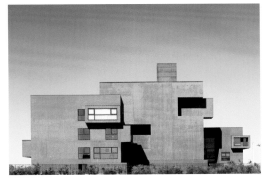

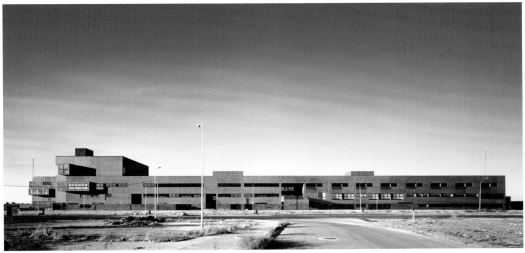

Rust-red colouring of the iron-sulphate pigment in the render | Foyer |
Light-flooded access corridor | Building volumes seen from the east |
The elongated building seen from the north

the Mancha, a somewhat barren and bizarre land-scape whose wide expanses are interrupted by ranges and valleys alternating with a gridded patch-work of vineyards and olive groves.

Despite its strategic location on the direct rail route between Madrid and the Mediterranean, the city has managed to withstand outside influences and maintain its traditions and rural character. The his-toric town centre is home to baroque churches and monasteries as well as the tower of the "Alcázar", the Moorish fortress that gives the town its name. The elongated volume of the "Asilo de Ancianos" is arranged at right angles to the grain of the city and

clearly demarcates the edge of the town: to its west open landscape, an industrial estate to the north, a bullring and hospital to the east and the local by-pass road to the south.

The sizeable volume of the building has a distinct, uniform rust-red colouring achieved by mixing iron-sulphate pigment into the external render. This coloration creates a visual connection to the sandstone, of which the majority of the old town is built, and to the characteristic colour of the Man-cha. It also lends the building a readily identifiable and consistent appearance, helping the staff and residents relate to it as "their" building.

To fulfil the aforementioned requirements, the architects Ignacio Vicens and José Antonio Ramos proposed a straightforward arrangement of two par-allel strips punctuated with spaces and open areas of different characters. A larger rectangular section containing the chapel – open to both residents and the local inhabitants – connects the two strips and also relates through its size to the eastern edge of the town.

The rules of the Catholic order, which has a follow-ing in Spain and South America, decree that single men, single women and married couples have their own separate living areas. The internal structure

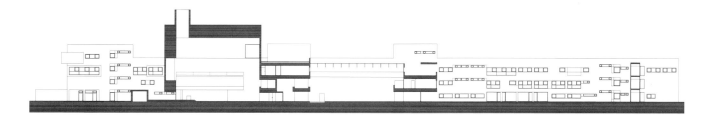

Section – elevation

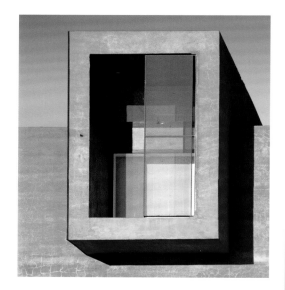

Façade detail | Two slightly-offset parallel buildings from an internal courtyard

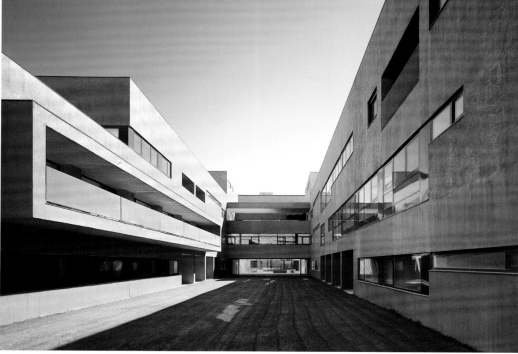

of the building therefore has to provide two sets of canteens, common rooms and patients' rooms, separated according to gender. In addition, there is a separate wing for the sisters of the order, for therapy rooms, the kitchens, laundry and other ancillary facilities. All these areas are clearly delineated architectonically, while at the same time the architects have attempted to link them via the external spaces. The living areas and corridors open out onto entrance lobbies, sometimes one storey high, sometimes three, so that old people with impaired mobility can still enjoy the natural surroundings and sunlight. These are complemented by a series of variously-sized patios cut out of the volume of the

building, and walled gardens and terraces on the upper floors that are linked to the spaces within. The chapel likewise opens onto a small courtyard whose seasonally changing vegetation forms a background to the altar. The interlocking nature of indoor and outdoor spaces also applies to the colour and texture of the building and gardens, which are planted with local species. Cypresses and olive trees provide shade, while rosemary, thyme and lavender stimulate the senses with their aroma.

In the interior, the ochre-coloured brick flooring contrasts with the whitewashed walls which reflect the changing sunlight over the course of the day.

The linearity of the corridors is interrupted by perpendicular views into the open lobby areas; the opposite sides of the walls are structured with stretches of birch veneer doors and panelling.

The simple treatment of the surfaces and the homogenous appearance of the exterior of the building contrast with the spatial richness of the interior and reflect the notion of monastic sacrifice. The contrasting rich materiality of the chapel is therefore all the more impressive. The use of Roman travertine, Venetian stucco lustro and gold leaf within the strict geometry and rectangular forms can be seen as a contemporary interpretation of

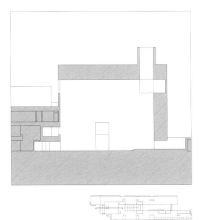
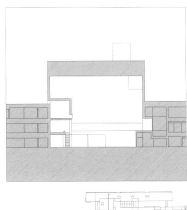
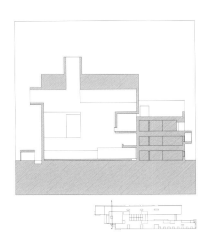
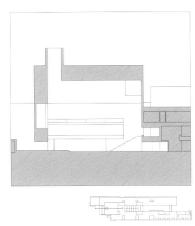

Cross section through the chapel

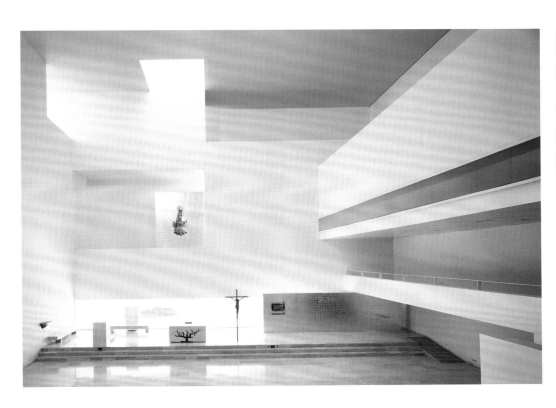

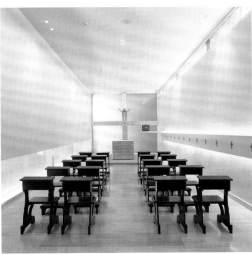

Interior of the chapel | Oratory

baroque altar spaces. The architects pay particular attention to the powerful effect of light whose physical presence is symbolised and heightened in the glistening gold of the surfaces.

The sculptural treatment of the wall behind the altar in the chapel forms an abstract cross out of shafts of light and projections and recesses in the wall. A small oratory for private worship, accessible only from the sister's living quarters on the third floor, projects into the interior of the chapel. This room appears to float above the gallery, allowing daylight to spill into the chapel through a glazing strip just above floor level. For the architects this is an ex-

pression of a central principle of the order founded in 1873: in the same way that the work of the nuns is dedicated to the well-being of the old people living in their care, here too the oratory designed especially for the sisters of the order also gives light to the residents of the home.

Although without doubt the architecture of the building provides a good environment for living in, the question remains as to whether this form of care for the elderly is able to give people a real sense of home and whether old age is the right phase in life with which to subordinate oneself to such a strict regime so unlike one's previous way of life.

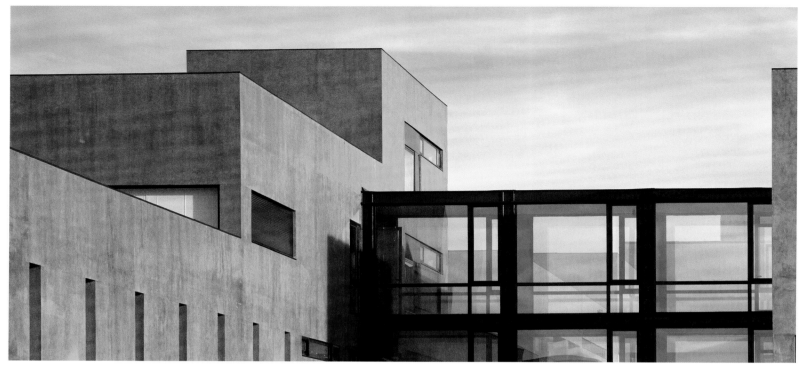

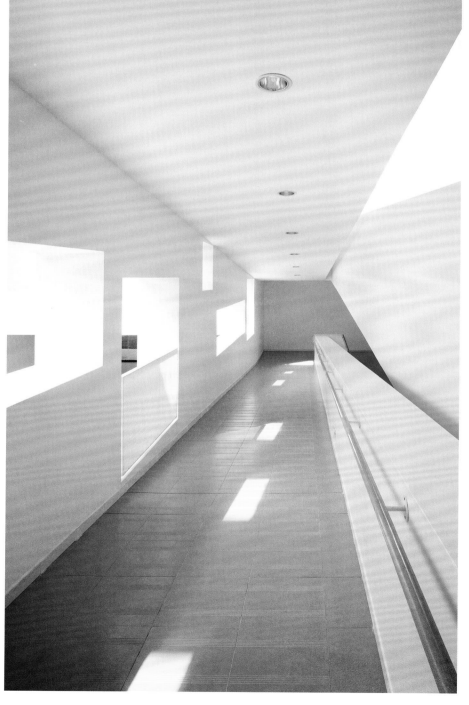

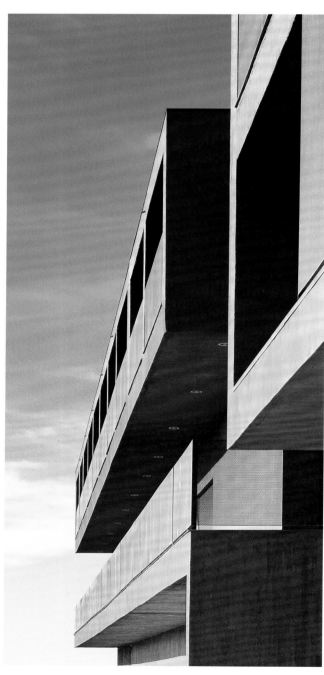

Light and almost transparent connecting walkways | Linear corridor with views out to the side | Rigorous geometric articulation of the façades

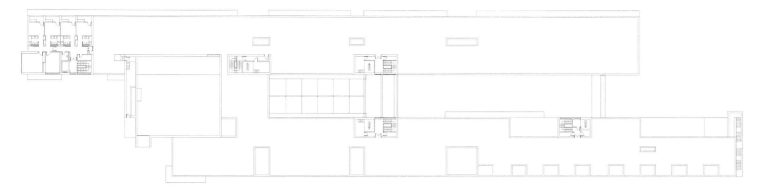

Rooftop plan

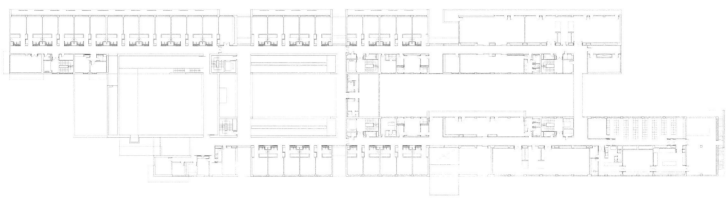

Second floor plan

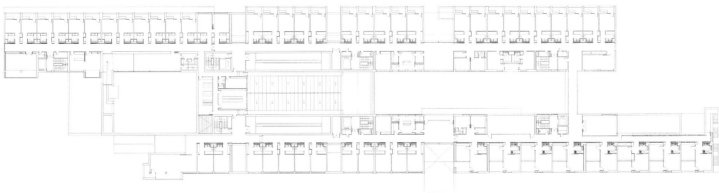

First floor plan

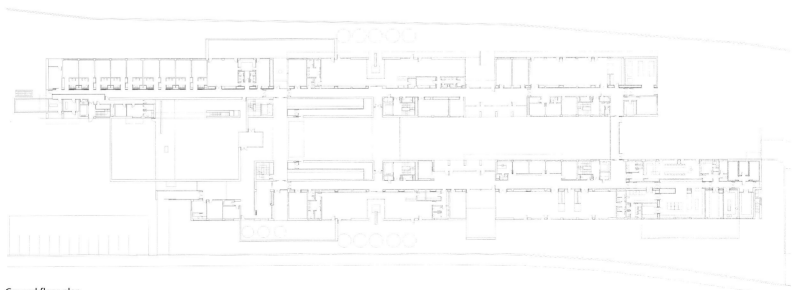

Ground floor plan

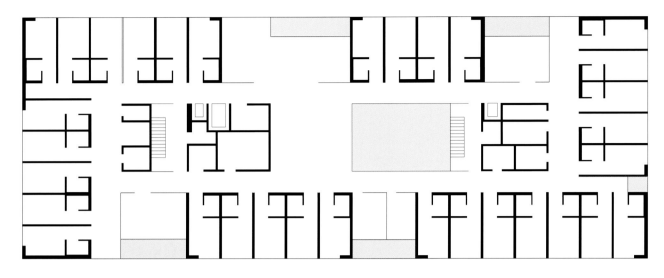

Second floor plan

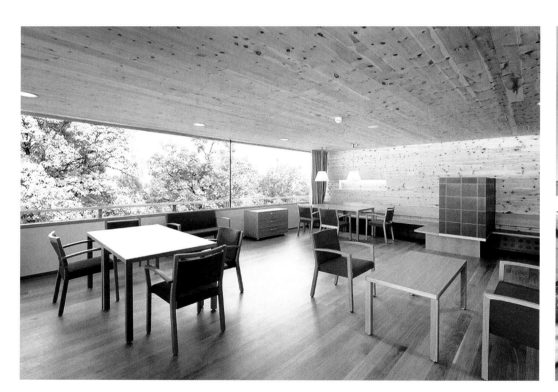

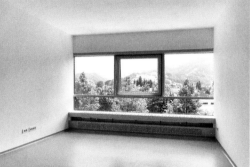

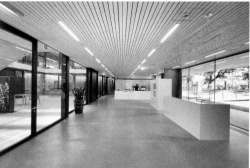

Nursing home

Dornbirn, Austria

Architect	ARGE Riepl Riepl Architekten Johannes Kaufmann Architektur
Client/Operator	City of Dornbirn
Completion	2005
Useable floor area	7,316 m²
Units/Capacity	108 residents

Commissioned by the City of Dornbirn, the building stands alongside an existing nursing home in a park-like landscape and exhibits in its architectural design both clarity and openness as well as spatial variety and differentiation. The alternating arrangement of flush-fitted window bands and the raised parapets of the communal terraces lend the façades of the clear-cut, rectangular volume a certain tension. The precise, narrow incisions of the terraces heighten this impression, creating a vibrant play of light and shadow in the otherwise balanced arrangement of the façade. In the construction of the four-storey timber structure, special attention was given to the

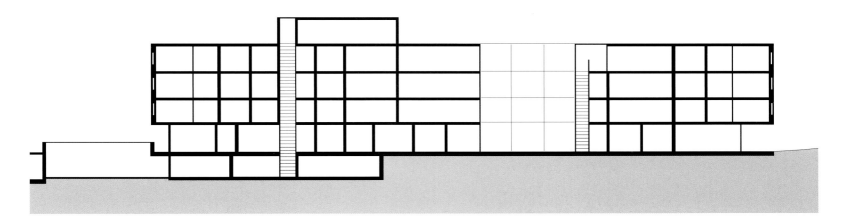

Longitudinal section

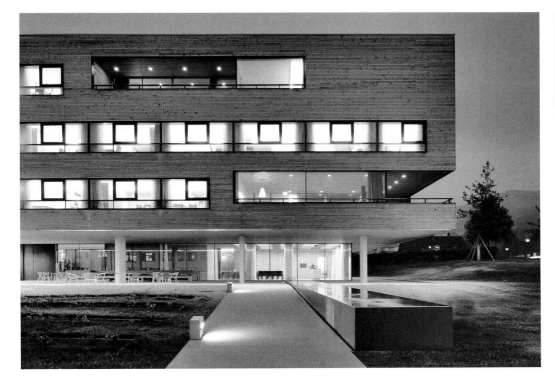

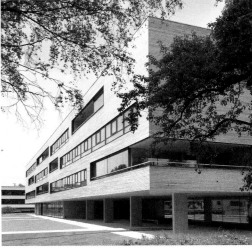

Generous use of wood in the interiors | Very low window sills in the resident's rooms | Strongly linear directionality of the spacious entrance area | A timber structure with window strips arranged flush with the façade | Narrow, precise incisions in the façade mark the position of the communal terraces on each floor

selection of ecologically friendly materials as well as a well-insulated building envelope to create a building that is efficient for both client and user alike. For the architects it was also important to create as much openness as possible through the use of extensive glazing, breaking down the boundary between indoors and outdoors. The French windows in the residents' rooms extend almost to the floor, affording a view out over the park from the bed or a chair.

The three upper floors of the building rest on a glazed plinth set back from the façade so that the building appears to float delicately above the

ground. The exceptionally spacious design of the ground floor is punctuated by open areas which allow residents to go outdoors and move about even in unfavourable weather conditions. Room-like courtyards in the interior offer countless views across the complex and a full-height atrium lends the home transparency and provides an overview. The generous use of wood throughout for the walls and ceilings as well as the furniture, all made by a local joiner, respond to the residents' need for security and comfort.

The individual clusters of rooms are each gathered around a central area – the "market square"

– which features large-format photos of familiar scenes in and around Dornbirn.

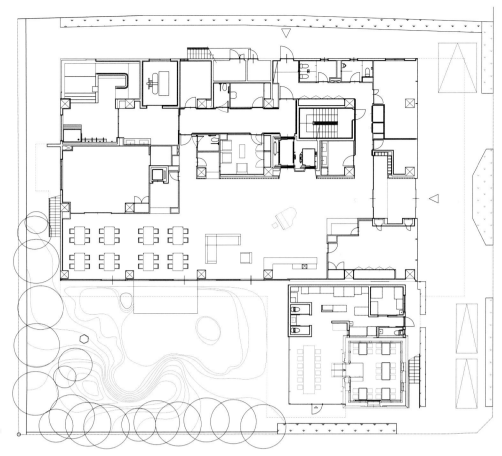

First floor plan

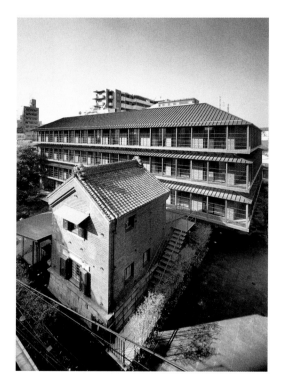

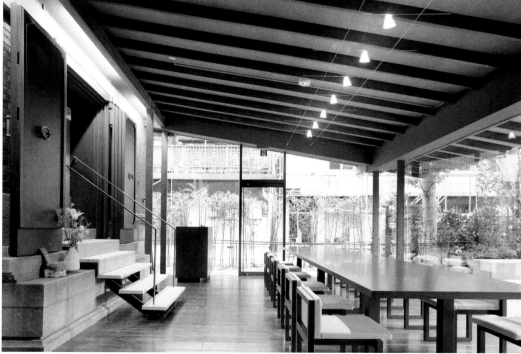

Nezu Withus

Nezu, Tokyo, Japan

Architect	Kengo Kuma & Associates
Building contractor	Kuboco
Completion Date	2005
Useable floor area	2,940 m²
Units/Capacity	47 single rooms, 4 twin rooms

The Withus is a senior citizens' residence offering nursing care. The building faces a narrow lane in Nezu, an old district in downtown Tokyo where one still finds old wooden houses standing in rows. The aim of the design for Withus Nezu was to retain the specific atmosphere of the wooden Tajima residence that had existed on the site from the Meiji Period (1868-1912).

The building is centred around the garden, which belonged to the old residence and was preserved as it was. In a densely populated area like Nezu, such a garden rich in greenery and birds was an indispensable asset for the community. Siding board façades face the street and the

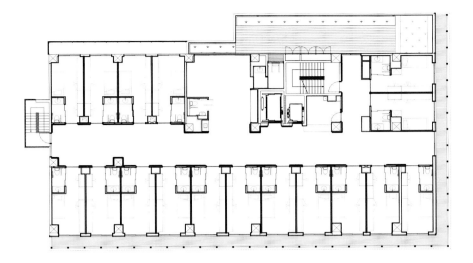

Roof level floor plan

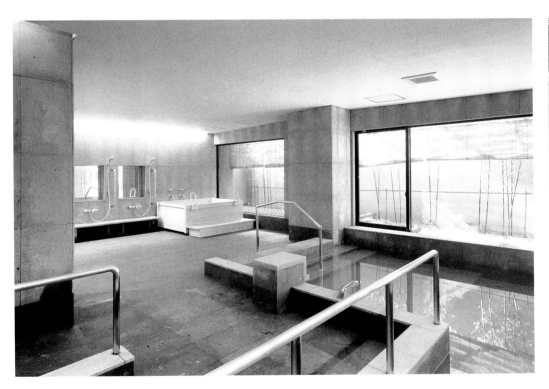

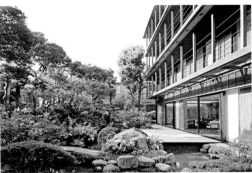

Entrance area with historical warehouse building which houses a noodle restaurant open to the public | Dining room with view towards the entrance | Bathing area | Sumptuous greenery of the Japanese Garden

garden. An existing brick warehouse situated in the north-west was moved to the corner of the site to serve as a semi-public dining space, where people from outside are welcome. In this way the residents have the opportunity to mix with their neighbours from the area.

Materials and remains from the former residence were used for the new building: the old pillars support the exterior eaves, shoji screens function as mobile partitions. The stone slab in the entrance became a bench. The integration of these elements helped to create the unique atmosphere of traditional Japanese houses.

Shading plays a significant role in Japanese houses. Formerly, the deep eaves and roof of the Tajima house resulted in a succession of shading elements that protected the interior from strong sunlight. The same idea was applied in the new residence. Broad shading elements protect the openings. The pebbles and water in the garden reflect natural light deep inside the room.

A large hall on the first floor facing the garden, another important element of traditional Japanese houses, offers a place to welcome visitors, enjoy seasonal events and dine. The hall connects to the rehabilitation facilities around it. Access to the bathroom, members' room and barber, ar-

ranged to the north of the hall, is separated from the other facilities in order to maintain the residents' privacy. Their living rooms are arranged in two different sections – one for patients with cognitive difficulties and the other for general residents. The patients have easy access to communal space and are allowed to walk around freely in order to alleviate the symptoms of their condition.

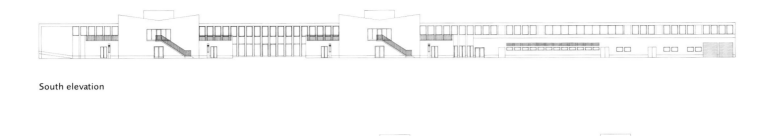

South elevation

North elevation

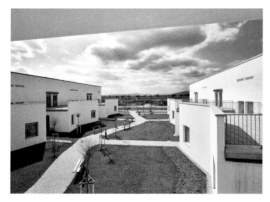

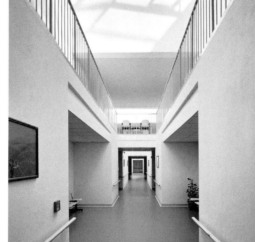

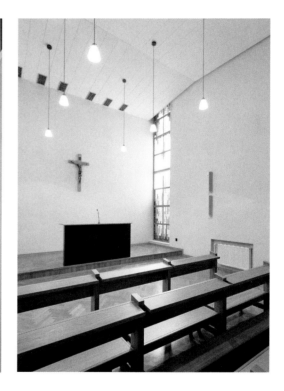

Two parallel residential rows | Naturally lit internal corridor
with small niches in front of each group of residents' rooms |
Interior of the chapel | Two residential wings are "skewered"
by a long service wing | The entire complex forms a "white
village" | Pairs of splayed gable walls face each other

Jezárka Home
for the Elderly

Strakonice, Czech Republic

Architect	Libor Monhart, Vladímir Krajíc
Client	Vojenské Stavby a.s., Protom s.r.o. (Company representing client)
Operator	City of Strakonice
Completion	2000
Useable floor area	6,975 m²
Units/Capacity	120 residents

The small white "village" built in the rolling hills of
south Bohemia by the municipality of Strakonice
for its elderly citizens clearly responds to a need for
peace and seclusion while avoiding creating a sense
of isolation among its residents. On the one hand
there is a school, hotel and residential estate of detached houses in its immediate vicinity, on the other
some of the home's outdoor facilities and common
rooms as well as the café and the chapel in the main
wing are open to the public.

The guiding principle or design idea that informed
the planning, which began in 1995, was to unite
tradition and modernism both in its architecture as

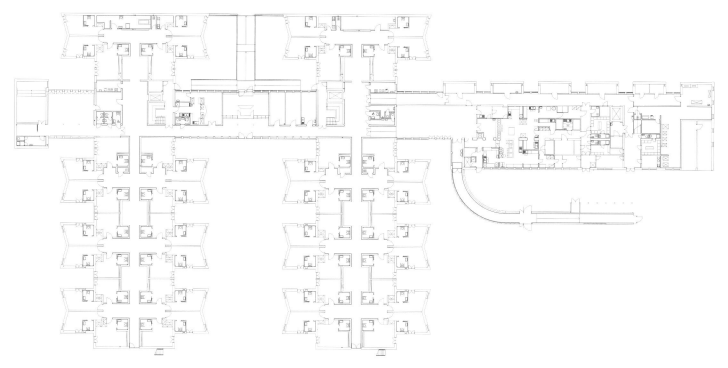

First floor plan

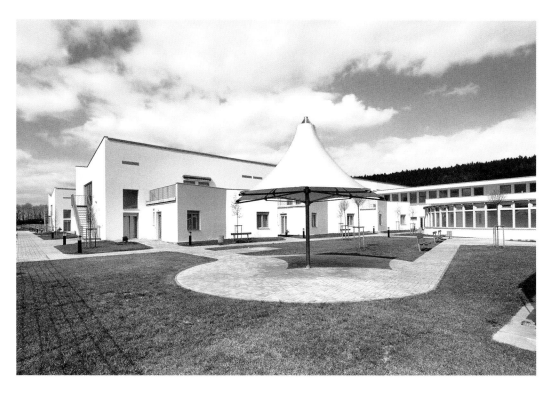

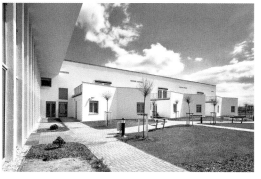

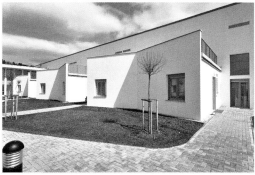

well as concept. The result is an example of "classical modernism" that reveres unadorned exteriors and inner functionalism while simultaneously upholding traditional notions of security, solidity and comfort. The architects therefore consciously avoided extensive glazing, metal elements and the like, building the complex as a brick construction and rendering the façades with a white plaster.

The complex consists of two parallel two-storey rows of apartments, divided into four segments which are pierced at right angles by a long building to the north that runs the length of the site. From the main entrance hall in this section, one can reach the administrative offices and all the common rooms as well as the two residential wings. The ground-floor apartments are arranged in pairs so that two doorways share a common entrance niche. This is reflected on the outside in the splayed frontages of the two apartments that face one another.

The upper storey is reserved for residents with more limited mobility who leave the building only rarely. Each of the single rooms on this floor adjoins a generous terrace so that the residents have immediate and easy access to the world outside. Residents who stay outdoors for any length of time are rewarded by changing patterns of light and shadow thrown across the white walls by the alternately open and solid balustrades, the projecting fire escape or the green of the lawns, which reflects gently off the walls as the day progresses.

The outdoor areas are criss-crossed with an unusually dense network of pathways between the individual sections of the building and segments of the residential wings. For the architects Libor Monhart and Vladimír Krajíc, this was particularly important in order to provide maximum access to the lawns, trees, benches and paths, in short to everything that makes life pleasant in the surroundings of one's home.

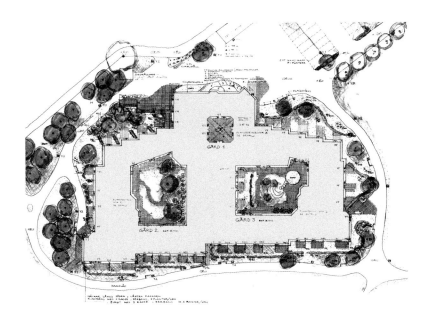

Site plan

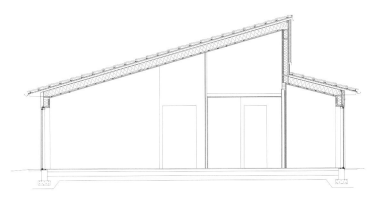

Section through terraced house

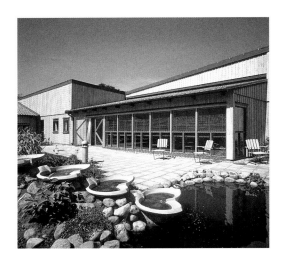

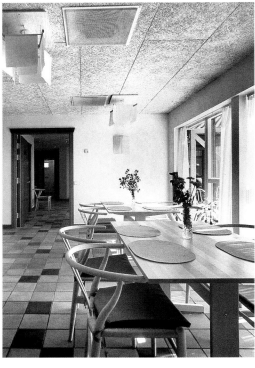

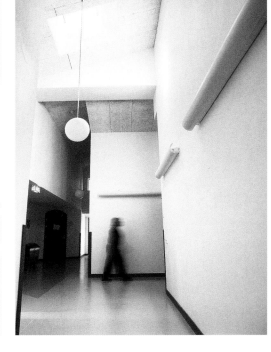

Communal areas face onto the interior courtyard | Natural colours and materials characterise the interiors and furnishings | Large doorway openings and wide bays in the corridors create a sense of space and openness | The residents are free to live their lives according to their own rhythm

Vigs Ängar

Köpingebro, Sweden

Architect	Husberg Architects office AB / Lillemor Husberg Architect SAR/MSA
Client / Operator	Ystad Municipality
Completion date	1995
Useable floor area	2,700 m²
Units / Places	32 units and 36 places

Listed as one of the most interesting social buildings in the world by the United Nations in 2000, the project draws inspiration from the anthroposophical belief that every human being is a unique and constantly developing individual. Of the 32 dwellings, which house up to 36 residents, half were originally intended as serviced flats, the other half as two residential housing units with adjacent communal facilities.

The establishment enjoys an expansive view over the valley of the Nybro River and is arranged on one level around two enclosed courtyards. The flats are like little terraced houses most of which

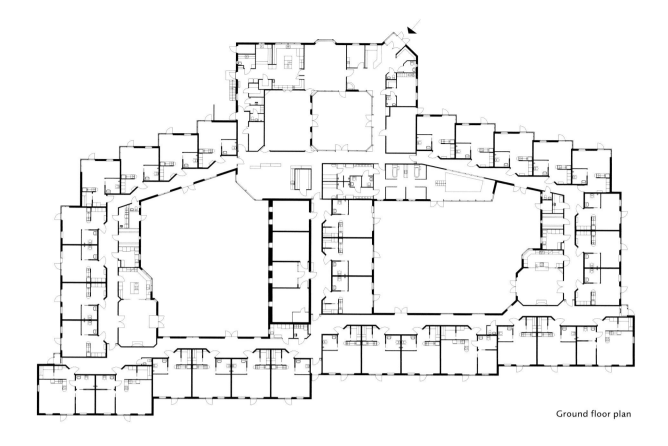

Ground floor plan

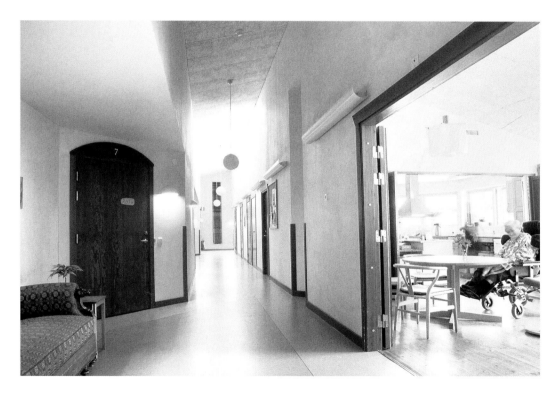

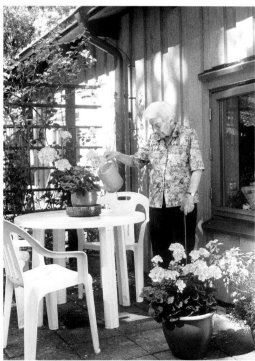

face out onto the countryside. On the inside they are connected by an inner walkway. The dwellings are arranged in three residential groups with sixteen 35 m² flats, twelve 40 m² and four 60 m² flats with two rooms and a kitchen. Today all the flats are residential housing. There are two communal areas with an open fireplace and a farmhouse kitchen as well as an additional lounge. The public areas are arranged around a small courtyard and include a restaurant-café and a pool which are also open to non-residents. There is a room for talks and other cultural programmes. Generously dimensioned outdoor areas allow easy access for wheelchair-bound persons.

The ecological building concept includes the use of natural materials, paints with natural pigments, energy-saving measures, environmentally-friendly drainage, sewage and water purification plus underfloor heating which extracts heat from ground water via a heat exchanger.

The residents can furnish their flats with their own belongings. A special unit is designed for people with dementia. Here, the lounge serves as an actual living-room because the residents spend most of their waking hours inside the house. The inhabitants are able to live according to their own daily rhythm and do not need to

adhere to a common timetable – for example, there is no set time for getting up in the morning. Music, movement and creative activities are as much part of everyday life as warm baths and massages. All meals are made from fresh ingredients using organic and nutritional produce that is free of additives wherever possible. Food is particularly important as its aromas evoke experiences and memories. All residents have their individual contact person among the staff.

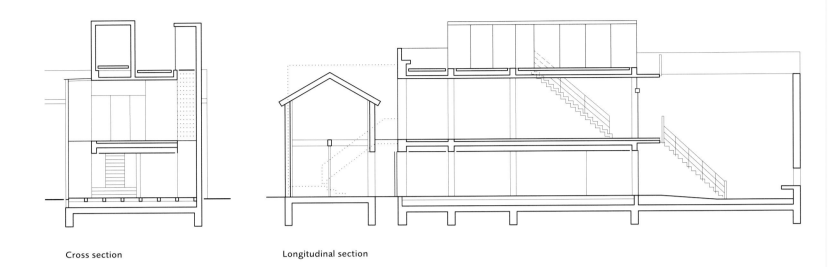

Cross section   Longitudinal section

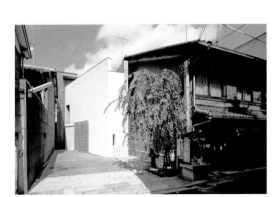

A white-rendered diagonal wall announces the building in an opening between historical buildings | The central space with view of the interior courtyard | Stark contrast between materials in the circulation spaces on the first floor and ground floor | Japanese rice-paper and bamboo matting in the meditation and tea ceremony rooms

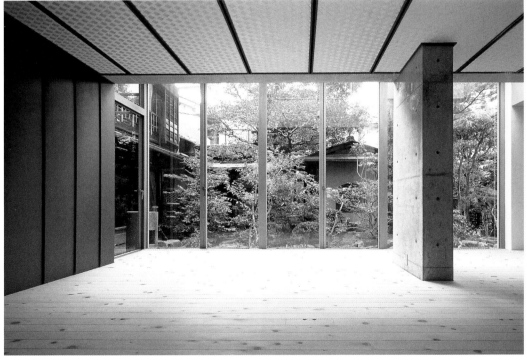

Kamigyo
Day-Care Centre

Kyoto, Japan

Architect	Toshiaki Kawai (Kawai Architects)
Building contractor	Makoto Construction
Operator	Mitsuhashi Takashi
Completion	2000
Useable floor area	new building: 203 m² existing building: 380 m² total: 584 m²
Units/Capacity	according to demand

Located in the narrow alleyways of the historic quarter of Kamigyo in Kyoto, the day-care centre provides a place for the elderly and infirm to visit during the day with full disabled access. The centre's concept caters primarily for the basic needs of old people in Japan, providing help with bathing, eating and individual rehabilitation exercises.

Inserted into a gap in the dense urban fabric of traditional Japanese timber houses, the bright white-rendered building is easy to find, although all that is visible is a narrow skew wall set back from the street. Although conspicuous in its formal reduction, the architect Toshiaki Kawai

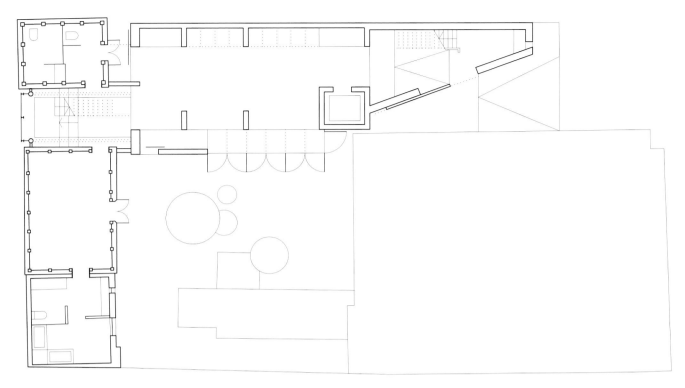

Ground floor plan

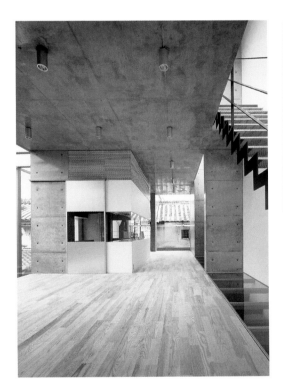 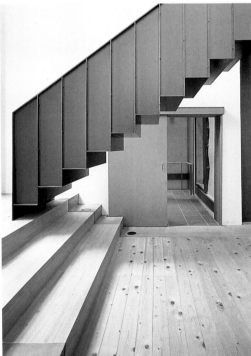 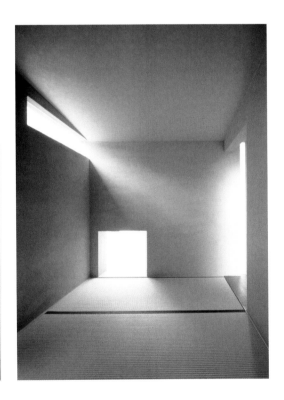

integrates the building into its surroundings by creating a subtle but effective interplay of contrasting materials, historical details and succession of spaces.

Visitors arrive via a forecourt and pass through an entrance with a sliding timber screen, similar to those in old tea houses, before progressing into an inner courtyard. Open to the sky, this pebble-floored space provides access via a ramp to the central space where the elderly are greeted and cared for according to their needs. From there, a lift provides access to the upper floor. In the main spaces on the ground and upper floor, fair-faced concrete walling and black steel stairs contrast with the timber floors and the bamboo matting and Japanese paper of the suspended ceilings. A two-storey glass façade affords a view from both floors onto a courtyard garden planted in the traditional manner.

While the surrounding buildings have pitched tile roofs, the day-care centre has a flat roof with two tea ceremony rooms, accessed via a single straight stair. Here elderly Japanese guests can enjoy this traditional comfort, seated on rice-straw tatami matting with a view over their city.

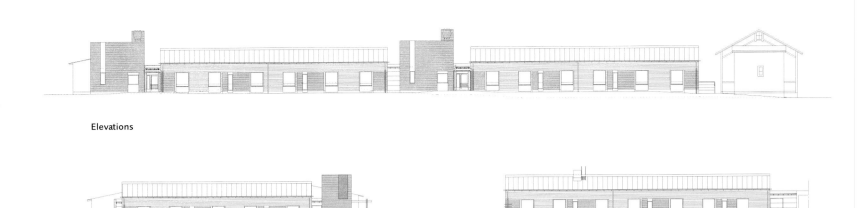

Elevations

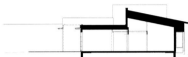 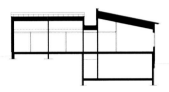

Side elevations

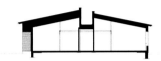

Sections

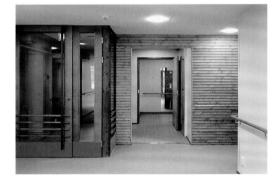

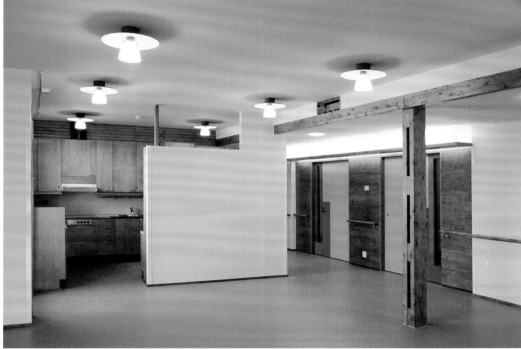

Two entrances, to the sauna block on the right and to one of the group houses on the left | The doors of the private rooms open directly onto the communal living and dining area

Ulrika Eleonora Home for the Elderly

Loviisa, Finland

Architect	L&M Sievänen architects / Liisa & Markku Sievänen with Meiri Siivola
Client / Operator	Loviisa District Service Home Foundation
Completion	2002
Size	1,950 m²
Units / Capacity	under planning: housing complex with 56 units and seven groups homes; built: 32 units

Situated in a small town on the southern coast of Finland about 100 km east of Helsinki, this project comprises group homes for elderly people who are physically debilitated or suffering from dementia. The group home is akin to a large family, with between seven and nine inhabitants in each unit, in which the care staff acts as "parents".

In 1999, the Loviisa District Service Home Foundation together with Loviisa City, the STAKES National Research and Development Centre for Welfare and Health, and the Central Organisation for the Care of the Elderly arranged an architec-

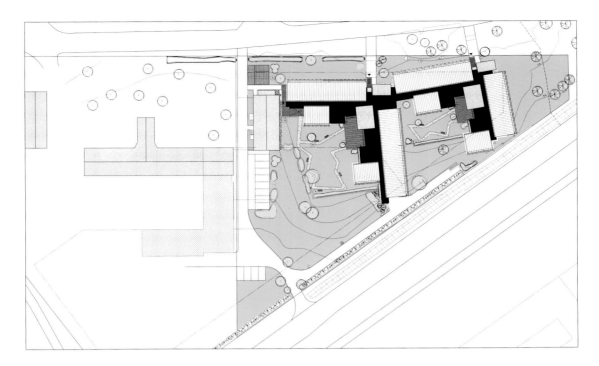

Site plan

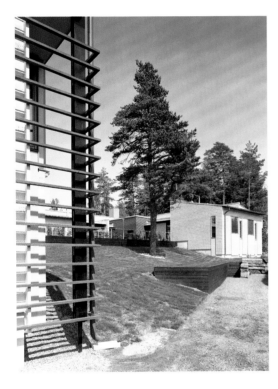

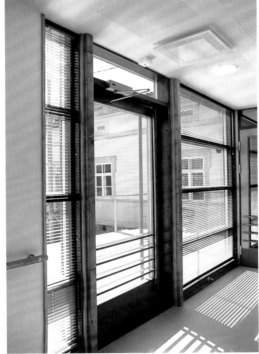

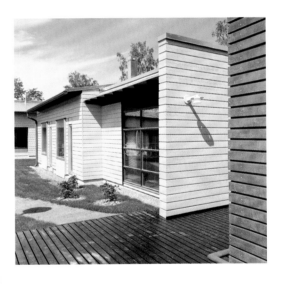

Small-scale housing units organised around courtyards | A corridor with a view of the existing Ukkola building | A connecting terrace between two residential units and the sauna block

tural competition for a 56-unit complex to be built in conjunction with the Ulrikakoti Home for the Elderly. The existing Ulrikakoti, a 19th-century wooden residence for the elderly, has already been extended twice and comprises a main building with two symmetrically arranged wings, one for storage purposes, the other the Ukkola Men's Residence. The main structure is listed as a historically significant building.

The winning competition entry was based on the architectural premise of continuing the old timber traditions of Loviisa. In addition, the massing of the new buildings is designed so that the prin-

cipal building retains its status as the dominant component, and the symmetry of the existing layout is not disturbed. At the same time, the intention was to break up the mass of the building in order to avoid any institutional associations. The building thus forms a "village" of small-scale housing units with semi-detached and terraced "houses" and a low-rise apartment building (the latter is not yet built).

In an effort to continue the small-scale dimensions and intimacy of the streetscape, the extended volumes of the building were reduced by resorting to the formation of angles, so that the

view of the road would vary as is common along older, winding roads. The fairly large building complex is fitted into the terrain by employing a fan-shaped articulation and terracing of the site. The office areas adjoining the entrance and a sauna section linked to outdoor patios are clearly visible in the massing of the whole. Special colours distinguish them from the rest of the building.

The wooden building matches the context of the landscape and local tradition, employing a contemporary means of expression without resorting to a strongly contrasting theme. Features of the external cladding such as the width of the

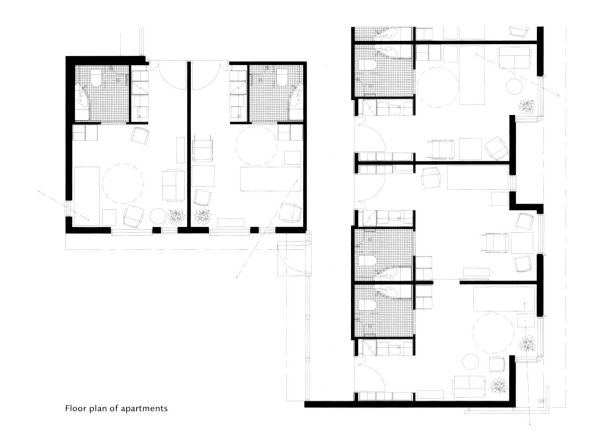

Floor plan of apartments

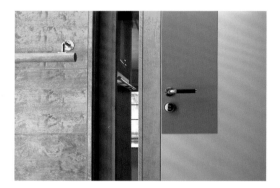

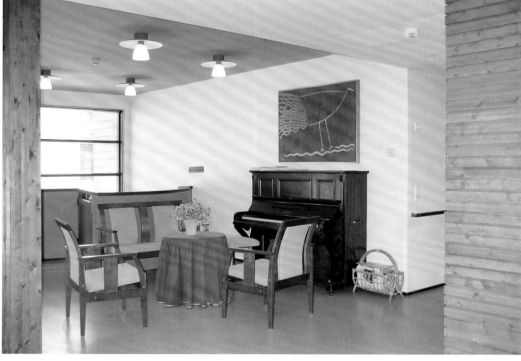

Detail of doorway to a private room | Example of furnishings in one of the living rooms | Courtyard with walking circuit

boarding, paint, colours and so on relate to the long-standing building tradition in Loviisa. Much wood is also used in the interior, creating a warm and colourful atmosphere of domesticity. The external colours are partly echoed in the interior, while the entrances to the living units are enhanced with colours and stained boarding. Domestic appliance rooms and saunas are finished with wooden panelling, and the dayrooms have stained columns and beams. Each resident has a private room opening onto the group's common living and dining areas, ensuring that care staff and the residents are always in contact with one another. The doors to the private rooms open

inwards so that they can be left open. The aim is to enhance a sense of community. These doors are also glazed, with louvred blinds so that the occupants can regulate visibility in and out of the room themselves. Furthermore, the private rooms were designed to be airy and have high ceilings, inspired by the character of the old building. Rooms with sloped ceilings vary in height from 2.8 m along the window wall to 3.6 m along the inner wall. Corner windows in the private rooms create a connection with the world outside. Two group homes share domestic appliance rooms and sauna areas that are connected to patios, as are the living areas.

The building is equipped with underfloor heating which, like the air conditioning, can be adjusted for each room separately. Each private room has a bathroom, the "Gaius brand", a product developed by the architectural office in conjunction with the Central Organisation for the Care of the Elderly: although smaller than the Finnish standards for disabled persons, they provide enough space for two helpers to attend. The technical solutions used in the building support the basic aims of the planning concept to encourage independent living for the elderly, and to increase their sense of well-being.

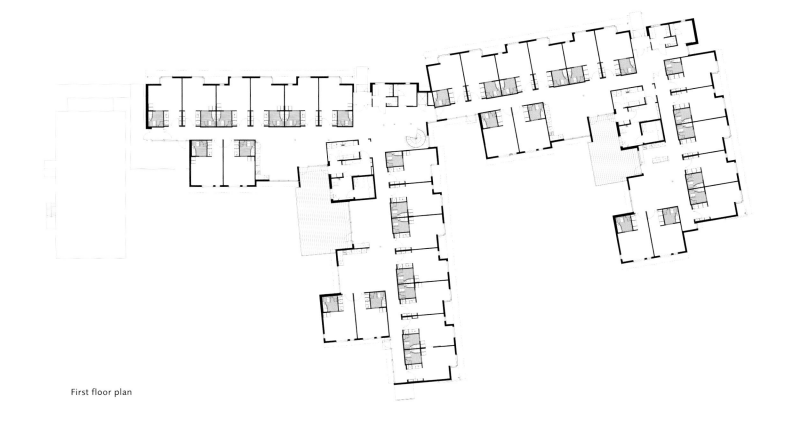

First floor plan

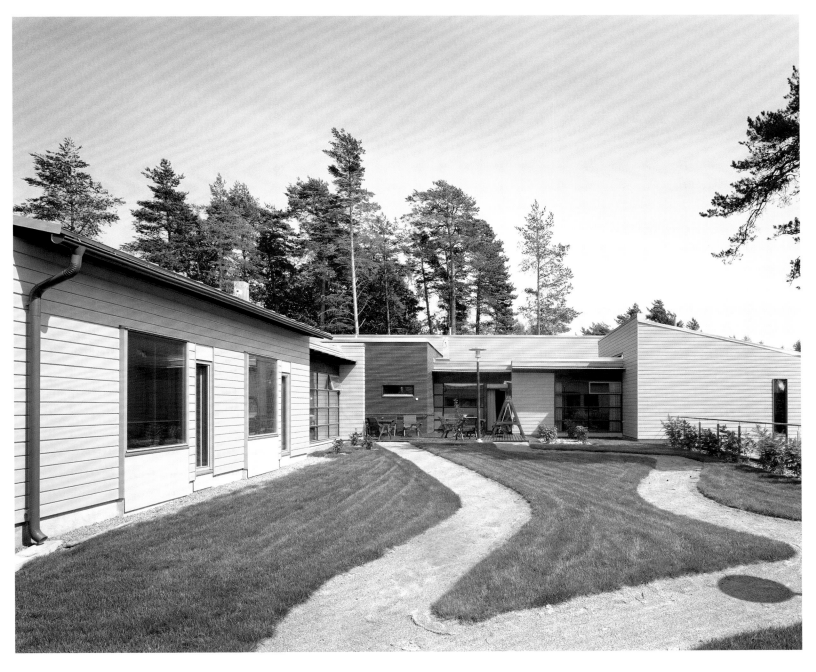

Integrated housing
and neighbourhood concepts

Integrative approaches often arise in combination with other functions in the neighbourhood, such as a children's nursery, advisory centre or community centre.

Different social groups live together in larger residential complexes. For the most part, these are initiated by special operators or associations rather than by the residents themselves. The projects aim to strengthen mutual neighbourly assistance and interaction between different generations and residential groups with differing needs – fostering this interaction both internally, within the complex, as well as externally in the surrounding neighbourhood.

Mutual support and assistance helps compensate the personal limitations of individual residents, while at the same time counteracting the risk of isolation and strengthening synergies, both inbound and outbound. To encourage communal living, such concepts should provide spaces for coming together, consultation and services/infrastructure, accompanied in part by trained staff.

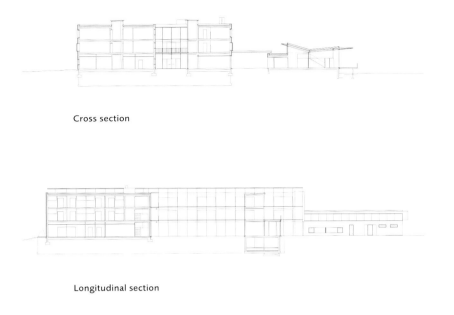

Cross section

Longitudinal section

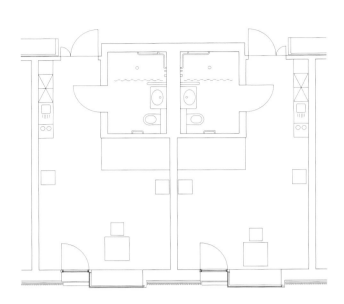

Floor plan of resident's rooms

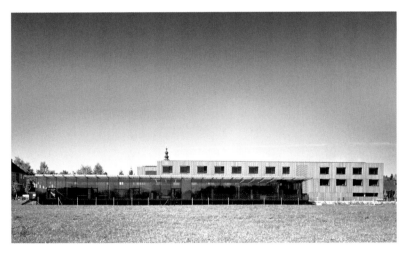

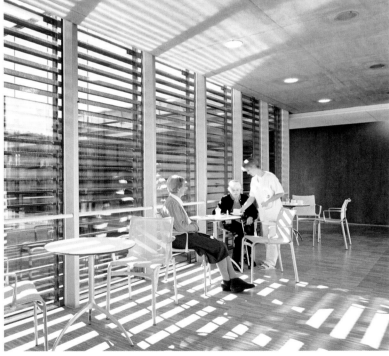

Overall view | Communal space

Home for the Elderly and Children's Nursery

Thalgau, State of Salzburg, Austria

Architect	kadawittfeldarchitektur GbR, Klaus Kada, Gerhard Wittfeld
Client	Marktgemeinde Thalgau
Operator	MFOR Bundesverband Pro Humanitate e. V.
Completion	2002
Useable floor area	5,000 m²
Units/Capacity	56 units; 75 children's nursery places

Inter-generational contact between the youngest and the oldest members of our society is the driving idea behind the competition-winning design of this project. The combination of a home for the elderly and children's nursery is intended to create synergies beneficial for both groups: in an age in which family structures are dissolving, both old people as well as children have an opportunity to establish cross-generational relationships based on affinity.

The arrangement of three parallel strips of buildings slightly offset to one another in a north-south direction creates an entrance terrace on the south side. The terrace adjoins both the three-storey home for

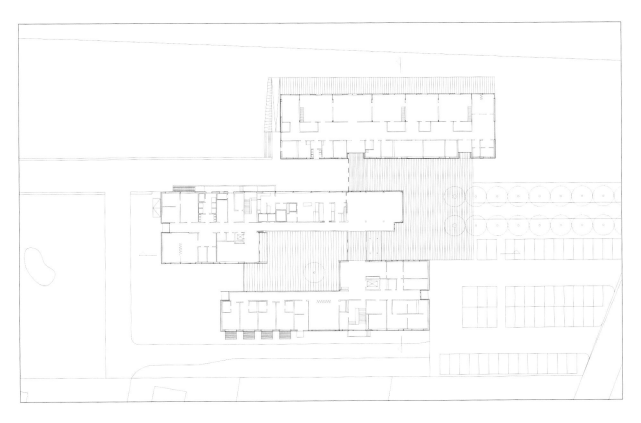

Ground floor plan

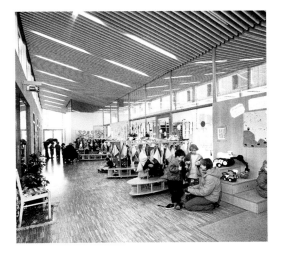
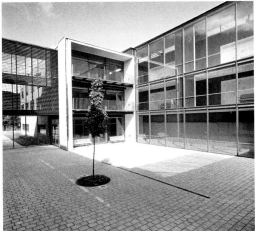
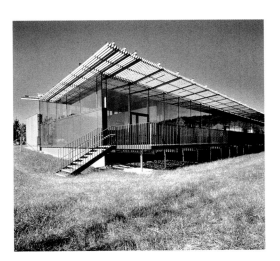

Children's play area | View of the entrance courtyard |
Children's nursery

the elderly and the single-storey children's nursery and also serves as a terrace for the dining room. A connecting element runs crossways acting as a clasp that joins the buildings with one another. Over and above its function as circulation, this also provides a stimulating route that alternates between inside and outside: at one end the large windows in the foyer of the home afford a view out towards the church while the dining room and the entrance to the children's nursery have an inward focus. The far end of the corridor looks out over the Alpine landscape.

The home for the elderly is organised as a series of paths and public spaces analogous to a small town.

The heart of the building is a central courtyard formed by a parting between two of the building's strips. Walkways lead around the courtyard. The ground level houses the care facilities, offices and staff rooms as well as the residents' common room. Both of the upper storeys contain apartments with a care station on each floor.

The residents' rooms are reached via small seating niches in the walkways, which face out onto the courtyard and serve as places to meet. Every room also has direct contact to the world outside in the form of a French window that is part of a box-framed window. This can serve as a place to sit in the sun

or as a window box for flowers. A balcony window on one side provides ventilation and fresh air. Earth tones and warm colours characterise the atmosphere within the interiors and provide orientation.

Despite its integrative approach, the contrasting forms and elaboration of the façades reveal characteristic differences between the section for the young and for the old. The home for the elderly, with its homogenous cladding of horizontal larch weatherboarding, rhythmic pattern of windows and rectangular shape, appears weighty while the glass façades and sailing roofs of the children's nursery, reminiscent of flapping wings, embody a sense of lightness.

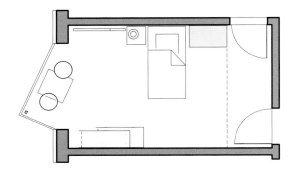

Floor plan of care room with south-facing bay window

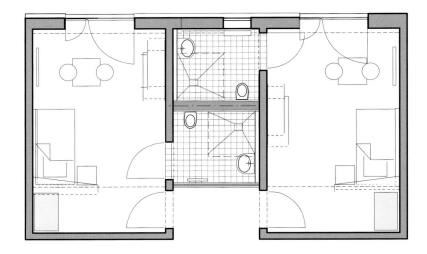

Floor plan of north-facing care rooms

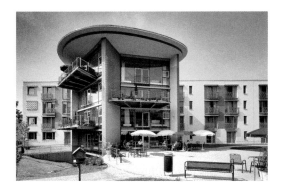

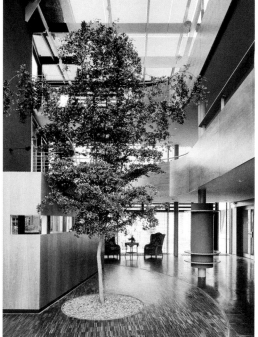

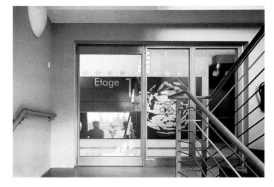

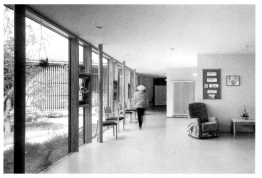

South façade of the nursing complex with the the "tower" fan-
ning outwards | Interior of the foyer building connecting the
existing building and new extension | Stairwell with colour-
coded and clear wayfinding system | Community space of
pavilion for dementia residents

Burgbreite
Home for the Elderly

Wernigerode, Germany

Architect	Kauffmann Theilig & Partner Freie Architekten BDA
Client / Operator	GSW Gemeinnützige Gesellschaft für Sozialeinrichtungen Wernigerode mbH
Completion	2000
Useable floor area	6,440 m²
Units / Capacity	8 apartments, 92 residents 12 dementia residents

Since the reunification of Germany, the renovation of prefabricated buildings made with slab or
element construction methods has been a recurring task for planners. So too in the architectural
competition held in 1996 for the modernisation and
extension of the former "pensioner's home" to a
contemporary home for the elderly. The proposal
also needed to contribute to improving the overall
amenities of the "Burgbreite" housing estate.

The architects Kauffmann Theilig & Partner responded by designing new building volumes that
differ markedly from the linear perpendicularity of
the surrounding buildings in order to give the home

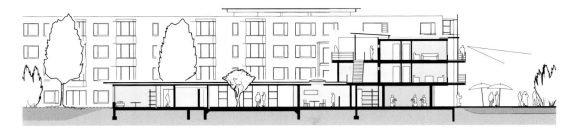

East-west section

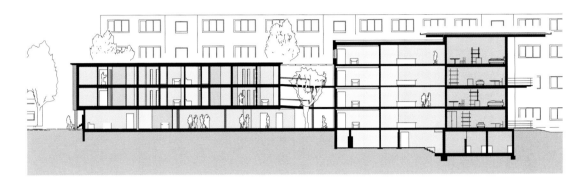

North-south section

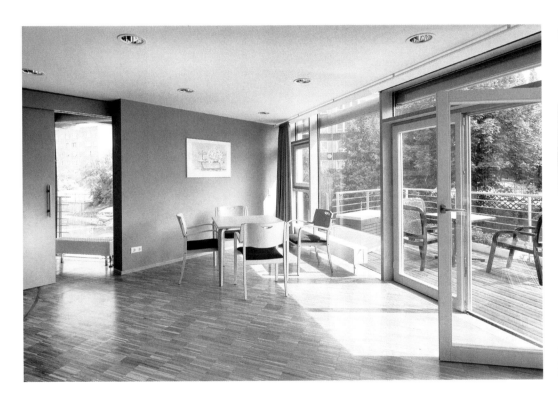

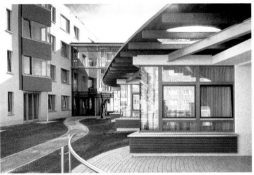

Dining room with balcony on the first floor | North façade, pavilion with outdoor circuit, with glazed foyer between the two at the rear

for the elderly a distinct profile in the predominantly multi-storey surroundings of the housing estate. In particular, the glazed tower on the south side that fans out from the façade creates a new centre and a point of identification. It contains a dining room on each floor and a common room for up to 20 people, which on the first and the third floor are augmented by sunny balconies.

The existing four-storey building from the 1970s, which contains the main nursing facilities for 92 residents, remains recognisable in its original form but is enlivened by a series of interventions in its façades. Full-height windows on the south side,

each with a delicate wood-grille balustrade, as well as angled bay windows that puncture the plane of the façade on the north side, allow plenty of light into the building and lend the façade – together with its colour scheme – a completely new appearance.

The foyer – a glass hallway that serves as main entrance, meeting area and communal space – functions as a connector between the old and the new building and is the venue for a variety of diverse events. From here one reaches the main nursing wing in the old building as well as the single-storey, horseshoe-shaped new building containing the pa-

vilion for people with dementia. The physiotherapy rooms and meeting areas.

The residential wing contains eight barrier-free two-bedroom apartments ranging from 45 to 57 m² whose living rooms and balconies face onto the public space outside. Diagonally-placed walls allow the living area to widen towards the west façade, providing maximum daylight illumination.

The pavilion with its fully-glazed façade facing onto the internal courtyard provides a brightly lit communal room as well as a sheltered outdoor circuit for residents suffering from dementia.

Detail showing projecting bays as modulation for the façade | Barrier-free apartments in the extension

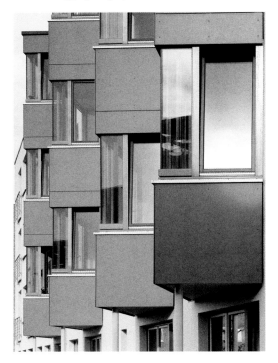
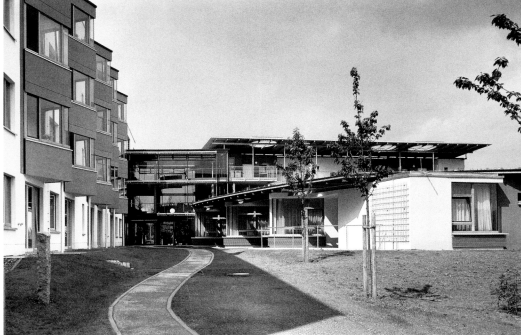

View from the south of the entire complex and its surroundings

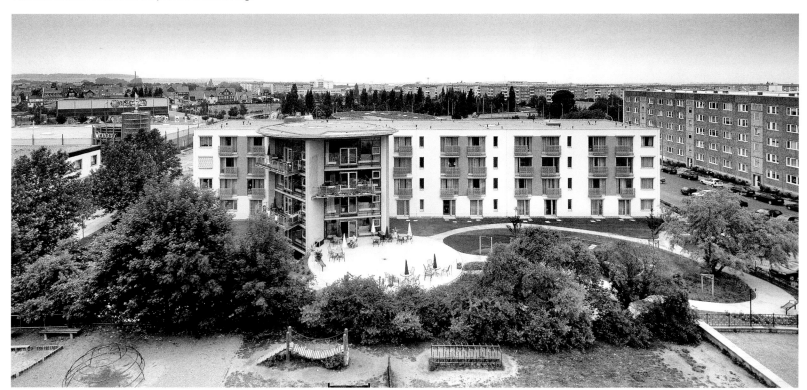

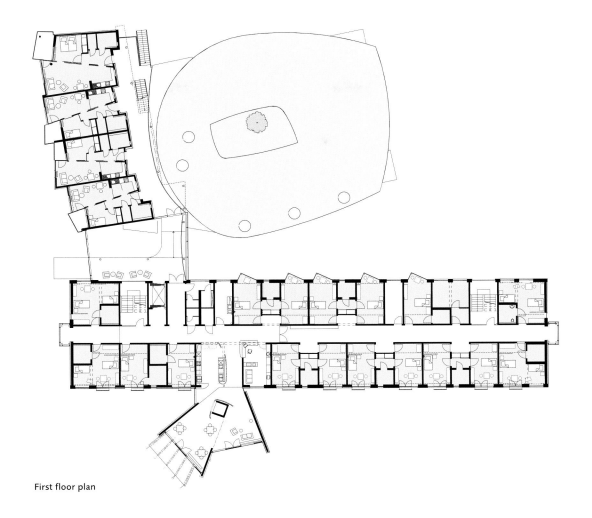

First floor plan

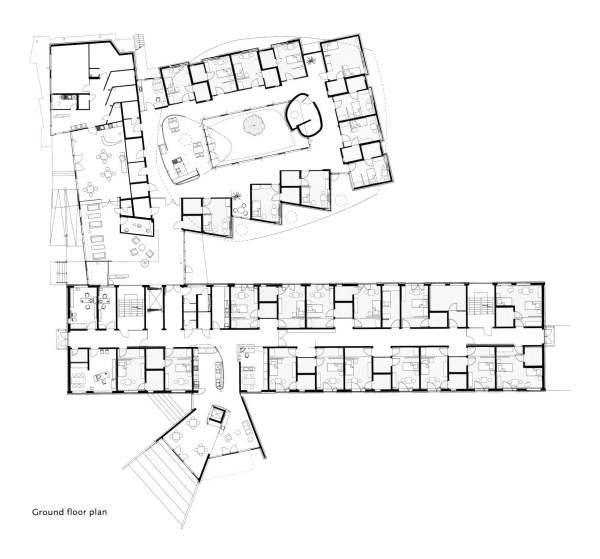

Ground floor plan

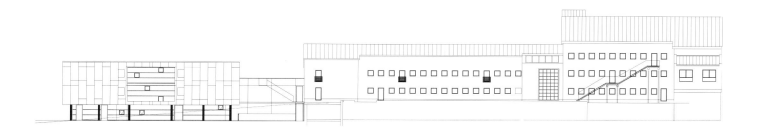

North elevation

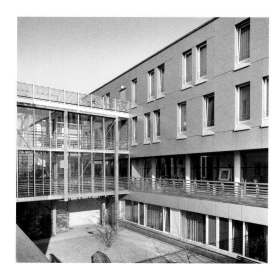

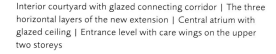

Interior courtyard with glazed connecting corridor | The three horizontal layers of the new extension | Central atrium with glazed ceiling | Entrance level with care wings on the upper two storeys

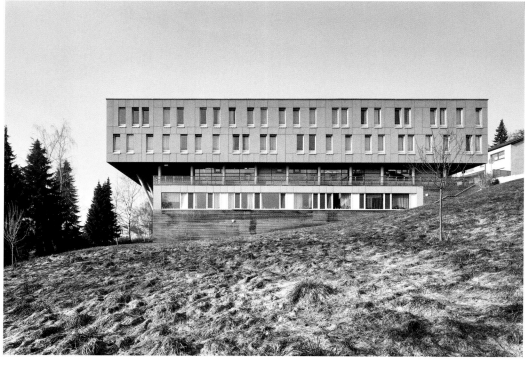

"Haus am Steinnocken"

Ennepetal, Germany

Architect	Enno Schneider Architekten
Client /Operator	Heimverband der Inneren Mission im Ev. Johanneswerk e.V.
Completion	2003
Useable floor area	2,350 m²
Units /Capacity	18 serviced apartments
	6 short-stay care places
	72 care residents

In 1999, the German Federal Ministry of Family Affairs, Senior Citizens, Women and Youth (BMFSFJ) initiated a pilot project entitled "The Cost-effective Building of High-quality Care Facilities for the Elderly" which aims at the implementation of new developments in housing and care provision through forward-looking architectural design. The pilot project was initiated in the form of a competition in four locations. The winning design by Enno Schneider Architekten for the "Haus am Steinnocken" home for the elderly adopts a two-pronged approach in which the highly functional areas for nursing care are housed in a new building and the living areas with less intensive care requirements in an

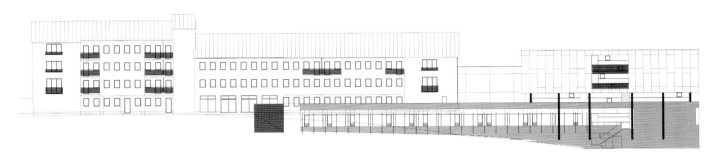

South elevation

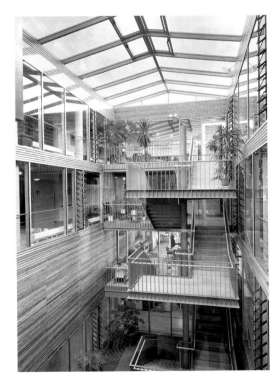

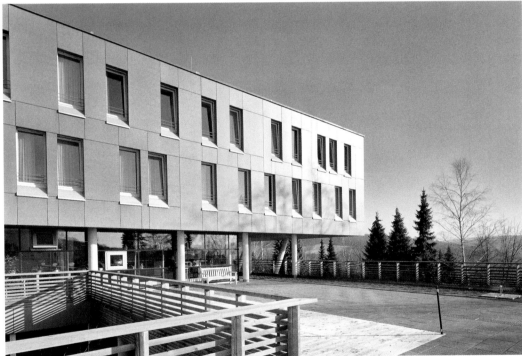

existing building from 1964. The result – built while the home was in operation – is a synthesis of sophisticated new architecture and the sensitive modernisation of an existing building. Careful attention was given to reducing the volume of the building by embedding it in the slope of the site.

Divided into three sections, the horizontal layering of the new building responds to the topography of the site. It consists of a three-storey volume alongside the road which cantilevers outwards on diagonal columns over the plinth level below, which in turn runs the length of the front of the existing building. The two-storey plinth with two care areas

connects the old and new buildings via a glazed walkway, while the glazed treatment of the ground floor emphasises its more public function as a social gathering point with entrance area, cafeteria and terrace. The two upper storeys, each containing two care areas, are treated as an independent, apparently free-floating volume. The new extension picks up the floor levels of the existing building and connects with it via bridges on each floor.

The central atrium with glazed ceiling and open staircase provides not only vertical circulation and greater orientation but also allows natural light to flood into the building. The hall also serves as a

distributor for fresh air drawn in from the garden, which then passes along the corridors and into the rooms and their individual bathrooms. The serial repetition of the rooms allows a high degree of prefabrication and the building shell is consequently made of precast concrete elements clad with fibre-cement panelling.

The strict arrangement of the floor plan of the extension differentiates between two kinds of care areas: "neighbourhoods" and "communities". The 16.3 m²-large single rooms on the south side are accordingly grouped around a common living and dining area, while those on the north side are

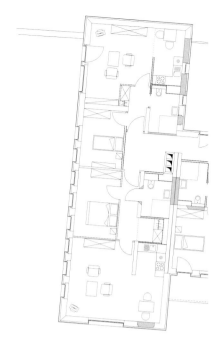

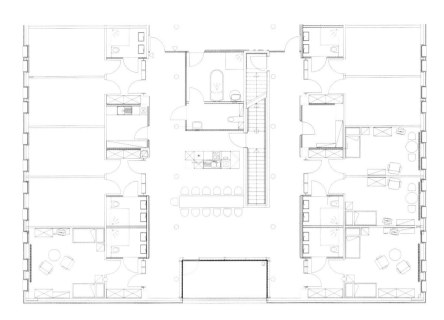

Detail of floor plan   Detail of floor plan

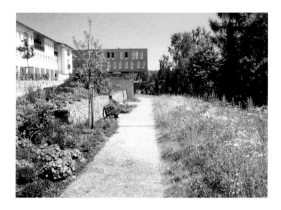

Dry stone wall at the southern boundary of the site

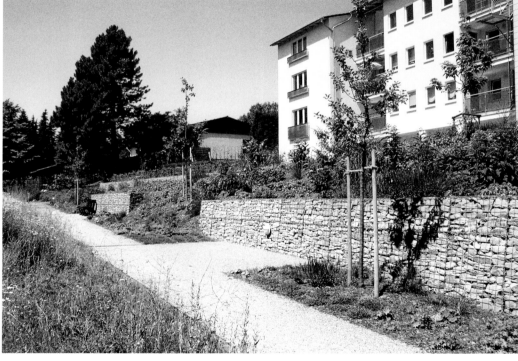

arranged around the stairwell atrium. Here too there is a communal living and dining room so that these areas can also be used as "communities" if required.

The nursing home provides a total of six living areas with individually adaptable care concepts, with people with dementia forming the primary care group. The design of the living and kitchen areas aims, therefore, to create the sense of a joint household and they have been made as comfortable and homely as possible.

The rooms for residents who are in constant need of nursing care are located in the plinth. The rooms

have wide doors and face outwards over the green landscape, as do the common areas which are augmented via a sheltered interior courtyard.

The architectural character of the existing building has been largely retained and converted to comply with barrier-free DIN norms, without needing to make major changes to the structure of the building. The plinth and ground level accommodate the service centre, administration, staff rooms and utility areas as well as six short-stay care beds. On the upper floors, the former single and twin rooms have been combined to form 18 barrier-free 45.3 m²-large serviced apartments with completely redesigned

bathrooms and a 5.1 m²-large loggia. While the care and administration areas can be accessed from the new entrance in the new building, the tenants in the serviced apartments are free to use the barrier-free entrance in the existing building.

The entire complex and the planning of its outdoor areas relates to the landscape. The orchard at the lower end of the site has been revived and replanted and a dry-stone wall now marks the boundary of the site to the south.

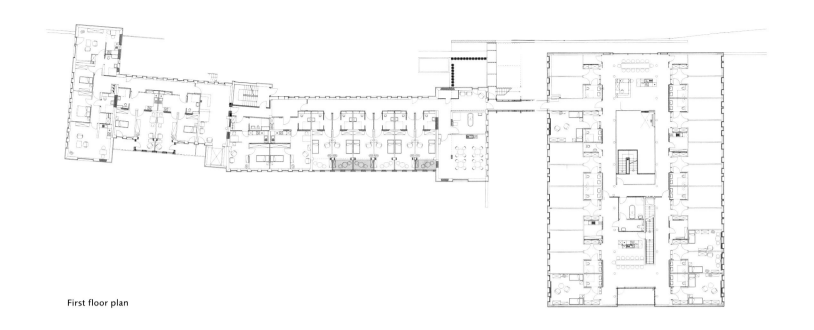

First floor plan

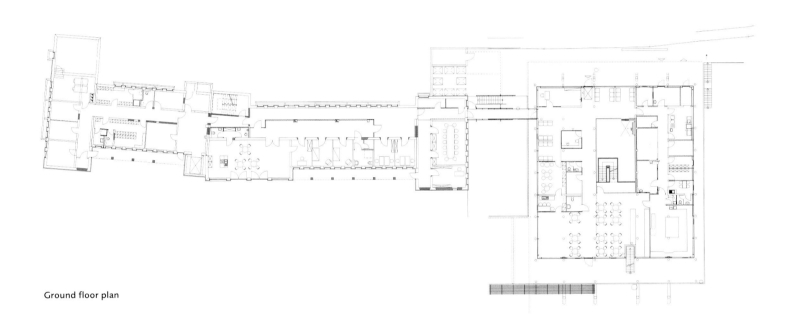

Ground floor plan

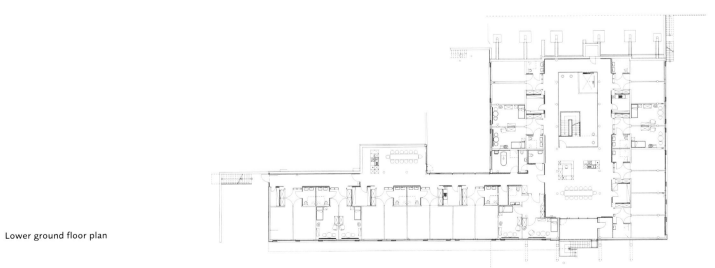

Lower ground floor plan

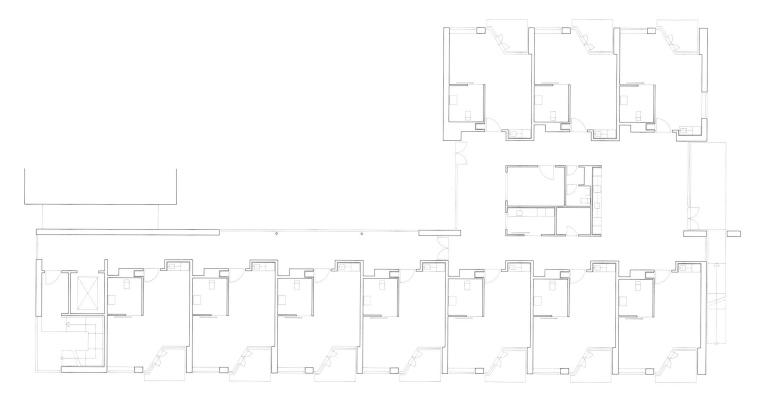

Ground floor plan of new building

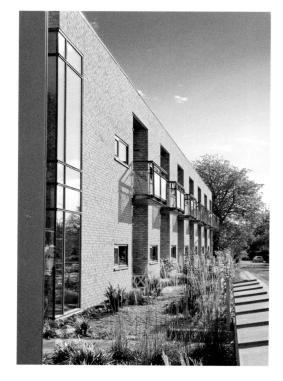

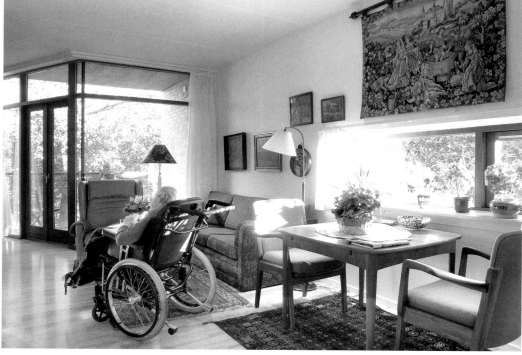

Toftehaven
Nursing Home

Ballerup, Denmark

Architect	Vilhelm Lauritzen Architects
Client/Operator	Ballerup Municipality and Baldersbo Housing Dept.
Completion	2004
Useable floor area	new building 1.450 m², conversion 3.000 m²
Units/Capacity	20 units, 68 residents altogether

The extension of this nursing home in an outlying suburb of Copenhagen involved the building of a new wing and the extensive modernisation of the existing buildings from 1967. The project aims to upgrade the existing narrow, single-storey buildings, arranged in a grid pattern around two patios, to fulfil contemporary Danish standards as well as to improve the visibility of the entire complex in the neighbourhood and to link it to a larger and more visible rehabilitation centre with a day-care facility.

An architectural competition in 2002 was won by the architect Vilhelm Lauritzen who converted the

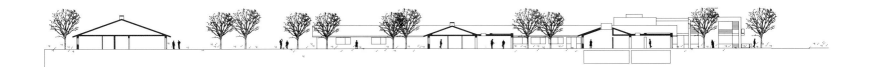

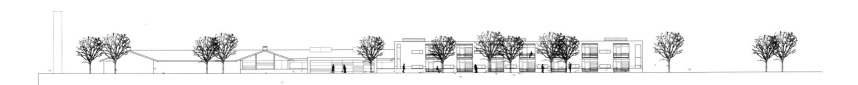

Sections

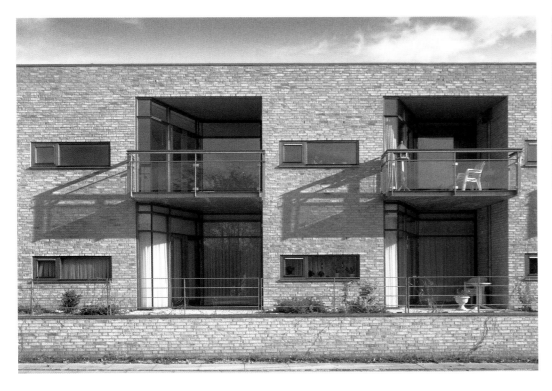

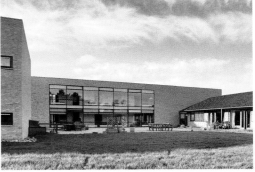

Street façade of the new wing | Individually personalised studio | Ochre facing brickwork of the new building picks up the materiality of the existing buildings | L-shaped new extension with existing building on the right

existing 18 m² rooms into 35-36 m²-large studios and two-room flats. This conversion was achieved without major alterations to the building structure and while keeping the arrangement into sections of ten units each. Each flat has a kitchenette and disabled-access bathroom as well as direct access to an outdoor terrace, balcony or small garden. Differences in floor levels and door thresholds are bridged using gridded metal ramps and metal floor plates. A new two-storey L-shaped wing, whose yellow brickwork picks up the colour of the surrounding buildings, was built along the road on the west edge of the site to provide a further 26 apartments. As part of a restructuring of the

complex, the architect also relocated the main entrance and a forecourt on the west side. The public functions such as administration, physiotherapy rooms, hairdresser and meeting areas are arranged along the extension of this axis. An attractive courtyard provides orientation within the building itself, and adjoins the dining hall and café.

The design of the wing for Alzheimer sufferers, accommodating 12 residents, retains the original 18 m² rooms and follows the Cantou concept. This includes clearly visible signage and orientation aids, a colour scheme conceived especially for dementia sufferers and the provision of a

therapeutic kitchen. The latter is designed so that the residents can be involved in the preparation of meals or laying the table if they so wish. While cupboard doors are transparent so that crockery and cutlery is always visible and easy to find, switches for electrical equipment are concealed for safety's sake. As is typical throughout Denmark, all the residents at Toftehaven can participate in day-to-day tasks in the home and the gardens.

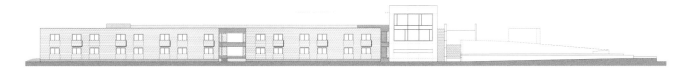

East elevation

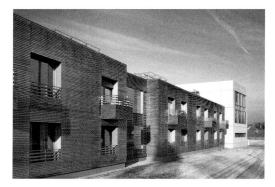

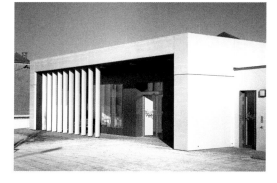

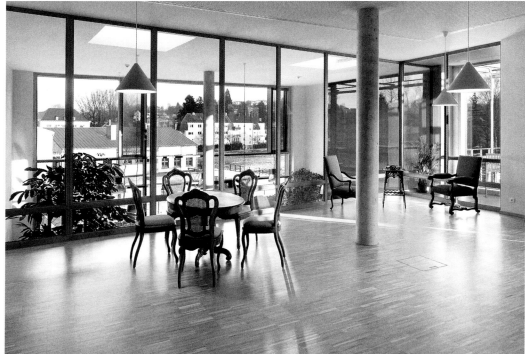

CIPA Residential and Nursing Home

Junglinster, Luxembourg

Architect	witry & witry architecture urbanisme with Atelier d'architecture et de design Jim Clemes
Client	Red Cross Luxembourg
Completion	2004
Useable floor area	8,889 m²
Units/Capacity	100 residents

In 1999, the Red Cross in Luxembourg organised an architectural competition for the design of residential accommodation for 100 old people with all the necessary associated care and service facilities for everyday life. In addition, the CIPA (Centre intégré pour personnes âgées) needed to fit into the structure of the village of Junglinster and maximise interactions with its surroundings at all levels.

The winning design by Witry & Witry architects and Jim Clemes follows the topography of the site, a meadow that falls away gradually. The three-storey wings to the west and north there-

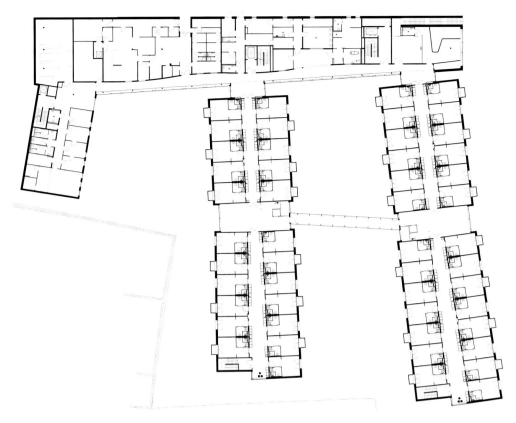

Plan of the entire complex

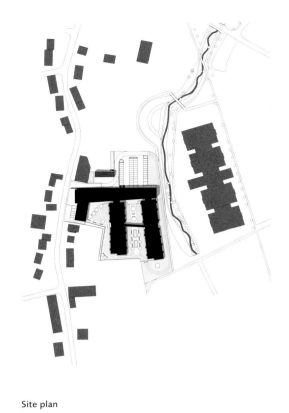

Site plan

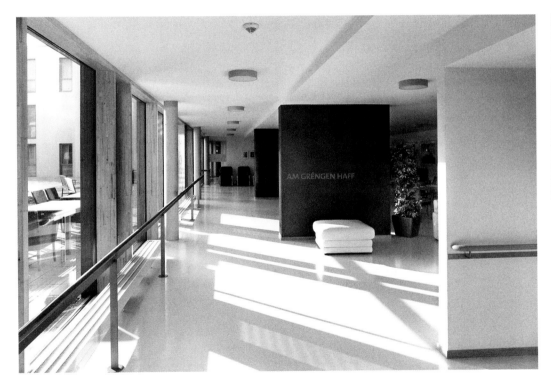

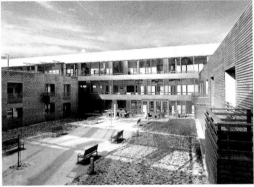

Residential wing with larch cladding | Entrance to the social day-care centre for the elderly | Communal space with view of the surrounding village | A coordinated colour scheme helps provide orientation for the residents | South-facing residential wings

fore adjoin the Rue Rham, while both of the two-storey larch-clad residential wings look southwards over orchards along the banks of the River Ernz Noire, a scenery typical for the region. Separated into four sections, the complex offers successive degrees of privacy: beginning with the public entrance area at street level on the Rue Rham, progressing via the restaurant, café, multi-purpose hall and small shops to the privacy of the clearly-designed residential wings, with their cheerful red-orange window jambs. The integrative concept also extends to the roof gardens on the residential wings – thematically grouped according to colours and aromas derived from

the surrounding orchards – which can also be reached from street level.

Stairs and lifts allow visitors to reach the semi-public areas in the west wing, which is arranged parallel to the residential wings. This wing houses medical services on the second floor and social and geriatric day-care facilities at garden level. Further services and facilities are also contained in the north wing.

The residential wings are divided into four independently organised units and provide accommodation for both healthy and active elderly

residents as well as those suffering from dementia. The common rooms in the centre of each level are designed as small, modern living rooms for residents and visitors to meet, talk and be together. Throughout the complex, especially where paths cross and different areas meet, small squares and seating niches provide additional semi-private places to meet, rest and enjoy the view.

Project data

Béguinage

Address
BeginenWerk, Erkelenzdamm 51, D-10999 Berlin

Architect
PPL Barbara Brakenhoff, Chopinstraße 9B,
D-04103 Leipzig

Brookside House

Address
46 Brookside Avenue, Knotty Ash,
Liverpool L14 7LN UK

Architect
shedkm, 61a Bold Street, Liverpool L1 4EZ UK

Client
Liverpool Housing Action Trust, Housing 21

Consultants
Green roof
erisco bauder, Bauder Limited, Ipswich
Concrete sleeves
Buchan Concrete Solutions, Middlewich

Lifts
Otis Elevator Company, Otis Ltd., London
Windows
velfac ltd, Hildersham
Render
sto ltd., Glasgow
Glazing
reglit glass, Rutherglen

Landscape planner
Brodie McAllister, McAllister Landscape, Bristol

Brouwersgracht and L.A. Rieshuis

Address
Brouwersgracht 280-282,
NL-1013 HG Amsterdam;
L.A. Rieshuis, Vinkenstraat 175-181,
NL-1013 JX Amsterdam

Architect
mecanoo architecten, Oude Delft 203,
P.O. Box 3277, NL-2601 DG Delft

Contractor
Aannemersbedrijf Scheurer BV, Kamerling
Onneslaan 40, NL-1097 DH Amsterdam

Consultant
Strackee Bouwadviesbureau b.v.

CIPA Residential and Nursing Home

Address
Rue Rham, L-6142 Junglinster

Architect
witry & witry architecture urbanisme,
32 rue du Pont, L-6402 Echternach;
Atelier d'Architecture et de design Jim Clemes,
120 rue de Luxembourg, L-4221 Esch-sur-
Alzette

Client
Croix Rouge Luxembourgeoise,
44 Bvd. Joseph II, L-1840 Luxembourg

Consultants
Structural engineer
TR Engineering SA
HVAC
Goblet Lavandier & Associés
Ingénieurs-Conseils SA

Landscape planner
witry & witry architecture urbanisme

Art installation
Burg Giebichenstein Hochschule für Kunst
und Design Halle, Prof. Klaus Michel;
Luc Wolff

Competence Centre for People with Dementia

Address
Wallensteinstraße 65, D-90431 Nuremberg

Architect
feddersenarchitekten,
Reuchlinstraße 10-11, D-10553 Berlin

Client
Evangelisch-Lutherisches Diakoniewerk
Neuendettelsau, Wilhelm-Löhe-Straße 16,
D-91564 Neuendettelsau

Consultants
Site supervision
Rückert Architekten & Ackermann + Weiss
Architekten GmbH, Munich
Structural engineer
Pichler Ingenieure GmbH, Beratende Ingenieure
VBI, Berlin

HVAC
Energieplan GmbH, Augsburg
Electrical engineer
Energieplan GmbH, Nördlingen
Geological engineer
LGA Bautechnik, Nuremberg
Fire safety
Peter Stanek, Berlin
Health and safety coordinator
Genesis – Umwelt Consult GmbH & Co KG,
Schwabach
Colour concept
Friederike Tebbe, Berlin

Landscape planner
Harms Wulf, Berlin

"Haus am Steinnocken"

Address
Steinnockenstraße 43, D-58256 Ennepetal

Architect
Enno Schneider Architekten,
Bahnhofstraße 8, D-32756 Detmold,
und Gipsstraße 6, D-10119 Berlin

Client
Heimverband der Inneren Mission im Ev. Jo-
hanneswerk e.V., Schildescher Straße 101-103,
D-33611 Bielefeld

Consultants
HVAC
Ingenieurbüro Tölke, Detmold
Structural engineer
Ingenieur-Büro Bunte, Detmold
Electrical engineer
Ingenieur-Büro Kloberdanz, Detmold

Landscape planner
ARGE Bimberg / Weber, Iserlohn

Home for Pensioners and Nursing Home

Address
Niederösterreichisches Landes-Pensionisten-
heim mit Tagesbetreuungsstation, Hermann-
Gmeiner-Gasse 4, A-3100 St. Pölten

Architect
Dipl.-Ing. Georg W. Reinberg,
Lindengasse 39/10, A-1070 Vienna

Client
Pinus in Konzern der niederösterreichischen
Hypoleasing; Fachabteilungen der niederöster-
reichischen Landesregierung: Abt. 2HB2, Abt.
4.HB4, GS7 Nutzer; Neugebäudeplatz 1, A-3101
St. Pölten

Consultants
Structural engineer
Dipl.-Ing. Kurt Schuh, Vienna
Construction performance
Dipl.-Ing. Günter Feit, Klosterneuburg

Technical installations
KWI Planungs- und Beratungsgesellschaft mbH
& Co. KG, St. Pölten
Lighting planning
Lighting Design Austria, Eichgraben
Air quality assessment
Institut für Baubiologie und Ökologie, Vienna

Landscape planner
Dipl.-Ing. Anna Detzlhofer, Vienna

Home for the Elderly and Children's Nursery

Address
Ferdinand Zuckerstätter Straße 19, A-5303
Thalgau

Architect
kadawittfeldarchitektur,
Aureliusstraße 2, D-52064 Aachen

Client
Marktgemeinde Thalgau,
Wartenfelder Str. 2, A-5303 Thalgau

Consultants
Structural engineer
Sommerauer u. Gaderer Ziviltechniker GesmbH,
Mondsee
Construction performance
Technisches Büro für Bauphysik
Dipl.-Ing. Reiner Rothbacher, Zell am See
Technical installations
Technisches Büro, Dipl.-Ing. Axel Burggraf,
Salzburg
Electrical engineer
Technisches Büro Ing. Friedrich Müller-Uri,
Thalgau

Landscape planner
kadawittfeldarchitektur

Burgbreite Senior Centre

Address
Platz des Friedens 7, D-38855 Wernigerode

Architect
Kauffmann Theilig & Partner, Freie Architekten BDA, Prof. Andreas Theilig, Dieter Ben Kauffmann, Rainer Lenz; Zeppelinstraße 10, D-73760 Ostfildern

Client
GSW, Alzbergstraße 6b, D-38855 Wernigerode

Consultants
Structural engineer
Pfefferkorn Ingenieure, Stuttgart with Ing.-Büro Dr. Ehelebe, Wernigerode
Construction performance
Horstmann + Berger, Altensteig
HVAC, Electrical Engineer
ArGe Haustechnik, Wernigerode;
Gattermann, Schock & Schubbert, Wieckert
Nursing care consultancy
Sibylle Heeg, University of Stuttgart

Landscape planner
Kauffmann Theilig & Partner
with Thorsten Scholze, Helmstedt

Carmelite Monastery

Address
Karmeliterstraße 1, D-53229 Bonn

Architect
Fischer – von Kietzell – Architekten BDA Partnerschaftsgesellschaft (until 04/2008), Am Karmelkloster 1, D-53229 Bonn

Client
gwk neubau gmbh, Am Karmelkloster 14, D-53229 Bonn

Consultants
Structural engineer
Dipl.-Ing. Büro Abed Isa

Landscape planner
Fischer – von Kietzell – Architekten BDA Partnerschaftsgesellschaft,
Architect: Jürgen von Kietzell

Cronstetten House

Address
Speicherstraße 39-47, D-60327 Frankfurt am Main

Architect
Frick.Reichert Architekten,
Lange Straße 31, D-60311 Frankfurt am Main

Client
Cronstett- und Hynspergische Evangelische Stiftung, Lindenstraße 19, D-60325 Frankfurt am Main

Consultants
Structural engineer
Kannemacher + Dr. Sturm, Frankfurt am Main
HVAC, Electrical engineer
Ingenieurbüro Borchert, Willingshausen

Landscape planner
Ipach und Dreisbusch, Neu-Isenburg

Day-care Centre
with Therapeutic Garden

Address
Accueil de jour de l'Éhpad départementale du Creusot, 75 rue Jouffroy, F-Le Creusot (71)

Architect
Philippe Dehan Architecte – Urbaniste,
17 rue des Gobelins, F-75013 Paris

Client
Éhpad du Creusot, BP 55, F-71202 Le Creusot

Consultants
Foundations
E2F, Lyon
Contractor
Vadrot/C3B, Macon
Scaffolding
Pelletier, Paray-le-Monial
Exterior carpentry
Pieralu, Chasselay
HVAC
Quesada, Le Creusot

Landscape planner
Stéphanie Mallier, Dampierre

Elbschloss Residences

Address
Elbschloss Residenz GmbH,
Elbchaussee 374, D-22609 Hamburg

Elbschloss Residences

Architect
Kleffel Köhnholdt Papay Warncke Architekten, Michaelisstraße 22, D-20459 Hamburg

Client
Pensionskasse Hoechst,
Philipp-Reis-Straße 2, D-65795 Hattersheim

Consultants
Structural engineer
Manz + Kruse, Buxtehude
Technical installations
Rodde & Partner, Hamburg
Façade
KKPW Architekten
Lighting engineer
P. Raasch, Hamburg

Landscape planner
H. O. Dieter Schoppe Landschaftsarchitekt BDLA, Hamburg

Wellness area

Architect
geising + böker gmbh,
Schulterblatt 58B, D-20357 Hamburg

Dementia Day-Care Area

Architect
feddersenarchitekten,
Reuchlinstraße 10-11, D-10553 Berlin

Landscape planner (terrace)
Harms Wulf Garten- und Landschaftsarchitekten, Berlin

Jezárka Home for the Elderly

Address
Rybniční 1282, CZ - 386 01 Strakonice

Architect
FACT v.o.s., Podolska 401/50,
CZ-147 00 Prague 4

Contractor
Protom s.r.o., Pisecka 290,
CZ-386 01 Strakonice

Construction engineer
Ing. Jiri Treybal, TMS Projekt Strakonice

Landscape planner
Ing. Hajek

Kamigyo Day-Care Centre

Address
686 Daikoku-cho, Kamitachiuri-agaru, Jouhugu-ji, Kamigyo-ku, Kyoto, Japan

Architect
Toshiaki Kawai (Kawai architects), 490 Tateshin-mei-cho, Inokuma-dori, Motoseiganji-sagaru, Kamigyo-ku, Kyoto, Japan

Contractor
Makoto Construction, 2-17-8 Kitahorie,
Nishi-ku, Osaka, Japan

Consultant
Takashi Mitsuhashi

Kenyuen Home for the Elderly

Address
Esumi, ka mi-mihirami 800, Susami-cho, Nishimuro-gun, Wakayama, Japan

Architect
Muramatsu Architects, 4-8-18-504 Kitashinjuku, Shinjuku-ku, Tokyo 169-0074, Japan

Client
Tobishima corporation, 2banch 3banncho, Chiyoda-ku, Tokyo 102-8332, Japan

Consultants
Site supervision, façade construction, lighting planning, interior design
Motoyasu Muramatsu
Structural engineer
Masato Araya
Technical installations
Akio Chiku, Shigeyuki Ishiwata,
Yoshihiro Kimura, Seiichi Mukuo

Landscape planner
Motoyasu Muramatsu

"Miss Sargfabrik"

Address
Missindorfstraße 10, A-1140 Vienna

Architect
MISSARGE / BKK-3 / BK,
Missindorfstraße 10, A-1140 Vienna

Client
Verein für integrative Lebensgestaltung, Goldschlagstraße 169, A-1140 Vienna

Consultants
Structural engineer
ARGE Fröhlich / Lorcher ZT GmbH, Vienna
Construction performance
D.I. Walter Prause, Vienna
HVAC
BPS Engineering Brunner & Partner OEG, Vienna

Landscape planner
Fa. Traumgarten, Georg Guggenberger, Vienna

Project data

Nedregaard Boligområde Senior Residences

Address
Langelandsveien 40-42, N-6010 Ålesund

Architect
Longva arkitekter AS, Rosenborggaten 19,
Pb. 5939 Majorstuen, N-0308 Oslo

Client
Daaeskogen Eiendom AS,
Langelandsveien 17, N-6010 Ålesund

Consultants
Structural engineer
Siv.ing. Rolf Olset AS
Electrical engineer
Karl Kvalsund AS
HVAC
Technoconsult AS

Landscape planner
Longva arkitekter AS

Nezu Withus

Address
2-14-18 Nezu, Bunkyo-ku, Tokyo

Architect
Kengo Kuma & Associates,
2-24-8 Minamiaoyama, Minato-ku, Tokyo

Contractor
Kuboco, 1-16-10 Uchikanda, chiyoda-ku, Tokyo

Landscape planner
Kengo Kuma & Associates, Kuboco

Nursing Home

Address
Höchsterstraße 30, A-6850 Dornbirn

Architect
Riepl Riepl Architekten,
OK Platz 1A, A-4020 Linz;
Johannes Kaufmann Architektur,
Sägerstraße 4, A-6850 Dornbirn

Client
City of Dornbirn,
Rathausplatz 2, A-6580 Dornbirn

Consultants
Structural engineer
Moosbrugger Ingenieure, Dornbirn
Construction performance
Lothar Künz, Hard
Timber construction
Fussenegger und Rümmele, Dornbirn

Technical installations
Ökoplan, Altach
Electrical engineer
Ing. Peter Hämmerle, Lustenau
Lighting planning
Charles Keller, St. Gallen

Landscape planner
Dipl.-Ing. Barbara Bacher, Linz

Santa Rita Geriatric Centre

Address
c/ Marius Verdaguer s/n Ciutadella de Menorca

Architect
Manuel Ocaña del Valle, c/Sagasta 23,
7° izda E-28004 Madrid

Client
CIME Conseil Insular de Menorca,
Plaza de la Biosfera 5

Consultants
Contractor
OHL
Technical installations
Joan Camps and Julio Grau

Landscape planner
Teresa Gali Izard

Sheltered Housing Complex

Address
Laan der zeven Linden 175,
NL-Emerald, Delfgauw/Pijnacker

Architect
KCAP Architects & Planners,
Piekstraat 27, NL-3071 EL Rotterdam

Client
Ceres Projects, Rijswijk

Consultants
Van Eck, Rijswijk

Sonnweid Nursing Home Extension

Address
Sonnweid AG,
Bachtelstrasse 68, CH-8620 Wetzikon

Architect
Bernasconi + Partner Architekten AG,
Langensandstrasse 23, CH-6005 Lucerne

Consultants
Electrical engineer
Jules Häfliger AG, Lucerne
HVAC
Inag-Nievergelt AG, Zurich

Landscape planner
Beglinger Söhne AG, Mollis

"Stadtcarré"

Address
Bahnhofstraße 4-10, D-74906 Bad Rappenau

Architect
ASIRarchitekten, Prof. I. Roecker,
Mittelstraße 10, D-70180 Stuttgart

Client
Kruck + Partner, Wohnbau- und Projektentwick-
lung GmbH und Co. KG, Bismarckstraße 107,
D-74074 Heilbronn

Consultants
Structural engineer
Schlaich, Bergermann und Partner, Stuttgart;
Dipl.-Ing.(FH) Benz GmbH, Geislingen
HVAC
TEB GmbH, Vaihingen/Enz;
Zeeh, Schreyer und Partner, Ludwigsburg
Electrical engineer
SIB GmbH & Co. KG, Von-Witzleben-Straße 22,
Heilbronn

Landscape planner
Dupper Landschaftsarchitekten,
Bad Friedrichshall

Interior planting
Strohm Innenbegrünungen, Widdern

The Tradition of the Palm Beaches

Architect
Perkins Eastman, 115 Fifth Avenue, New York,
NY 10003, USA

Contractor
The Whiting-Turner Company, 300 East Joppa
Road, Baltimore, MD 21286

Consultants
Technical installations and fire safety
Johnson, Levinson, Ragan, Davila, Inc.
Construction engineer
Michael B. Schorah & Associates, Inc.
Structural engineer
Slider Engineering Group

Landscape planner
Cotleur & Hearing

Toftehaven Nursing Home

Address
Nygårdsvej 35, DK-2750 Ballerup

Architect
Vilhelm Lauritzen Architects, Wildersgade 41,
DK-1408 Copenhagen

Client
Ballerup Municipality, Hold-an Vej 7,
DK-2750 Ballerup;
Baldersbo Housing Association, Præstevænget
46, Postbox 124, DK-2750 Ballerup

Consultant
Teytaud A/S

Landscape planner
Henrik Jørgensen, MDL

Ulrika Eleonora Home for the Elderly

Address
Vanha Viipurintie 7, FIN-07900 Loviisa

Architect
L&M Sievänen, architects / Liisa and Markku
Sievänen and assistant architect Meiri Siivola,
Länsiportti 1 B - C, FIN-02210 Espoo

Client
Loviisa District Service Home Foundation,
Kuningattarenkatu 7, FIN-07900 Loviisa

Consultant
Construction Office Hinkkanen

Landscape planner
L&M Sievänen with Gunilla Törnblom,
Loviisa town gardens authority

Vigs Ängar

Address
Vigavägen 18, S-27074 Köpingebro

Architect
Husberg Architects office AB /
Lillemor Husberg Architect SAR/MSA, Box 64,
S-27222 Simrishamn

Client
Ystadt Municipality

Consultant
Byggteknikgruppen, Malmoe AB, Box 17509,
S-20010 Malmö

Landscape planner
Kerstin Lundén Architect LAR/MSA

Palladiumflat

Address
Siersteenlaan 418-424, NL-9743 ES Groningen

Architect
Johannes Kappler Architekten,
Wilhelm-Marx-Straße 9, D-90419 Nuremberg

Client
Chr. Woningstichting Patrimonium,
Peizerweg 36, NL-9727 AP Groningen

Consultants
Structural engineer
Ingenieursbureau Dijkhuis, Groningen
Technical and electrical installations
Zonderman, Groningen
HVAC
Feenstra, Groningen

"Plaine de Scarpe" Nursing Home and Home for the Elderly

Address
La Plaine de Scarpe, Rue Jehanne de Lallaing,
BP 9, F-59167 Lallaing

Architect
Yann Brunel Architecte, 20 Rue Voltaire,
F-93100 Montreuil sous Bois

Client
Société de Secours Minière du Nord, 771 Boule-
vard Ambroise Croizat, F-59287 Saint Guesnain

Consultant
Saunier et Associés, Lens

RainbowVision

Address
500 Rodeo Road, Santa Fe, NM 87505, USA

Architect
LLOYD & ASSOCIATES ARCHITECTS, 501
Halona St., Santa Fe, NM 87505, USA

Client
RainbowVision Properties, Joy Silver, President;
Contractor Weis Construction, 7645 Lyndale
Ave, Minneapolis, MN 55423, USA

Landscape planner
David Lovero, Santa Fe, NM, USA

Residencia Alcázar Juan Hermanitas Ancianos

Address
Desamparados Provincia, Avd. Teresa Forner,
s/n, E-13600 Alcazar Juan Ciudad Real

Architect
Vicens + Ramos, c/ Barquillo N° 29,
2° IZQ, E-28004 Madrid

Client
Congregación de la Hermanitas
de los Ancianos Desamparados

Consultant
Construcciones LAIN

Landscape planner
Vicens + Ramos

Steinacker Residential Complex

Address
Trichtenhausenstrasse 120-128,
CH-8053 Zurich-Witikon

Architect
Hasler Schlatter Partner,
Am Schanzengraben 15, CH-8002 Zurich

Client
Baugenossenschaft Zürich,
Dreispitz 21, CH-8050 Zurich;
Wohn- und Siedlungsgenossenschaft Zürich,
Dörflistrasse 50, CH-8050 Zürich

Consultants
Structural engineer
Ernst Winkler + Partner AG, Effretikon
Heating, ventilation
Müller-Bucher, Zurich
Sanitary installations
Ariag A. Rindlisbacher AG, Zurich
Electrical engineer
Schneider Engineering + Partner, Zurich

Landscape planner
Zschokke & Gloor, Kempraten

Art installations
Pascale Wiedemann, Chur

St. Anna Nursing Home

Address
Rüppurrer Straße 29, D-76137 Karlsruhe

Architect
PIA – Architekten,
Dessauer Straße 3, D-76139 Karlsruhe

Client
Orden der barmherzigen Schwestern vom
hl. Vincenz von Paul, Freiburg,
Habsburgstraße 120, D-79104 Freiburg

Consultants
HVAC
Krebser und Freyler, Teningen
Structural engineer
Hartmann, Jung, Ruck GmbH, Karlsruhe

Landscape planner
Prof. Kokenge, Dresden

St. Michael Centre for the Elderly

Address
Höhensteig 1, D-12526 Berlin

Architect
GAP mbH Gesellschaft für Architektur und
Projektmanagement, Schöneberger Straße 15,
D-10963 Berlin

Client
St. Hedwig Krankenhaus, Anstalt des öffent-
lichen Rechts, Große Hamburger Straße 2-5,
D-10115 Berlin

Consultants
HVAC, Electrical engineer
Genius Ingenieurbüro GmbH, Berlin
Structural engineer
GSE Ingenieur-Gesellschaft mbH Saar-Enseleit
und Partner, Berlin

Landscape planner
ST raum a Gesellschaft von Landschaftsarchitekten mbH, Berlin

Tårnåsen Housing and Activity Centre

Address
Valhallaveien 62/64, N-1413 Tårnåsen

Architect
KVERNAAS ARKITEKTER AS,
Kolbotnveien 7, N-1410 Kolbotn

Client
Oppegård Municipality,
Rosenholmveien 40, N-1414 Trollåsen

Consultant
Dr. Techn. Kristoffer Apeland AS

Landscape planner
Multiconsult, avd. 13.3 Landskapsarkitektur /
KVERNAAS ARKITEKTER AS

West View Manor

Address
1715 Mechanicsburg Road, Wooster, OH 44691,
USA

Architect
JMM Architects, Inc, 4685 Larwell Drive,
Columbus, OH 43220, USA

Contractor
BCMC Inc, P.O. Box 422, Wooster, OH 44691,
USA

Landscape planner
JMM Architects, Inc.

Will Mark Kashiihama Senior Residences

Address
3-2-1 Kashiihama, Higashi-ku, Fukuoka-City,
Fukuoka Prefecture, Japan

Architect
KUME SEKKEI Co. Ltd., 2-1-22, Shiomi, Kotoku,
Tokyo 135-8567, Japan

Client
Fukuoka Jisho Senior Life Co., Ltd.

Contractor
Taisei Corporation, 1-25-1, Nishi-Shinjuku,
Shinjuku-ku, Tokyo 163-0606, Japan

Consultants
Interior design
KUME SEKKEI Co., Ltd. + ILYA Co., Ltd.

Landscape planner
KUME SEKKEI Co., Ltd. + Design Network
Co., Ltd.

"Wohnfabrik Solinsieme"

Address
Solinsieme, Tschudistrasse 43,
CH-9000 St. Gallen

Architect
ARCHPLAN AG, Wallstrasse 5,
CH-9000 St. Gallen

Client
Solinsieme – Genossenschaft für neue Wohn-
form, Tschudistrasse 43, CH-9000 St. Gallen

Consultants
Structural engineer
Bänziger + Köppel Dipl.-Ingenieure ETH,
St. Gallen
Electrical engineer
Ingenieur-Büro Thomas Camenisch, St. Gallen

Sanitary installations
Ingenieur-Büro Kurt Staub, St. Gallen
Construction performance
Kühn + Blickle Institut für Lärmschutz,
Unterägeri
HVAC
Gallusser + Partner AG, St. Gallen

Landscape planner
Rudolf Lüthi Landschaftsarchitekt HTL BSLA,
Wittenbach

Authors

Eckhard Feddersen

born in 1946, sees himself as a mediator. After studying architecture in Karlsruhe, the USA and Berlin, he became a member of the faculty of architecture at the Technical University of Berlin and later tutor for design and building construction. Since 1973, Eckhard Feddersen has designed and realised buildings in the social sector, for old people, people with disabilities and children. In the same year he set up an architectural office together with Wolfgang von Herder, followed in 2002 by the office feddersenarchitekten, focusing further on property concepts for the social sector. In 1999 he was Director of Planning for the Berlin Building Exhibition; in 2003 he initiated the Competency Network for Health, Care and Disabilities in Berlin with participants from politics, medicine and welfare organisations. In 2008, together with Insa Lüdtke, he founded Cocon Concept Feddersen Lüdtke Consulting which focuses on transformations in the housing sector. He has lectured and published widely.

Insa Lüdtke

born in 1972, studied as an architect at the Technical University of Darmstadt (Dipl.-Ing.) and works as a freelance journalist for diverse media with a special focus on architecture and health. In 2002 she took over responsibility for public relations at feddersenarchitekten; she is also an initiator and member of a network of professionals in the field of architecture and publicity. In 2006 she became a member of the advisory committee at the German Architecture Museum (DAM) for an exhibition on "Living in the Future" and is a member of the advisory board for the magazine *MedAmbiente*. Born out of her publicity work at feddersenarchitekten, in 2008 she founded Cocon Concept Feddersen Lüdtke Consulting together with Eckhard Feddersen, a company which focusses on transformations in the housing sector. She lectures widely, chairs discussions and has written for numerous publications.

Dr. Helmut Braun

born in 1948, is a qualified social education worker and social gerontologist. His doctoral thesis examined determining parameters for the care provision requirements of elderly people (Kassel 1992). After working in the planning unit of the Social Welfare Department and as head of department for the Welfare of the Elderly at the City of Munich, he became managing director of the KWA (Kuratorium Wohnen im Alter), one of the largest operators of senior residences in Germany, and chairman of the board. In 2008 he also became chairman of the board of Procurand AG, one of the largest nursing home providers in Germany. In a voluntary capacity, Helmut Braun was vice president of the German Association for Gerontology and Geriatrics (DGGG) between 1988 and 1994 and a board member of the national conference on quality assurance in the care and health industries (BUKO-QS). He has been a lecturer in Munich, Kassel, Dortmund and Heidelberg and has published numerous articles on care for the elderly, social policies and planning for the elderly.

Dr. Stefan Dreßke

studied sociology in Berlin and London and is an academic assistant at the Institute for Social Policy and Social Services Administration at the University of Kassel. His fields of expertise include the organisation of different aspects of health care provision, including outpatient care, psychosocial care in hospitals, palliative care and disabilities.

Maria Dwight

is president and founder of Gerontological Services, Inc., a 25-year-old market research and consulting firm in Santa Monica, California. Her 42 years of experience include the initiation of the first Geriatric Authority in the USA, as well as research, consulting services, lectures, seminars and speeches throughout the United States, Europe and Asia. She has taught at the summer institute at Harvard Graduate School of Design for 26 years.

Dietmar Eberle

born in 1952, is professor of architecture and design at the Swiss Federal Institute of Technology (ETH) in Zurich. After studying in Vienna, from 1979 onwards he was one of the initiators of a new architectural scene in Vorarlberg, Austria. His architectural practice with Carlo Baumschlager operates internationally and has offices in Lochau, Vaduz, Vienna, Beijing, St. Gallen, Zurich and Hong Kong, which together have realised more than 300 buildings.

Angelika Hausenbiegl

born in 1964, has a master's degree in nursing theory from the University of Vienna. Her diploma project examined the healing properties of laughter and humour in geriatric care. She trained to become a certified hospital manager at Vienna University of Economics and Business Administration, earning an E.D.E. Certificate as Home Manager as well as an Eden Associate Certification (Eden Europe, Eden-Alternative TM). She is currently writing her sociology dissertation at the University of Vienna on the living and housing requirements of an increasingly older society.

Bernhard H. Heiming

born in 1963, is a structural engineer and has worked for 25 years in London, Frankfurt and Berlin as a project coordinator, director, technical director and managing director in the property sector. He is currently managing partner at Terragon GmbH in Berlin and is involved in the development, project management, project controlling as well as project supervision, consultation and marketing of property projects in the social sector and housing for the elderly. He is chairman of the Housing for the Elderly Task Group at the Federal Association of Independent Property and Housing Associations (BFW) and represents this association at the U.E.P.C. Union Européenne des Promoteurs-Constructeurs.

Matthias Hürlimann

is a partner in the consulting practice Demenzplus and studied architecture and planning at the Swiss Federal Institute of Technology (ETH) in Zurich. He has worked in the offices of Colin St. John Wilson in London, headed the research project "Gestaltungsplan" at the ORL Institute and was involved in the Swiss National Fund research project on identifying barriers for the disabled and elderly in building constructions, undertaken at the Institute for Construction Research at the ETH Zurich. Matthias Hürlimann is founder and co-owner of the architectural office archi-NETZ which focuses on projects in housing, social facilities, buildings for the disabled and the elderly as well as agriculture. He is also co-founder of the Swiss Centre for Construction for the Disabled. Together with Dr. Rudolf Welter, he provides consultation and project supervision for construction and organisational development and renovation/conversion projects in the disabled and elderly housing sectors. He writes for specialist publications and runs further education courses.

Katharina Hürlimann-Siebke

is a partner in the consulting practice Demenzplus and studied economics at Merseburg University of Applied Sciences. After working for many years in public relations for universities and as a journalist, she joined Matthias Hürlimann and archi-NETZ in Zurich in 2000 as a project partner. Together they undertook the project "Idea a + b" on self-sufficient living for older and disabled people commissioned by benabita. She is author of professional publications as well as a research report on approaches to overcoming steps and changes of level in old buildings commissioned by the Swiss Centre for Building for the Disabled.

Dr. rer. phil. Marie-Therese Krings-Heckemeier
is chair of the executive board of empirica ag Research and Consulting in Berlin and a partner in empirica Qualitative Marktforschung, Struktur- und Stadtforschung GmbH in Bonn. In addition she is a member of the Council of Real Estate Experts, vice-chair of the Expert Commission for the Second National Social Report on the Elderly and a member of the DIN German Institute for Standardisation Project Committee on Services for Sheltered Housing for the Elderly. Since 1976, Marie-Therese Krings-Heckemeier has worked in research and consulting for national and federal state ministries, local municipalities, housing associations, investors, banks, life insurers and building societies among others. Her work focuses on urban and regional development, property markets and special types of real estate including real estate abroad, town planning policy, lifestyle research and sociospatial analysis and project controlling as part of the "Soziale Stadt" programme for socially integrative cities.

Yasmine Mahmoudieh
born in 1961, studied art history in Florence, architecture in Geneva, interior design in Belmont and received her Bachelor of Arts in Architecture and Design in 1985 from the University of California, Los Angeles (UCLA). After founding offices in Los Angeles and Berlin, mahmoudiehdesign operates since 1999 from Berlin and London and conceives and realises projects in the hotel, restaurant, retail and workplace sectors. Her office has won numerous awards for interior design projects including parts of the Coconut Grove Plaza in Miami, an office building for Tishman Speyer, the Radisson SAS in Copenhagen, the Radisson SAS DomAquarée in Berlin, and Haus Rheinsberg. Yasmine Mahmoudieh teaches as a guest lecturer at the École Hôtelière de Lausanne, one of the most highly regarded schools in the hotel trade.

Johanna Myllymäki-Neuhoff
is an educationalist (Dipl.-Päd.) and gerontologist (Dipl.-Pyschogerontol.) and studied social policy and social services at the Universities of Siegen, Erlangen-Nuremberg and Kuopio in Finland (Lic.SSc. (Fin)). Since the 1990s she has worked as a teacher and lecturer at universities in Germany and Finland. After many years in the academic realm, as project coordinator for a pilot project centre for dementia and as a gerontologist for a large social welfare provider, Johanna Myllymäki-Neuhoff currently works as a gerontologist and coordinator in the Centre for Geriatric Medicine at Nuremberg Clinic. She has published widely on the topic of dementia and care for the elderly.

Georg W. Reinberg
born in 1950, studied as an architect at the Technical University of Vienna (Arch. Ing.) and at Syracuse University in New York (M. Arch.). His office, Architekturbüro Reinberg, which he runs together with his wife Marta Enriquez-Reinberg, has operated since 1982 as a planning office, and since 1985 as a design engineering office, with special focus on planning and realisation as well as cost controlling and construction management. In addition to his Visiting Professorship for Solar Architecture at the Danube University Krems and a position as lecturer in the postgraduate MSc programme "Renewable Energy in Central and Eastern Europe" at the Technical University of Vienna, Reinberg has also lectured internationally in Mexico, the USA, Panama, Italy, France, England, Spain, the Czech Republic, Belgium, Sweden and Germany. His publications include the book *Ecological Architecture – Design, Planning, Realization*, authored together with Matthias Boeckl and published by Springer Verlag in 2008.

Beth Tauke
is an Associate Professor of Architecture and former Associate Dean in the School of Architecture and Planning at the University at Buffalo – State University of New York. She directs university education activities for the Center for Inclusive Design and Environmental Access (IDEA) and is the director of the Universal Design International University Education Consortium. Professor Tauke is one of the co-editors of *Universal Design Education Online* and co-editor of *Diversity and Design: The Journal of Inclusive Design Education*. She has published many journal articles and has co-edited the book *Universal Design: New York* with Dr. G. Scott Danford.

Nikolaos Tavridis
born in 1969, studied business economics and is a consultant for the operation and running of residential schemes for the elderly. After working in management for care providers as a controller, financial director and member of the management team at Casa Reha Betriebs- und Beteiligungsgesellschaft mbH and as managing director of ProVita Betriebsgesellschaft mbH, in 2001 he became a partner in Axion Consult GmbH in Bad Homburg. In addition, he is also operator and managing director of the Elbschloss Residenz GmbH and Patria Residenzen GmbH.

Dr. Rudolf Welter
is a partner in the consulting practice Demenzplus, an architect and an environmental and organisational psychologist. He studied at the University of Michigan and the Swiss Federal Institute of Technology (ETH) in Zurich, and wrote his dissertation on adaptive building for hospitalised long-term patients. Rudolf Welter develops and implements innovative planning methods and ways of increasing user participation in social organisations and health institutions (hospitals, clinics, care homes) with a view to designing living and working environments. Since 1980 he has worked as a freelance project consultant, supervisor and coach for project teams working on the construction or organisation of development or renovation/conversion projects. He is the author of numerous articles, teaches in universities and runs further education courses.

Harms Wulf
born in 1958, is a landscape architect. Since founding Harms Wulf Landschaftsarchitekten in 1992, his office has increasingly focused on the design of barrier-free outdoor environments for private and public use in the health, education and elderly care sectors. To pursue his commitment to the design of barrier-free environments, Harms Wulf joined the Berlin Chamber of Architects' Committee for the Barrier-Free Design of Cities and Buildings in 2001, and was elected chair of the committee in 2006.

Bibliography

General

Bauer, Michael; Mösle, Peter; Schwarz, Michael, *Green Building: Guidebook for Sustainable Architecture*, Berlin, Heidelberg, New York: Springer, 2009.

Bollnow, Otto Friedrich, *Human Space*, London: Hyphen Press, 1997.

Brauer, Kerry-U., *Wohnen, Wohnformen, Wohnbedürfnisse. Soziologische und psychologische Aspekte in der Planung und Vermarktung von Wohnimmobilien*, Wiesbaden: IZ Immobilien Zeitung Verlagsgesellschaft, 2008.

Caduff, Corina; Pfaff-Czarnecka, Joanna (Ed.), *Rituale heute. Theorien – Kontroversen – Entwürfe*, Berlin: Dietrich Reimer Verlag, 2001.

Crosbie, Michael J.; Steven Winter Associates, *Home Rehab Handbook*, New York: McGraw-Hill Professional, 2002.

Gilg, Mark; Schaeppi, Werner, *Lebensräume. Auf der Suche nach zeitgemäßem Wohnen*, Zurich: Niggli, 2007.

Opaschewski, Horst W., *Deutschland 2020. Wie wir morgen leben – Prognosen der Wissenschaft*, Wiesbaden: VS Verlag für Sozialwissenschaften / GWV Fachverlage, 2006.

Schneider, Friederike (Ed.), *Floor Plan Manual Housing*, 3rd revised and expanded edition, Basel, Boston, Berlin: Birkhäuser, 2004.

Old age and the elderly

Colvez, Alain et al, *Cantou et long séjour hospitalier*, Paris: Inserm/FNG, 1994.

KEUCO GmbH & Co. KG (Ed.), *Third Age – Third Skin. Social Infrastructure in a Time of Change*, Wuppertal: Verlag Müller + Busmann, 2007.

Lakotta, Beate; Schels, Walter, *Noch mal Leben vor dem Tod. Wenn Menschen sterben*, Munich: Deutsche Verlags-Anstalt, 2004.

National Collaboration Centre for Mental Health; Social Care Institute for Excellence; National Institute for Health and Clinical Excellence (Ed.), *Dementia: the NICE-SCIE Guideline on Supporting People with Dementia and their Carers in Health and Social Care (National Clinical Practice Guideline)*, Leicester: British Psychological Society, 2007.

Niejahr, Elisabeth, *Alt sind nur die anderen. So werden wir leben, lieben und arbeiten*, Frankfurt am Main: S. Fischer, 2004.

Nübel, Gerhard; Kuhlmann, Heinz-Peter; Meißnest, Bernd (Ed.), *Leben bis zuletzt. Das Ende neu entdecken*, Frankfurt am Main: Mabuse-Verlag, 2007.

Victor, Christina, *The Social Context of Ageing*, London, New York: Routledge, 2005.

Universal Design

Clarkson, John; Coleman, Roger; Keates, Simeon; Lebbon, Cherie (Ed.), *Inclusive Design: Design for the Whole Population*, London: Springer, 2003.

Confino-Rehder, Shirley, Universal Design. *Planning today for tomorrow: a Study on Livable Communities*, lecture in Casale Monferato, 1998 and Montreal, 1999.

Danford, G. Scott; Tauke, Beth (Ed.), *Universal Design: New York*, New York: Mayor's Office for People with Disabilities, 2001.

Goldsmith, Selwyn; Dezart, Jeannette, PRP Architects, *Universal Design. A Manual of Practical Guidance for Architects*, Jordan Hill, GB, and Woburn, MA: Architectural Press, 2000.

Herwig, Oliver, *Universal Design. Solutions for Barrier-Free Living*, Birkhäuser, Birkhäuser, Basel, Boston, Berlin, 2008.

Jordan, Wendy A., *Universal Design for the Home. Great-Looking, Great-Living Designs for all Ages, Abilities and Circumstances. Barrier-Free Living for all Generations*, Beverly, MA: Rockport, 2008.

Lidwell, William; Holden, Kristina; Butler, Jill, *Universal Principles of Design. A Cross-Disciplinary Reference. 100 Ways to Enhance Usability, Influence Reception, Increase Appeal, Make Better Design Decisions, and Teach through Design*, Beverly, MA: Rockport, 2003.

Pinto Guimarães, Marcelo, *Understanding Universal Design by Simulations about Socially Inclusive Environments*, Saarbrücken: VDM, 2008.

Preiser, Wolfgang F.E.; Ostroff, Elaine (Ed.), *Universal Design Handbook*, New York: McGraw-Hill Professional, 2001.

Living for the elderly

Andritzky, Michael; Hauer, Thomas; BauWohnberatung Karlsruhe; Schader-Stiftung Darmstadt (Ed.), *Neues Wohnen im Alter: Was geht und wie es geht*, Frankfurt am Main: Anabas, 2004.

Baucom, Alfred H., *Hospitality Design for the Graying Generation. Meeting the Needs of a Growing Market*, Hoboken, NJ: John Wiley & Sons, 1996.

Brawley, Elisabeth C., *Designing for Alzheimer's desease*, New York: John Wiley & Sons, 1997.

Chaline, Brigitte; Boussahba, Sophie, *Unités d'accueil spécialisées Alzheimer: Manuel de conception architecturale*, Paris: Pfizer France, 2001.

Coleman, Roger; Clarkson, John; Dong, Hua; Cassim, Julia, *Design for Inclusivity: A Practical Guide to Accessible, Innovative and User-centred Design (Design for Social Responsibility)*, Aldershot: Gower Publishing, 2007.

Cooper, Marcus; Barnes, Claire; Barnes, Marvin, *Healing Gardens. Therapeutic Benefits and Design Recommendations*, New York: John Wiley & Sons, 1999.

Dehan, Philippe, *L'habitat des personnes âgées. Du logement adapté aux Êhpad, USLD et unités Alzheimer*, Paris: Editions du Moniteur, 2007.

Durrett, Charles, *The Senior Cohousing Handbook, 2nd Edition. A Community Approach to Independent Living*, Gabriola Island: New Society Publishers, 2009.

Fabach, Robert; Hebenstreit, Martin (Ed.), *Pflegeheime und Architektur. Ein Leitfaden für eine bewohner- und pflegegerechte Planung*, connexia – Gesellschaft für Gesundheit und Pflege, 2008.

Grosbois, Louis-Pierre, *Handicap physique et construction*, Paris: Editions du Moniteur, 2001.

Harrigan, John E.; Raise, Jennifer M., Senior Residences. *Designing Retirement Communities for the Future*, New York: John Wiley & Sons, 1998.

Heinze, Rolf G.; Eichener, Volker; Naegele, Gerhard; Bucksteeg, Mathias; Schauerte, Martin, *Neue Wohnung auch im Alter. Folgerungen aus dem demographischen Wandel für Wohnungspolitik und Wohnungswirtschaft*, Darmstadt: Schader-Stiftung, 1997.

Heumann, Leonard F.; McCall, Mary E.; Boldy, Duncan P. (Ed.), *Opportunities and Impediments in Housing, Health, and Support Service Delivery*, Westport, CT: Greenwood Press, 2001.

Huber, Andreas (Ed.), *New Approaches to Housing in the Second Half of Life*, Basel, Boston, Berlin: Birkhäuser, 2008.

Imrie, Robert, *Accessible Housing. Quality, Disability, and Design*, London/New York: Taylor & Francis, 2006.

Kuratorium Deutsche Altershilfe (Ed.), *Farbe ins Heim. Farbvorschläge des Kuratoriums Deutsche Altershilfe*, Cologne: Kuratorium Deutsche Altershilfe, 2002.

Kuratorium Deutsche Altershilfe (Ed.), *Das Einzelzimmer – Standard in der stationären Altenhilfe?* (Architektur+Gerontologie 4), Cologne: Kuratorium Deutsche Altershilfe, 2005.

Leibrock, Cynthia A., *Design Details for Health. Making the Most of Interior Design's Healing Potential*, New York: John Wiley & Sons, 1999.

Marberry, Sam O., *Healthcare Design*, New York: John Wiley & Sons, 1997.

McGee, Paula (Ed.), *Respecting Cultural Diversity in Health Care. The Way Forward for the 21st Century. Proceedings of the Third National Conference of the Transcultural Nursing and Healthcare Associates*, Sheffield: UCE Centre for Health & and Social Care Research, 2001.

Narten, Renate, *Wohnen im Alter. Bausteine für die Wohnungswirtschaft*, Hanover: vdw Verband der Wohnungswirtschaft Niedersachsen-Bremen, 2004.

Peace, Sheila M.; Holland, Caroline, *Inclusive housing in an ageing society*, Bristol: The Policy Press, 2001.

Pearce, Benjamin W., *Senior Living Communities. Operations Management and Marketing for Assisted Living, Congregate, and Continuing-Care Retirement Communities*, Baltimore, MD: John Hopkins University Press, 1998.

Perkins, Bradford; Kliment, Stephen A.; King, Douglas, *Building Type Basics for Senior Living*, Hoboken, NJ: John Wiley & Sons, 2004.

Purves, Geffrey, *Healthy Living Centres. A Guide to Primary Health Care Design*, Oxford: Elsevier, 2002.

Rau, Ulrike (Ed.), *barrierefrei – bauen für die zukunft*, Berlin: Bauwerk Verlag, 2008.

Reinberg, Georg W.; Boeckl, M. (Ed.): *Reinberg – Ecological Architecture – Design – Planning – Realization*, Berlin, Heidelberg, New York: Springer, 2008.

Rühm, Bettina, *Unbeschwert Wohnen im Alter. Neue Lebensformen und Architekturkonzepte*, Munich: Deutsche Verlags-Anstalt, 2003.

Schittich, Christian (Ed.), *Housing for People of all Ages: Flexible, Unrestricted, Senior-Friendly*, Munich: Institute for International Architecture Documentation, and Basel, Boston, Berlin: Birkhäuser, 2007.

Steven Winter Associates, *Accessible Housing by Design. Universal Design Principles in Practice*, New York: McGraw-Hill Professional, 1997.

Stoneham, Jane; Thoday, Peter, *Landscape Design for Elderly and Disabled People*, Woodbridge, Suffolk: Garden art press, 1996.

Torrington, Judith, *Upgrading Buildings for Older People*, London: RIBA Publishing, 2004.

Torrington, Judith; Tregenza, P., "Lighting for People with dementia", in: *Lighting Research and Technology*, 39, 1/2007, p. 81-97.

Vercauteren, Richard; Predazzi, Marco; Loriaux, Michel, *Une architecture nouvelle pour l'habitat des personnes âgées*, Ramonville-Saint-Agne: Érès, 2000

Vercauteren, Richard, *Construire le projet de vie en maison de retraite ou L'animation dans les établissements pour personnes âgées*, Ramonville-Saint-Agne: Érès, 2000.

Welter, Rudolf; Hürlimann, Matthias; Hürlimann-Siebke, Katharina (Ed.), *Gestaltung von Betreuungseinrichtungen für Menschen mit Demenzerkrankungen*, Zurich: Demenzplus, 2006.

Wüstenrot Stiftung (Ed.), *Wohnen im Alter*, Stuttgart and Zurich: Karl Krämer Verlag, 2006.

Zeisel, John, Inquiry by Design: *Evinronments / Behavior / Neuroscience in Architecture. Interiors, Landscape and Planning*, revised edition, New York: W.W. Norton, 2005.

Eckhard Feddersen and Insa Lüdtke

Feddersen, Eckhard (interview), "Wir brauchen einen integrierten Ansatz im Wohnungsbau", in: *Detail*, 03/ 2006, p. 226.

Feddersen, Eckhard, "Der demografische Knick. Statements zum Wohnen im Alter", in: *DBZ*, 08/2006, p. 60-61.

Feddersen, Eckhard, "Silver Living – jeder nach seiner Façon – Wohnen der Generation 50-Plus", in: *Die Wohnungswirtschaft (DW)*, 07/2003, p. 42-44.

Feddersen, Eckhard, "Von der Spezialimmobilie zum multifunktionalen Normalgebäude", in: *Die Wohnungswirtschaft (DW)*, 11/ 2003, p. 42-45.

Feddersen, Eckhard; Lüdtke, Insa; Rau, Ulrike; Wulf, Harms, *"Wohnen mit Zukunft", in: Barrierefrei – Bauen für die Zukunft*, Bauwerk Verlag, Berlin 2008, p. 237 ff.

feddersenarchitekten (Ed.), *Demenz + Architektur*, Berlin 2006.

Lüdtke, Insa, "Bauplanungsmodell: Steine, Sterne, Standards", in: *Care Invest*, 01+02/2008, p. 12-13.

Lüdtke, Insa, "Eine neue Familie basteln", in: *Der Tagesspiegel*, Berlin, 27.09.2002.

Lüdtke, Insa, "High-Tech bis High-Touch. Über Möglichkeiten des Technikeinsatzes für Menschen mit Demenz", in: *MedAmbiente*, 5/2008, p. 4-5.

Lüdtke, Insa, "Vielfalt als Gütezeichen", in: *Altenheim*, 10/2007, p. 22-24.

Lüdtke, Insa, "Wohnen für alle – jeder nach seiner Façon", *VDW-Magazin*, 01/2006, p. 19-20.

Journals and magazines

Altenheim

AIT, theme "Bauten für Gesundheit & Soziales", 11/2005, 11/2006, 11/2007, 11/2008.

Architektur + Wettbewerbe, theme "Seniorenresidenzen", 197/March 2004.

Baumeister, theme "Einfach alt werden", 5/2006.

CARE konkret.

CARE Invest.

Deutsche Bauzeitschrift (DBZ), theme "Wohnen im Alter", 7/2003, 8/2006.

Deutsche Bauzeitung (db), theme "Barrierefreies Bauen", 03/2005.

form. theme "Neue Ideen für Alte", Sept./Oct. 2005.

kma – das Gesundheitswirtschaftsmagazin.

MedAmbiente.

Werk, Bauen und Wohnen, theme "Wohnen im Alter/Housing for the Elderly", 1+2/2004.

Websites

www.aeldresagen.dk (Danish DaneAge Association)

www.age.org.uk (The Age Concern)

www.age-award.ch

www.anfarch.org (Academy of Neuroscience for Architecture)

www.ap.buffalo.edu/idea/diversityindesign/ (The Journal of Inclusive Design Education)

www.baunetz.de (platform for architects and planners)

www.barrierefrei.de (portal for barrier-free living and building for the disabled)

www.bmfsfj.de (German Federal Ministry of Family, Senior Citizens, Women and Youth)

www.bertelsmann-stiftung.de

www.bosch-stiftung.de

www.deutsche-alzheimer.de/

www.design4all.ch

www.designforall.at

www.design.ncsu.edu/cud/ (Center for Universal Design)

www.generationendialog.de (Initiative for promoting intergenerational dialogue)

www.gerontechnology.info/Journal/

www.housingcare.org (Information on different forms of living for the elderly)

Index of names

Index of places

Photo credits

All plans and construction drawings were provided by the respective architectural offices.

10,11 Diagrams Beth Tauke

12 Hotel Fox, Dänemark

14 **top left, bottom right**
Reinhard Görner
top centre, right
feddersenarchitekten
bottom left, centre
Theodor Fliedner Stiftung

15 **left** Joachim Loch
right feddersenarchitekten

16 **top** Angelika Hausenbiegl
bottom Kengo Kuma & Associates

17 **top**
Kengo Kuma & Associates
bottom Toru Waki

18 Ronald Grunert-Held

19 **top** Markku Sievänen
centre Barbara Thieme
(www.buero-ix.de)
bottom Annette Lozinski

20 **top** Angelika Hausenbiegl
bottom Ronald Grunert-Held

21 **left** Angelika Hausenbiegl
right Ronald Grunert-Held

26 Peter Mason

29 Pacific Retirement Services
of Medford Oregon

30, 31 Ronald Grunert-Held

32 **left** Michael Holz
right Ronald Grunert-Held

33 **top**
Vilhelm Lauritzen Architects
bottom feddersenarchitekten

34 Werner Krüper

35, 36 Michael Radig

38 Will McBride

43, 44 ©Eduard Hueber /
archphoto.com

46 Linus Lintner

47 mahmoudiehdesign

48 **top** Linus Lintner
bottom mahmoudiehdesign

49 mahmoudiehdesign

50 **top** Arne Piepereit
bottom Ronald Grunert-Held

51 **top** Ronald Grunert-Held
bottom lux Fotografen, Florian
Keller

52 **top left and centre left**
Ronald Grunert-Held
centre right Heike Overberg
right Piepereit

lower group:
top Harms Wulf
centre Ronald Grunert-Held
bottom Arne Piepereit

53 Ronald Grunert-Held

54, 55 ETH Zurich

64 Hegger, M.; Fuchs, M.;
Stark, Th.; Zeumer, M.,
Energy Manual, edition DETAIL,
Munich; page 34, Fig. A 6.5

66 Energy Manual, page 135,
Fig. B 4.96

67-69 Georg W. Reinberg

77 **top** Annette Scholz
bottom Marc Puchert

78 Marcus von Amsberg,
News & Media

79 Arne Hofmann

Typologies and projects

86 - 90 Johannes Marburg

92 - 94 Herta Hurnaus

96 Ralph Hut

97 **large** Ursula Meissen
Klein Ralph Hut

98 **top** Ralph Hut
bottom Ralph Hut

99 **left, large photo** Ralph Hut
small, top Ursula Meissen
small, bottom Ursula Meissen

104, 105
Foto-Design Waltraud Krase

106 Inge Miczka

107
Foto-Design Waltraud Krase

108 **upper group, left**
Inge Miczka
upper group, top right
Foto-Design Waltraud Krase
upper group, bottom right
Inge Miczka
bottom photo Brand Below

110, 111
KVERNAAS ARKITEKTER AS

112, 113 shedkm architects

114, 115 Johannes Vogt

116 **left** Johannes Vogt
right ASIRarchitekten

118 Johannes Vogt

119 **top left, centre left,
bottom** Johannes Vogt
top right ASIRarchitekten

120
KCAP Architects & Planners

121 Rob't Hart

122 Oliver Heissner

123 Aloys Kiefer

124 Michael Holz

126, 127 Oliver Heissner

128 - 130 Edward Massery

132, 133 David Emery

134 - 136 Hiroyuki Kawano

140, 141 Christian Richters

142, 143 Eibe Sönnecken

144, 145 Jiri Havran

146 **left** U. Meissner
right Urs Welter

147 **small photos, top**
Urs Welter
small photos, bottom
U. Meissner
large photo, right Urs Welter

148, 149 Steffen Großmann

150, 151 Wayne S. Lloyd, AIA

152 **left** Nacasa & Partners Inc.
right Shinkentiku-sha

153 **left** Shinkentiku-sha
right Nacasa & Partners Inc.

154 **left** Nacasa & Partners Inc.
right Shinkentiku-sha

156, 157
Nacasa & Partners Inc.

160 - 164
Ronald Grunert-Held

166 - 168 Olivier Wogenscky

170, 171
Dominique Meienberg

176 - 180 Pez Hejduk

182, 183 Stephan Baumann

184, 185 Dauid Aidan

186 - 188 Miguel de Guzman

190 - 192 Peter Kopitz

194 - 198 Eugeni Pons

200, 201 Bruno Klomfar

202, 203
Kengo Kuma & Associates

204, 205 Ester Havlova

206 **left** Bo Rosander
centre and right Peo Erikson

207 Peo Erikson

208, 209 Hiroyuki Hirai

210 Mikael Anttila

211 **left** Jussi Tiainen
centre Mikael Anttila
right Jussi Tiainen

212 **left** Mikael Anttila
right Markku Sievänen

213 Jussi Tiainen

216, 217 Willi Schnöll

218 - 220
©Roland Halbe/arturimages

222, 223 Jochen Stüber

224 Bimberg Landschaftsarchitekten

226, 227
Vilhelm Lauritzen Architects

228, 229
Lukas Huneke / Igel Studios

Products 239

Torre box grater
Manufacturer:
Silit-Werke GmbH & Co. KG,
Riedlingen
www.silit.de
Designer:
TEAMS Design GmbH,
Esslingen, Germany
www.teamsdesign.com
Winner of the universal design
award 09 www.ud-germany.de

KTR18P70 EasyStore,
Fridge with telescopic drawers
Manufacturer:
Robert Bosch Hausgeräte
GmbH, Munich
www.bosch-hausgeraete.com
Designer:
Robert Bosch Hausgeräte GmbH
Hans R. Janssen, Munich
www.bosch-hausgeraete.com
Winner of the universal design
award 09 www.ud-germany.de

PKG975N14E,
Glass ceramic cooker
Manufacturer:
Robert Bosch Hausgeräte
GmbH, Munich
www.bosch-hausgeraete.com
Designer:
Robert Bosch Hausgeräte GmbH
Robert Sachon, Bernd Kretsch-
mer, Ulrich Goss, Munich
www.bosch-hausgeraete.com
Winner of the universal design
award 09 www.ud-germany.de

Acknowledgements

Many people have contributed to the successful comple-
tion of this book. The following gave us numerous valuable
pointers for key topics addressed in this book: Dr. Helmut
Braun, ProCurand AG, Berlin; Wilfried Brexel, Senioren-
stiftung Prenzlauer Berg, Berlin; Prof. Dr. Klaus Hildemann,
Mülheim an der Ruhr; Waltraud Keuser, Keuser Consulting,
Mayen; Dr. Marie-Therese Krings-Heckemeier, empirica AG,
Berlin; Hans-Peter Winter, Kuratorium Deutsche Altershilfe,
Cologne; and Philipp M. Zemp, Senevita AG, Wabern.

We would like to thank all the contributing authors for providing such a variety of different and personal viewpoints
from their own experience in practice, which illustrate the
complexity of the topic of designing for the elderly. Our architectural colleagues from around the world have in turn responded with diverse and vibrant responses to the complexity of this subject. We wish to thank them too for providing
information and documentation on their respective projects.

In particular, we would like to thank our editor Christel Kapitzki, who helped us throughout the entire process with her
rich experience in book production, both in terms of content
and process. Likewise, we extend our thanks to Claudia Jäger
in our office for her extensive research and coordination with
the various architectural practices and contributors.

We are also indebted to our publisher Birkhäuser Verlag, to
the editor Andreas Müller for the fruitful collaboration and to
Oliver Kleinschmidt for the graphic design of this book.

Finally, we would like to thank all the institutions and firms
who like ourselves – each in their own field – continue to
demonstrate their enthusiasm for the topic of living for the
elderly.

Universal Design in an era of global demographic change

Initiated by "universal design e.V." in Hanover, conducted by the Chair of Industrial Design at the TU Munich and funded by the Robert Bosch Foundation, this research project investigated the challenges and opportunities facing the economy as a result of global demographic change. The authors of the study are Professor Fritz Frenkler from the Chair of Industrial Design at the TU Munich, Thomas Bade, founding member of universal design e.V., and Sandra Hirsch, academic assistant at the TU Munich.

The challenge of designing for future generations

Universal Design (UD) encompasses a catalogue of criteria that serve as a guideline for designing products for the future. If we are able to increasingly embrace the principles of Universal Design, global demographic changes could hold considerable potential for growth.

Fields of activity

Product design

Special emphasis should be given to products used in the public realm. The criteria of Universal Design should inform not only the design of products but also its directions for use, its packaging, marketing and distribution, and customer services.

Architecture and urban design

By applying Universal Design criteria such as flexibility, accessibility and widest possible usability, it should be possible to stabilise and even reinforce the population structure of cities, regions and municipalities.

Services

The design of services could offer considerable potential for creating added value among all consumer groups in the service sector.

Networking branches

According to prognoses, the networking of products with the building industry, including public buildings, and with the service sector will have particular potential.

The study is available as a PDF-file from the following address:
www.ud-germany.de/cms/ud/en/research_projects/research_project

At an expert conference entitled "Babylon – or holistic approaches to leveraging the economic potential of demographic change" organised by universal design e.V. and the Robert Bosch Stiftung in cooperation with the Bauhaus-Universität (12-14 November 2009), opinion leaders in industry will seek to establish a national Universal Design Alliance with experts from architecture and design.

Three winners of the universal design award 09 www.ud-germany.de:
Further information on the products shown is available in the illustration credits.

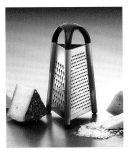

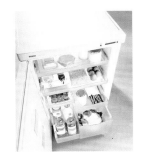

Torre box grater: The laser-cut grating surfaces are extremely sharp avoiding sticking or clogging

KTR18P70 EasyStore: A fridge with telescopic drawers

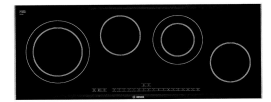

PKG975N14E
Glass ceramic cooker:
The easy reach hob is particularly suitable for wheelchair users or shorter people

Researching the design of care facilities for the elderly: improving orientation for people with dementia

The architecture of care facilities strongly influences the behaviour and well-being of residents with dementia and can be used to help them maintain mobility and independence. However, there is no scientific basis for many aspects of dementia-friendly architecture. At the Chair for Buildings for Health and Social Services at the Faculty of Architecture, TU Dresden, Professor Dr.-Ing. Peter Schmieg and Dr.-Ing. Gesine Marquardt have undertaken a study, funded by the Robert Bosch Foundation, to establish empirical criteria for the design of building structures that support the spatial orientation of dementia sufferers. The building structure of 30 care homes for the elderly were analysed along with data concerning the behavioural orientation of their residents. Using statistical significance tests they assessed the influence of built characteristics of the facilities on the orientation of the respective residents.

The results show that as the onset of dementia progresses, the residents' dependency on the design of their built environment increases. Significant factors included the number of residents in each living area, the access and circulation typology and the shape and design of common areas. Smaller facilities with up to 12 residents offered good orientation irrespective of their actual floor plan arrangement. Larger facilities can also offer a good environment depending on their arrangement. A key factor is the access and circulation typology: according to the study, linear typologies provide significantly better orientation than forms with one or more changes of direction in the circulation system (e.g. L-shaped corridors or circuits). Similar elements within a single facility or ward, for example several similarly designed living or dining areas, are detrimental to orientation. Accordingly, living environments for people with dementia must provide simple and clear spatial structures that are easy to comprehend. The study, which can be obtained from the authors, offers a series of recommendations in the form of a catalogue of design criteria.

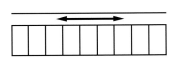

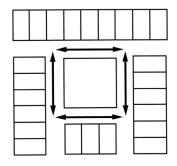

Linear circulation typology

Circuit around an atrium

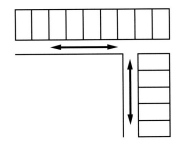

L-shaped circulation with a change of direction

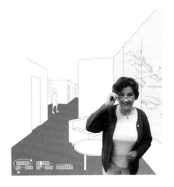

FUNDED BY THE

Robert Bosch Stiftung

Robert Bosch Stiftung GmbH | Heidehofstr. 31
D-70184 Stuttgart, Germany | www.bosch-stiftung.de

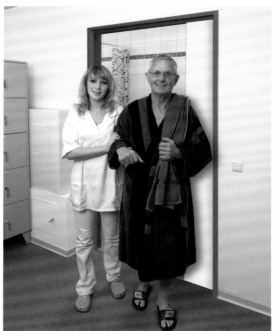

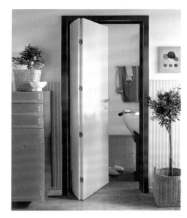

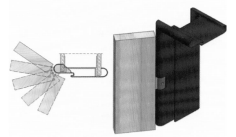

SafetyDesign – with finger protection system

Special frames for space-saving doors

Easy access due to an extra wide BOS steel frame – barrier-free living

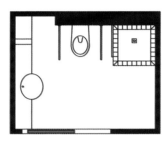

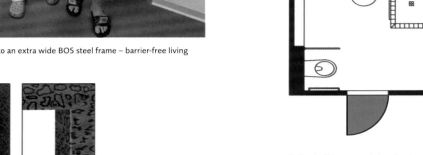

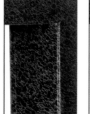 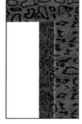

Dignified or fanciful – frames with special coatings for all tastes

Active leaf doors are obstructive in small rooms and take up a lot of space

LineaCompact sliding door frame: The area needed for an active leaf door is no longer necessary. This provides more freedom of movement and space, as the door disappears into the wall

Innovative steel frames for more comfort and quality of life

The steel frame specialist BOS Best Of Steel is a partner of the GGT Deutsche Gesellschaft für Gerontotechnik and develops frame systems for sophisticated demands. The areas of barrier-free living, residential homes, the generation 50plus and comfortable accessibility are consolidated in the concept "Living without Restrictions".

Sliding door frames:
Wider throughways for more comfort
The increasing popularity of sliding doors is unmistakable. The door disappears into the wall and the opening space required for an active leaf door is not needed. The LineaCompact sliding door frames are ideally suited for use in residential homes where for example two people share the use of one bathroom. There is nothing to obstruct entry into the bathroom and the throughway is wide enough to easily accommodate wheelchairs. BOS sliding door frames can also be equipped with electric door openers to meet sophisticated demands.

When space is limited, for example where an increased maneuverability for bed transportation is required, not only can sliding door frames be used, but BOS slanting soffit frames also offer an ideal solution. In this case the angle of entry is considerably larger making it much easier to push beds into the room. For exceptional situations, BOS special frames with integrated overhead tracks for folding doors are also available.

Professional areas of application
Specific functional uses impose particular demands on doors and frames, among others those of hygiene, radiation protection, corrosion resistance or extra-wide throughways. BOS Best Of Steel offers frames with anti-bacterial powder coating or in stainless steel, with a fungicide seal on request. For use in X-ray areas BOS frames are available with complete or partial lead linings, needless to say combined with all the advantages of wider throughways.

Safety and comfort
In conjunction with many certified door leaves, BOS steel frames fulfill the requirements for theft, fire and sound protection.

Steel frames for heavier door leaves, also in double rebated design, increase the soundproofing for interior doors. This is additionally optimized using the BOS latch adjustment, which allows for an easy adjustment of the contact pressure on the seal. In this way any possible difficulties regarding hard to open doors in areas used by disabled people can easily be improved via simple adjustment.

The visually attractive SafetyDesign steel frames protect against the possible trapping of fingers when opening or closing the door through the use of hinges which are integrated in the architrave.

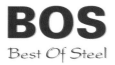

Best Of Steel

BOS GmbH Best Of Steel
Lütkenfelde 4 | D-48282 Emsdetten, Germany | Ph.: +49 (0)2572.203-0
www.BestOfSteel.de | info@BestOfSteel.de | www.BOS-Wohnen-ohne-Grenzen.de

Quality of life every step of the way

Living environments for the elderly should be tailored to the needs of older people to ensure maximum freedom of movement and independence. This applies especially to floor coverings, which should be non-slip, hard-wearing and hygienic while also offering a wide range of aesthetic qualities for creating comfortable environments. Floor coverings from Forbo, the world's largest manufacturer of linoleum floors and vinyl floor coverings, unite functionality and design for use in residential areas for the elderly.

Linoleum: Natural. Sustainable. Beautiful.

Linoleum embodies everything that nature has to offer: designs inspired by nature in beautiful, clear colours that radiate warmth and harmony. Linoleum is produced from natural, renewable resources and exhibits a range of positive qualities: it is hard-wearing, easy to clean, durable, permanently antistatic and warm to the touch. Ideal for use in health care environments, linoleum is well known for its bacteriostatic properties which reduce the spread of microorganisms and bacteria.

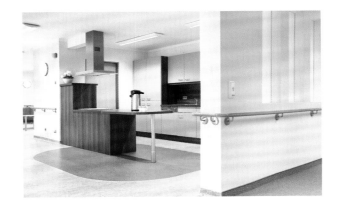

Vinyl: High tech under foot

The multi-ply structure of vinyl floor coverings incorporates an energy-absorbing layer that cushions impact on joints and is comfortable to walk on. A high-density base layer ensures a smooth rolling surface and provides indentation resistance. The filler-free calendered top layer has a high-quality surface finish providing a hard-wearing, pore-free surface that is easy to clean. In addition, technically optimised reproduction techniques allow for a wide variety of decorative effects and design possibilities. Surfaces with the appearance of natural wood, for example, create a homely atmosphere.

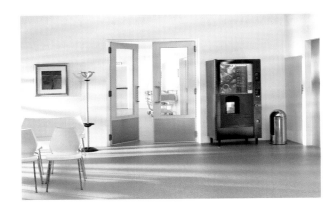

Premium quality for all generations

With the product ranges made of linoleum and vinyl, Forbo offers floor coverings made of natural, renewable materials and plastic floor surfaces in a wide range of designs, colours and patterns. Both product ranges include high-density floor surfaces that are hard-wearing, impact and indentation resistant and suitable for wheelchair users. Floor coverings are factory-sealed with a protective finish that provides lasting surface durability and makes them easier to clean. Accordingly, high-quality, easy-to-clean products not only minimise ongoing maintenance costs but also contribute through their lasting durability to the overall cost-benefit equation of buildings.

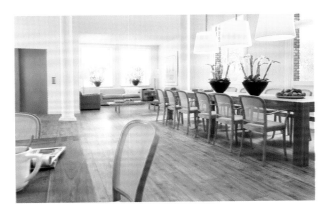

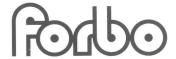

Forbo Flooring GmbH | Steubenstraße 27 | D-33100 Paderborn, Germany
www.forbo-flooring.de

Greater comfort in the bathroom with the barrier-free ErgoSystem® from FSB

The design of FSB's "diagonal-oval ErgoSystem" adheres rigorously to the ergonomics of grip. Over 128 years of expertise acquired in all aspects of "handle culture" by the Eastern Westphalian company FSB, a brand name in the design of door and window handles, have gone into the design of this product line of barrier-free products for sanitary installations. Its unique diagonally tilted oval cross-section provides optimal gripping comfort. For disabled people and the elderly in particular the comprehensive system of handles allows people to be self-sufficient without sacrificing design excellence. Barrier-free design need not compromise looks: in the ErgoSystem, functionality, aesthetics and ergonomics come together to form a convincing whole.

The ErgoSystem provides a helping hand in the bathroom without creating a clinical or overly technical or therapeutic impression. The basis is a range of handles in different variations for all conceivable areas of application. In combination with numerous accessories, Ergo becomes a universally applicable system. Whether a toilet roll holder, switch, arm rest or shower seat: the principle of the system informs them all. So too the new shower head: it can be adjusted easily with one hand; the retention mechanism can be released without having to either rotate one's hand or exert any appreciable force. Once released it lies naturally in the hand leaving the other hand free, for example to hold on to a handrail. The ErgoSystem's carefully thought-through concept has also earned it recognition from the jury members of renowned design awards.

Further information online: www.fsb.de/barrier-free

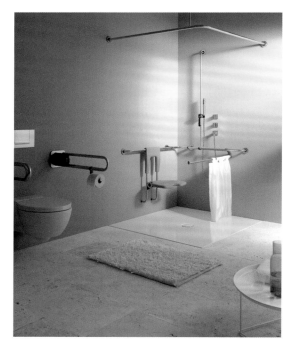
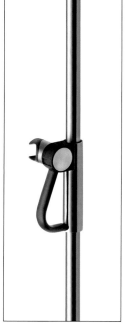
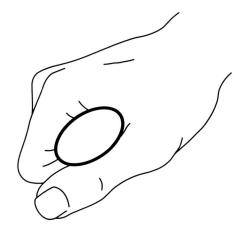

design award
winner
2003

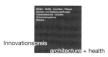
Innovationspreis
architecture + health

reddot design award
winner 2008

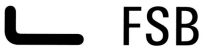 **FSB**

FSB - Franz Schneider Brakel GmbH + Co KG
Nieheimer Straße 38 | D-33034 Brakel, Germany | Ph. +49 (0)5272-6080
www.fsb.de | info@fsb.de

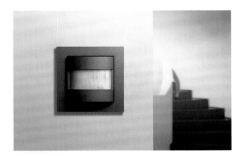

Automatic switches in hallways, staircases and corridors ensure that lights do not need to be turned on by hand

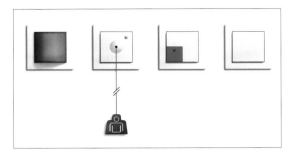

The Gira nurse call system 834 is an emergency call system that can be fitted, for example, in WCs for the handicapped

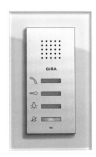

The Gira surface-mounted home station with hands-free function allows one to communicate safely and securely without having to open the door

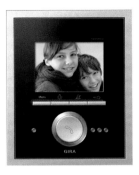

The Gira VideoTerminal has a large image, 5.7" active TFT colour display allowing one to control entry from indoors

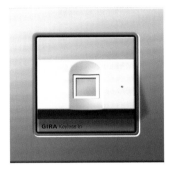

Gira Keyless In Fingerprint controls access using the biometric characteristics of the human fingerprint

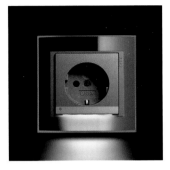

Socket outlets with LED orientation light serve the dual functions of safety and comfort

Continuing to live at home

Modern electrical installations help older people to live at home, in their familiar surroundings, for longer. The electronic systems offered by Gira include product ranges that cater especially for the residential needs of the elderly. Five of these have been awarded the "GGT-Siegel", a certification mark awarded by the Deutsche Gesellschaft für Gerontotechnik®.

As one's eyesight begins to deteriorate, Gira F 100 offer a particularly large rocker switch surface for easier operation. Likewise, in hallways, staircases and corridors, automatic light switches can be installed in place of conventional light switches and are immediately ready for use. Gira's radio-automatic control switches do not even need to be attached to the electricity supply.

Gira's illuminated SCHUKO socket outlets with integrated twilight sensor afford greater safety and comfort. An integral white LED orientation light beneath the socket projects a light corridor downwards providing indirect orientation lighting and signalling the location of switches or sockets without creating bothersome glare at night.

Nursing care for the elderly and infirm in the home is becoming increasingly widespread. Here pull-cord buttons in private bathrooms can be used to call a nurse. The cord is installed so that a person can activate it whether standing at the washbasin, sitting on the toilet, in the shower or bath, or lying on the floor. A light outside in the corridor in front of the bathroom provides a visual signal. The switch can also be linked to the telephone and in-house phone system to alert someone close by or outpatient care services. A switch outside the bathroom allows one to deactivate the call once help has arrived.

Forgetting, misplacing or losing one's keys is distressing not only for older people. Gira Keyless In Fingerprint controls entry by scanning the biometric characteristics of the human fingerprint. It can also adapt to the changing structure of skin over time as one grows older.

Door communication systems installed inside the home such as the Gira surface-mounted home station with hands-free feature facilitate simple and secure communication without having to open the door. A home station with additional video function offers even greater comfort. Home stations video with a 1.8" or 2.5" colour display are available for Gira's different switch ranges. A larger screen is available on the Gira VideoTerminal which features a 5.7" active TFT colour display.

In addition to these individual solutions, the installation of a KNX/EIB bus system provides a comprehensive, flexible and extendable solution. The Gira HomeServer 3 allows one to interconnect many related functions and provides a means of monitoring, changing and configuring the system from afar. This too contributes to greater security, comfort and quality of life for older people.

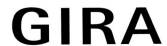

Gira Giersiepen GmbH & Co. KG | Dahlienstraße
D-42477 Radevormwald, Germany | www.gira.com

Social investments

When investing in nursing facilities, the operator should be an equal partner with whom one works together to achieve common goals. It is a partnership that continues for the agreed duration of the lease in which one strives side by side for the mutual benefit of both parties. Working on this basis, IMMAC has specialised in investments in the social sector for over a decade. IMMAC does not acquire property for the purposes of short-term speculation but instead builds a long-term portfolio.

IMMAC currently manages around 60 social investment properties throughout Germany. Numerous properties have been acquired through classic Sale-and-Lease-Back transactions or in the form of investment assistance in the takeover of facilities – for example when the running of facilities passes to the next generation, including within the family. To maintain and improve their competitiveness, necessary conversions, extensions or modernisation measures have been undertaken sensitively and with much attention to detail, sometimes during ongoing operation but always with minimum disruption for the residents.

When determining the purchase price, the most important aspect for IMMAC is not the return factor but its basis, the amount of the lease. IMMAC calculates the lease reasonably so that, after the difference between income from investment costs and the lease has been determined, the operator still has sufficient cash reserves for maintenance and ongoing replacement of inventory.

A sensible lease arrangement is key to ensuring a successful business basis for the benefit of all members in the chain. These include not only the investor and operator but also the staff and not least the residents living in a facility.

Your investment partner

As a market leader in social investments, IMMAC has over ten years experience as a reliable, specialised and competent partner and works directly with you to realise your project.

IMMAC provides nationwide, competent and effective assistance
- as an investor in care home facilities
- in Sale-and-Lease-Back transactions
- in the takeover of facilities
- in transactions following takeovers
- in the expansion of your company
- in the building of new facilities for the elderly/social facilities

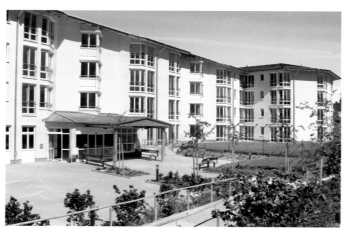
Ansbach

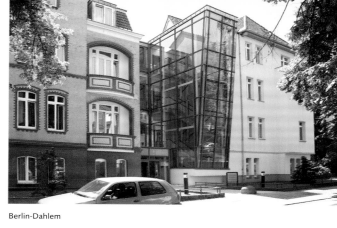
Berlin-Dahlem

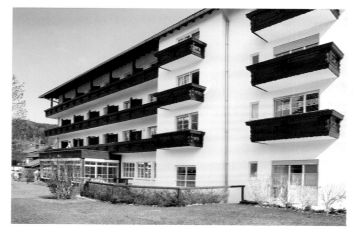
Mittenwald

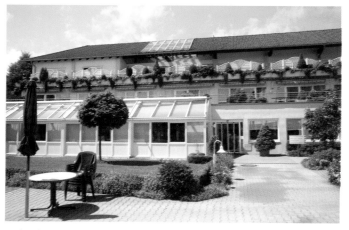
Marktredwitz

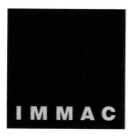

Hamburg Office | ABC – Straße 19 | D-20354 Hamburg, Germany
Ph.: +49 (0)40 - 34 99 40 0 | Fax: +49 (0)40 - 34 99 40 20
info@immac.de | www.immac.de

Welcome to IMMAC Institutional Client Service GmbH

Quality is the best foundation for any building project and the basis of every sound investment. This applies especially to the social investment market. As the leading funds investment group and specialist for investments in the social sector in Germany, IMMAC can capitalise on years of specialist knowledge.

IMMAC Institutional Client Service GmbH takes care of the entire process from the development and planning to the construction and renovation of facilities for the elderly, care homes and clinics. The result is a unique product portfolio built around profitability, stability and not least the most worthy of all aims: **quality of life**.

IMMAC's range of services includes:
On-site supervision and controlling during the construction phase | **Commercial project management** | **Acquisition/evaluation** | Conception | Contract management | Property securing | Controlling | Cost calculation | Arrangement of financing | Invoicing/reporting | Sales and marketing control | Consultation for operators and investors | Public relations | Investor relations | **Technical project management** | Acquisition/evaluation | Preliminary planning, preliminary planning inquiries, planning, specification, tender and contract awarding | Construction management and controlling | Contract management | Invoicing/reporting | Documentation | Consultation for operators and investors | Public relations | Investor relations | **Back office** | Administration | Organisation | Accounting

IMMAC creates opportunities for investors and operators interested in profitable investment properties in state-regulated markets.

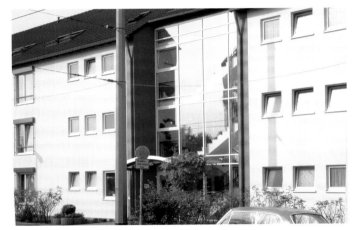

Duisburg-Marxloh after renovation of the façade.

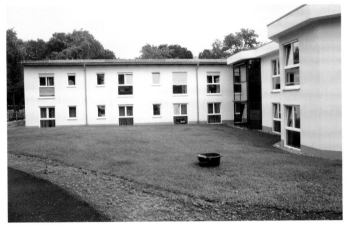

Oettingen

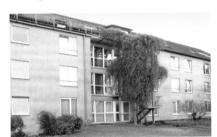

Duisburg-Marxloh before renovation of the façade.

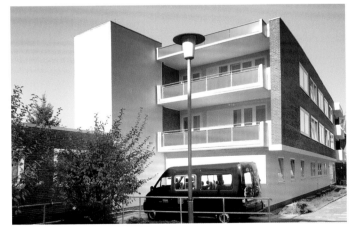

Hildesheim

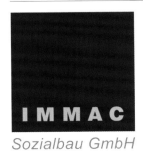

IMMAC
Sozialbau GmbH

Hamburg Office | ABC – Straße 19 | D-20354 Hamburg, Germany
Ph.: +49 (0)40 - 34 99 40 0 | Fax: +49 (0)40 - 34 99 40 20
info@immac.de | www.immac.de

Universal Design in the bathroom

In a study by the rheingold institute entitled "Baths and the Bathing Culture of the 50plus Generation" Kaldewei investigated the changing needs of older bathroom users and the resulting implications for bathtub and shower design. The result: the 50plus generation would like to see high-quality, well-designed products which unite innovative technology and an attractive appearance with a high degree of comfort and safety. Functionality designed specifically for the elderly should be as invisible as possible. As the leading European manufacturer of bath and shower units made of 3.5-mm-steel enamel, Kaldewei offers a wide range of Universal Design products, including 20 different baths and 25 shower trays.

Bathing relaxation for the 50plus generation

The 50plus generation is not limited to selected special products when choosing a bath tub but can select from a wide range of attractive designs with good ergonomics and generous sizes that are easy to get in and out of and are available with many comfortable extras such as easy-clean surfaces or exclusive whirlpool systems. The Rondo models with their timeless design fulfil all these requirements and are available in rectangular, hexagonal or octagonal forms. With its interlocking curved interior contours, this product family provides lots of room for the upper part of the body. Integrated arm rests provide optimal support when bathing. The Comfort-Level overflow outlet allows the water level to be increased by up to 50 mm. The Comfort-Level Plus includes an integrated filling function allowing one to dispense with obstructive tap fittings on the edge of the bath altogether.

Barrier-free showers for all ages

Among the shower designs, the large, super-shallow floor-level shower tray formats are particularly suited to the 50plus generation. Easy and safe entry is just as important as anti-slip surfaces and integrated seating. The Superplan XXL shower, which measures an exceptionally large 150 x 150 cm, offers maximum freedom of movement and can also be accessed with a wheelchair.

The material is particularly important for optimal durability and stability. Baths and shower trays made of Kaldewei 3.5 mm thick steel enamel are exceptionally durable, abrasion-, scratch- and impact-resistant and thanks to their easy-clean finish remain clean and hygienic. An anti-slip enamel surface finish ensures maximum safety in the shower. Kaldewei anti-slip and full anti-slip surfaces fulfil class B requirements for wet-loaded barefoot areas (German DIN 51097).

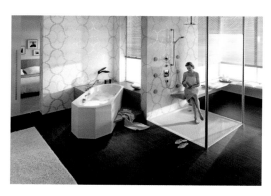

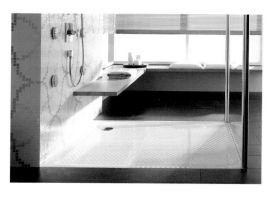

The 50plus bathroom is designed to allow unhindered use without outside help

Superplan XXL shower tray with full anti-slip enamel base

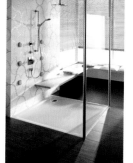

Rondo 8 Star bathtub

Superplan XXL shower tray with full anti-slip surface

Kaldewei baths and shower trays are produced in Ahlen, Westphalia, and shipped around the world. Kaldewei is a partner of the GGT Deutsche Gesellschaft für Gerontotechnik mbH.

KALDEWEI

Europe's No.1 for baths

Franz Kaldewei GmbH & Co. KG | Beckumer Str. 33-35
D-59229 Ahlen, Germany | www.kaldewei.com

Welcome to IMMAC Institutional Client Service GmbH

Quality is the best foundation for any building project and the basis of every sound investment. This applies especially to the social investment market. As the leading funds investment group and specialist for investments in the social sector in Germany, IMMAC can capitalise on years of specialist knowledge.

IMMAC Institutional Client Service GmbH takes care of the entire process from the development and planning to the construction and renovation of facilities for the elderly, care homes and clinics. The result is a unique product portfolio built around profitability, stability and not least the most worthy of all aims: **quality of life**.

IMMAC's range of services includes:
On-site supervision and controlling during the construction phase | **Commercial project management** | **Acquisition/evaluation** | Conception | Contract management | Property securing | Controlling | Cost calculation | Arrangement of financing | Invoicing/reporting | Sales and marketing control | Consultation for operators and investors | Public relations | Investor relations | **Technical project management** | Acquisition/evaluation | Preliminary planning, preliminary planning inquiries, planning, specification, tender and contract awarding | Construction management and controlling | Contract management | Invoicing/reporting | Documentation | Consultation for operators and investors | Public relations | Investor relations | **Back office** | Administration | Organisation | Accounting

IMMAC creates opportunities for investors and operators interested in profitable investment properties in state-regulated markets.

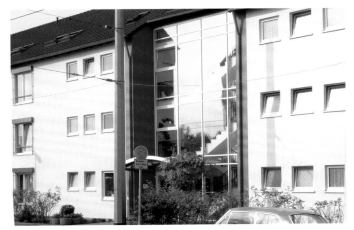

Duisburg-Marxloh after renovation of the façade.

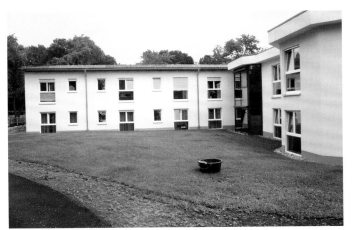

Oettingen

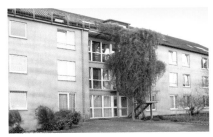

Duisburg-Marxloh before renovation of the façade.

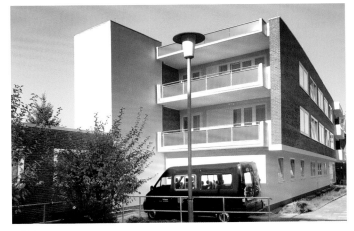

Hildesheim

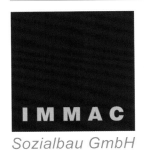

IMMAC
Sozialbau GmbH

Hamburg Office | ABC – Straße 19 | D-20354 Hamburg, Germany
Ph.: +49 (0)40 - 34 99 40 0 | Fax: +49 (0)40 - 34 99 40 20
info@immac.de | www.immac.de

Universal Design in the bathroom

In a study by the rheingold institute entitled "Baths and the Bathing Culture of the 50plus Generation" Kaldewei investigated the changing needs of older bathroom users and the resulting implications for bathtub and shower design. The result: the 50plus generation would like to see high-quality, well-designed products which unite innovative technology and an attractive appearance with a high degree of comfort and safety. Functionality designed specifically for the elderly should be as invisible as possible. As the leading European manufacturer of bath and shower units made of 3.5-mm-steel enamel, Kaldewei offers a wide range of Universal Design products, including 20 different baths and 25 shower trays.

Bathing relaxation for the 50plus generation

The 50plus generation is not limited to selected special products when choosing a bath tub but can select from a wide range of attractive designs with good ergonomics and generous sizes that are easy to get in and out of and are available with many comfortable extras such as easy-clean surfaces or exclusive whirlpool systems. The Rondo models with their timeless design fulfil all these requirements and are available in rectangular, hexagonal or octagonal forms. With its interlocking curved interior contours, this product family provides lots of room for the upper part of the body. Integrated arm rests provide optimal support when bathing. The Comfort-Level overflow outlet allows the water level to be increased by up to 50 mm. The Comfort-Level Plus includes an integrated filling function allowing one to dispense with obstructive tap fittings on the edge of the bath altogether.

Barrier-free showers for all ages

Among the shower designs, the large, super-shallow floor-level shower tray formats are particularly suited to the 50plus generation. Easy and safe entry is just as important as anti-slip surfaces and integrated seating. The Superplan XXL shower, which measures an exceptionally large 150 x 150 cm, offers maximum freedom of movement and can also be accessed with a wheelchair.

The material is particularly important for optimal durability and stability. Baths and shower trays made of Kaldewei 3.5 mm thick steel enamel are exceptionally durable, abrasion-, scratch- and impact-resistant and thanks to their easy-clean finish remain clean and hygienic. An anti-slip enamel surface finish ensures maximum safety in the shower. Kaldewei anti-slip and full anti-slip surfaces fulfil class B requirements for wet-loaded barefoot areas (German DIN 51097).

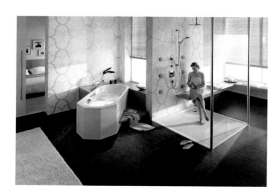

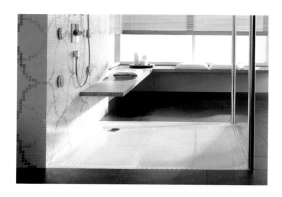

Superplan XXL shower tray with full anti-slip enamel base

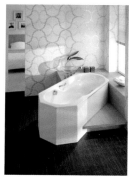

The 50plus bathroom is designed to allow unhindered use without outside help

Rondo 8 Star bathtub

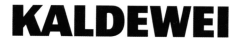

Superplan XXL shower tray with full anti-slip surface

Kaldewei baths and shower trays are produced in Ahlen, Westphalia, and shipped around the world. Kaldewei is a partner of the GGT Deutsche Gesellschaft für Gerontotechnik mbH.

KALDEWEI
Europe's No.1 for baths

Franz Kaldewei GmbH & Co. KG | Beckumer Str. 33-35
D-59229 Ahlen, Germany | www.kaldewei.com

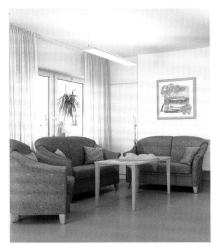

Dlite® amadea: harmonious, cosy lighting providing good visibility and safety

Good lighting enriches senior living

Light stimulates the mind, emotions, well-being as well as the circadian rhythm and helps us discern colours. As vision deteriorates with old age, it is the elderly who have most difficulty coping with the effects of inadequate lighting. Old people often use their eyes to compensate for hearing impairments, for example through lip-reading. An 80-year-old person requires a level of illumination on average ten times greater than that of a young adult. A lighting design concept that adequately addresses these needs is therefore essential to the successful realisation of interiors for the elderly.

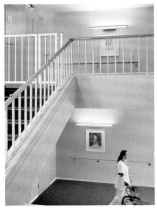

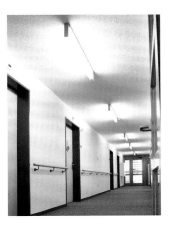

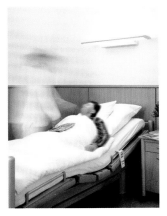

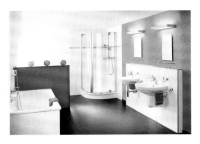

Dlite® vanera Bath: even, shadow-free lighting ensures that one can easily see the floor when stepping in and out of the shower

Visual Timing Light: simulates the cyclic progression of day and night by gradually changing brightness and colour

Dlite® vanera: special controls allow different lighting scenarios such as morning, midday, afternoon, evening and night light

Dlite® amadea Bed: light effects can be switched separately or can be dimmed

Issues:
Accidents and anxieties
Hard shadows and shiny reflections on floors are not uncommon in corridors and staircases. Residents sometimes perceive these as obstacles or threats causing them to lose their footing. Falls and accidents among old people are correspondingly widespread.

Lighting approach
Lighting solutions should employ a sufficiently high level of illumination, have a high proportion of indirect light and even distribution of the direct light component. Through a combination of wall and ceiling light fittings it is possible to accentuate different parts of the room.

Effects
Obstacles are recognised in good time.
Shadows and reflections are reduced and with it the risk of losing one's footing.
Spaces are perceived more easily, increasing safety.

Issue:
The disruption of the circadian rhythm
Experience has shown that patients with dementia have particular difficulties with spatiotemporal orientation. This can result in lethargy, bewilderment and depression.

Lighting approach
In recreation rooms, common rooms and corridors, Derungs Licht AG's innovative light management system "Visual Timing Light" can be used to simulate the twenty-four hour cycle, from sunrise to sundown and night time.

Effects
Twenty-four hour cycle of light lends rhythm and structure to the day.
Positively affects the day-night rhythm.
Regular sleeping and eating habits.
Positively affects mood and sense of well-being; invigorates the senses.
Significantly improves the articulation of patients with dementia.

Issue:
Catering for different needs in resident's rooms
Care staff need well-lit rooms to carry out their work. Residents on the other hand prefer lighting that is more pleasant and homely.

Lighting approach
The solution lies in a lighting system that can change to fulfil the respective needs: general/pleasant light, reading/working light, care/examination light and night time/guiding light.

Effects
Use of indirect light: provides patients and care providers with comfortable ambient lighting.
Use of direct light: provides the patient with a comfortable reading and work light.
Use of direct and indirect light: ensures that care providers have strong light for examinations. Sophisticated light direction systems prevent staff from casting a shadow on the work they are doing.
Night time LED: provides patients with a subtle night light to guide them safely in the dark and facilitates the work of care staff on their nightly rounds.

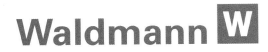

Marketing and Sales Germany | Herbert Waldmann GmbH & Co. KG
D-78056 Villingen-Schwenningen, Germany | Ph.: +49 (0)7720 601-100
info@waldmann.com | www.derungslicht.com

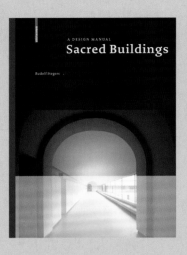
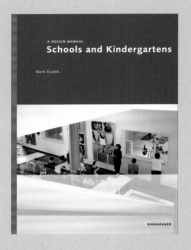
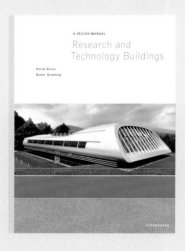
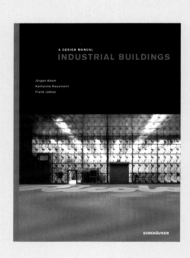